BIOFUNCTIONAL SURFACE ENGINEERING

edited by Martin Scholz

BIOFUNCTIONAL SURFACE ENGINEERING

PAN STANFORD PUBLISHING

Published by

Pan Stanford Publishing Pte. Ltd.
Penthouse Level, Suntec Tower 3
8 Temasek Boulevard
Singapore 038988

Email: editorial@panstanford.com
Web: www.panstanford.com

British Library Cataloguing-in-Publication Data
A catalogue record for this book is available from the British Library.

Biofunctional Surface Engineering

ISBN 978-981-4411-60-8 (Hardcover)
ISBN 978-981-4411-61-5 (eBook)

Printed in the USA

To my family

Contents

Preface xv

1. Regulatory Requirements for Medical Devices, Including Combinations with Biological Products or Drugs as an Integral Part **1**

Franziska Baumgarten

1.1 Definitions and Classification 2
1.2 Combi Products: Definitions and Classification 4
1.3 Evidence of Conformity to the Essential Requirements of the Directives 4
1.4 Specific Essential Requirements for Combi Products 4
1.5 Use of Harmonized Standards: Presumption of Conformity 5
1.6 Clinical Evaluation 6
1.7 Outlook: New Regulation for Medical Devices in the EU 9

2. Terminal Radiation Sterilization of Combination Products **11**

Kristina Kemter

2.1 Introduction 12
2.2 Interaction of Radiation with Biomolecules 13
2.2.1 Example 1: Sterilization of Herceptin 16
2.2.2 Example 2: Sterilization of Immobilized Antibodies in Three-Dimensional Carrier Foams 19
2.2.3 Example 3: Sterilization of Immobilized Viral Antigens on Vaccine Scaffolds 21
2.2.3.1 Influenza A functionality assay showing maintenance of antigenicity 21
2.2.3.2 Maintenance of antigenicity despite inactivation of virus upon irradiation 22

3. Polyelectrolyte Multilayers as Functional Coatings for Controlled Biomolecular Interactions **27**

Hanna Hartmann and Burkhard Schlosshauer

3.1 Controlled Interactions of PEMs with Cells 28
3.1.1 Physical PEM Parameters and Cell Adhesion 28
3.1.2 Biofactor-Dotted PEMs and Biomimetic PEMs 31
3.2 PEMs as Implant Coatings: Prerequisites for Applications 32
3.3 PEM as Biomaterial: Application Examples 33
3.3.1 Nucleic Acid Delivery 33
3.4 PEMs with Antimicrobial Activity 37

4. Polyelectrolyte Multilayers as Functional Coatings for Controlled Biomolecular Interactions **47**

Xin Xiong, Susanne Hossfeld, Simona Margutti, and Rumen Krastev

4.1 Introduction 48
4.2 Layer-by-Layer Technology and Preparation of PEMs 52
4.2.1 Polyelectrolytes 52
4.2.2 Formation of LbL Coatings 53
4.2.3 Methods for Deposition and Anchoring of PEMs 56
4.3 Structure of PEM and Its Relation to the Basic Components and Preparation Conditions 57
4.3.1 Film Stability 57
4.3.2 Exponential Versus Linear Growth 58
4.3.3 Polyelectrolyte Blends 59
4.3.4 Cross-Linking of Polyelectrolytes in PEMs 60
4.3.5 Mechanical Properties of PEMs 61
4.4 Summary and Outlook 62

5. Surface Characteristics and Biofilms **71**

Klaus Liefeith, Holger Rothe, Marion Frant, and Ronald Schade

5.1 Introduction 72
5.2 Interfacial Energy at Biointerfaces 73

5.3 Biofilm Formation 76
5.4 Antifouling Strategies 82
5.5 Passive Concepts That Do Not Interfere with the Adhering Microorganisms 83
5.6 Active Concepts That Interfere with the Adhering Microorganisms 89
5.7 Conclusion and Future Prospects 92
5.8 Biofilm Testing 93
5.9 Examples for in vitro Biofilm Testing 100
5.9.1 Dental Plaque Formation 100
5.9.2 Biofilm-Related Infections 104

6. Antimicrobial Implant Coating **121**

Klaus-Dieter Kühn

6.1 Introduction and Economical Aspects of Implant-Related Infection 122
6.2 Formation of Biofilm on Implant Surfaces 130
6.3 Germ Invasion 131
6.4 Colonization of an Implant Surface 132
6.5 Biofilm 134
6.6 Germ Detection 135
6.7 Medical Biofilms 136
6.8 Antimicrobial Agents 136
6.9 Antiseptic Agents 136
6.10 Heavy Metal Ions 137
6.11 Antiseptics Containing Halogen 137
6.12 Organic Ammonium Salts 138
6.13 Phenols and Phenol Derivatives 139
6.14 Alcohols 139
6.15 Chemotherapeutics/Anti-Infective Agents 139
6.15.1 Inhibition of Cell Wall Biosynthesis 140
6.15.2 Blocking of Protein Synthesis 140
6.15.3 Suppression of Nucleic Acid Synthesis 140
6.15.4 Interference with Permeability of Cytoplasma Membrane 141
6.16 Bacteriostasis/Bacteriocidal 141
6.17 Mechanism of Action of Antibiotics 141
6.18 Rifampicin 142
6.19 Resistance 142
6.20 Methicillin-Resistant *Staphylococcus Aureus* 145

6.21 Resistance in Biofilms 145
6.22 Small-Colony Variants and Persister Cells 146
6.23 Coating Strategies of Implants 146
6.24 Antimicrobial Protection of Biomaterials 147
6.25 Systemic Antibiotic Administration 148
6.26 Local Antibiotic Administration 148
6.27 PMMA Bone Cements as Local Carriers of Active Ingredients 151
6.28 Metallic Implants 152
6.29 Polymer-Layer-Forming Carrier System with Incorporated Antibiotics/Antiseptics 155
6.30 Antibiotics/Antiseptics Included in Porous Hydroxylapatite Coatings 159
6.31 Coating with Heavy Metal/Heavy Metal Salts 161
6.32 Coating with Self-Adhesive, Low-Soluble Antibiotic Salts 164
6.33 Other Implants 168
6.33.1 Vascular Grafts 168
6.33.2 Hernia Meshes 170
6.33.3 Sutures 172
6.33.4 Fleeces and Felts 173
6.33.5 Pacemaker/Defibrillator 174
6.34 Further Biomaterial Coatings 176

7. Small-Angle X-Ray Spectroscopy as a Method to Monitor the Three-Dimensional Structure of Immobilized Biomolecules on Medical Device Scaffolds during Production **191**

Rupert Tscheliessnig and Alois Jungbauer

7.1 Introduction 192
7.2 Nano-Coating 193
7.3 Small-Angle X-ray Scattering 196
7.4 Safety of Nano-Coating 201
7.5 Functionality of Nano-Coating 202

8. Aptamers as Biomimetic Surface Coatings for Blood-Contacting Implants **207**

Meltem Avci-Adali, Stefanie Krajewski, Nadja Perle, Nadja Wilhelm, Jan Niederländer, Heidi Stoll, Christian Schlensak, and Hans P. Wendel

8.1 Introduction 208

8.2 Aptamers 209
8.3 Execution of the SELEX Procedure 211
8.4 Coating Technology for Coupling of Aptamers to the Surface of Medical Devices 211
8.5 The Holy Grail: Small-Diameter Artificial Vascular Prostheses 212
8.5.1 Endothelial Progenitor Cells: A Fascinating Alternative Source of Cells for Endothelialization of Vascular Prostheses 213
8.6 Conclusion 218

9. Microneedles and Nanopatches for Transdermal Vaccination 223

Andreas Muschaweck, Martin Scholz, and Ulrike Protzer

9.1 Vaccination via the Dermal Route 223
9.2 Limitations of Standard Vaccination Procedures 224
9.3 Alternatives to Needles and Syringes 224
9.4 Microprojections for Transdermal Vaccination 225
9.5 Feasibility of Transdermal Vaccination with Microprojections 227
9.6 Challenges of Microprojections for Transdermal Vaccination 229
9.7 Conclusion 230

10. Autoantibodies as Biomarkers for Disease Diagnosis 233

Angelika Lueking, Heike Göhler, and Peter Schulz-Knappe

10.1 Autoantibodies as Biomarkers 234
10.2 Autoantibodies for Companion Diagnostics Enabling Personalized Medicine 237
10.3 Biomarker Discovery Strategies 238
10.4 Antigen/Autoantibody Interactions as Biomarker Candidates 242
10.5 Diagnostic Assays Based on Antigen/Autoantibody Interactions 245
10.6 Conclusion 246

11. Biofunctionalized Wound Dressings for Advanced Wound Care **251**

Martin Scholz

11.1 Need for Biofunctional Wound Dressings 252
11.2 Current Wound-Healing Procedures 253
11.2.1 Negative Pressure Wound Therapy/Vacuum-Assisted Closure 253
11.2.2 Silver-Coated Wound Dressings 253
11.2.3 Growth Factor Eluting Dressing (Regranex) 254
11.3 Possible Targets in Wound Healing and Phase-Specific Strategies 254
11.4 Stimulation of Myofibroblasts by Drug-Eluting Materials 256
11.5 Fabrication of a Drug-Eluting Platform Device as an Example 258
11.6 Stimulation of Myofibroblasts by Innovative Material Surfaces 262
11.7 Outlook 263

12. Circulating Tumor Cell: Trapping Devices **267**

Frank A. W. Coumans, Sjoerd T. Ligthart, Joost Swennenhuis, and Leon W. M. M. Terstappen

12.1 Introduction 268
12.2 Frequency and Clinical Relevance of CTC 268
12.3 CTC Enrichment and Staining with the CellTracksAutoPrep 273
12.4 Imaging and Enumeration of CTCs with CellTracks Analyzer 275
12.5 Immunomagnetic Enrichment 277
12.6 Detection of Treatment Targets on CTCs 280

13. Evidence Generation for Medical Devices: The Case of Cemented Joint Replacement Surgery in Arthroplasty Registries **291**

Antonis Kontekakis, Mareike Berghaus, Sebastian Gaiser, and Klaus-Dieter Kühn

13.1 Evidence-Based Medicine 291
13.2 What Is an Arthroplasty Registry? 292

13.3 What Data Are Captured within an Arthroplasty Register? 294
13.4 Methods 295
13.5 Cemented Total Knee Arthroplasty in Arthroplasty Registries 295
13.6 Cemented Total Hip Arthroplasty in Arthroplasty Registries 297
13.7 Economic Remark 300
13.8 Antibiotic-Loaded Bone Cement in Arthroplasty Registries 300
13.8.1 Hip 300
13.8.2 Knee 301
13.9 Different Types and Brands of Bone Cement in Arthroplasty Registries 302
13.10 How Do Registry Data Compare to the Information Provided by Clinical Trials? 304
13.11 Conclusion 306

Index 315

Preface

Biofunctional surface engineering and drug–device combination products will determine the future of medical devices such as orthopedic implants, stents, catheters, vaccine scaffolds, wound dressings, and extracorporeal circulation devices. Biologically functionalized combination devices constitute the interface between pharmaceutical products, medtech, and in vitro diagnostics and therefore are regulated by the authorities in a specific way (Chapter 1).

The field of biofunctional surface engineering is highly interdisciplinary, especially when considering in vivo applications of invasive medical devices as end products. Material scientists, chemists, biologists, and clinicians are involved and cooperate to cover all important aspects of safety and efficacy during the development and evaluation phase.

A basic requirement for the development of combination devices is the biocompatibility of the scaffold material and the surface characteristics. Today, tremendous experience exists already, related to the material of choice used for invasive approaches. Most commonly, titanium, stainless steel, several ceramics, and polymers (biodegradable polymers with embedded drugs are not addressed in this book) are used that have been shown to be biocompatible and safe. However, cellular and immune responses elicited by the foreign material are still a severe problem and may, for example, lead to aberrant tissue growth around the implant or to biofilm formation (see Chapters 5 and 6).

In addition to the implant material alone, the enabling biomolecule coupling chemistry and coating have to be biocompatible and safe. Moreover, the coupling chemistry should be feasible for coating of a broad range of materials. There are several standard coupling methods for covalent binding of biomolecules to implant materials, e.g., by using linkers selected from the silanes. In general, hydrophilic material surfaces are appreciated that provide sufficient reactivity with silanes or other linkers. The coupling of the biomolecules to the linkers in turn can be achieved by well described chemical steps such as click chemistry or maleimide chemistry. The choice of coupling chemistry and linker depends on the surface of the scaffold and the effector molecule.

An example of a promising new approach for the functionalization of implant material is the nano-coating with polyelectrolyte monolayers by means of the layer-by-layer method introduced by Decher et al. (1992, 1997). This technology is described in detail by H. Hartmann and B. Schlosshauer in Chapter 3 and by X. Xiong et al. in Chapter 4.

One of the major drawbacks in biofunctionalized surfaces involving irradiation or heat stress–sensitive biomolecules such as proteins is the need for terminally sterilized products (discussed in Chapter 2). The lack of effective sterilization techniques for biologics has spawned discussions about the reduction of regulatory requirements, which might impose significant safety risks. On the other hand, novel and safe technologies enable the coupling, stabilization, and protection of effector molecules in a way that allows terminal sterilization without loss of function. According to the FDA and the European pharmacopoeia, terminal sterilization is mandatory, whenever it is technically feasible.

The idea behind coating invasive materials was triggered some decades ago by the medical need to obtain better biocompatibility of the products. An example of the first coatings in the field of invasive medicine was the heparin coating of the inner surface of the heart–lung machine circuits. The rational of the heparin coating was to decrease the clotting of the blood, which occurs when platelets are activated by the artificial surface of the circuits. Unappreciated clotting entails the loss of patency of the circuits and results in increased risk for the patient to suffer from stroke. Today, heparin-, albumin-, or other coatings of invasive medical devices are broadly accepted.

Economically, the introduction of the heparin-coated devices had put an immense pressure on providers of extracorporeal circuits because they had to follow the concept behind this technology. Although no clear evidence existed for a clinical benefit of such a coating, clinicians and the hospitals rapidly adhered to this novel technology, simply because of its plausibility. In line with this plausibility, a higher price of the functionalized products was accepted by the customers.

Besides the clotting problem at the interface between blood and artificial materials, unappreciated immune responses constitute another significant risk to patients, e.g., undergoing cardiac surgery with support of the heart–lung machine or intensive care patients who are connected to apheresis circuits, dialysis, and any other devices with invasive access to the blood circulation.

The so-called systemic inflammatory response syndrome plays a significant role in severely ill patients, for example, in patients with severe and life-threatening injuries after multiple traumas. It is well known that the aberrant unspecific activation of polymorphous neutrophils contributes to the damage of tissues, which may lead to organ failure and death. Because artificial surfaces are recognized by neutrophils, which will be strongly activated upon contact with the foreign material, this surface-triggered neutrophil hyperactivation may further lead to disease progression. Ideas to limit or prevent material-mediated inflammation or even systemic inflammation by modifications of the surfaces currently exist. An example of such an innovative immunomodulating surface is the leukocyte inhibition module (LIM), which has been successfully evaluated in clinical studies. Recently, safety and efficacy of the nano-coating, an enabling technology for the LIM that consists of a neutrophil-inactivating surface involving covalently coupled agonistic anti-Fas (CD95) biomolecules, have been reported. The issue of stabilizing covalently immobilized anti-Fas IgM, a large and complex biomolecule, on a biocompatible open porous polyurethane surface is certainly a challenge, which has been solved by drying and reconstituting the biomolecule on the surface in a specifically adapted stabilizing solution. In the contribution of R. Tscheliessnig and A. Jungbauer (Chapter 7), the folding issues of the agonistic anti-Fas biomolecule undergoing drying, sterilization, and reconstitution have been analyzed by means of an adapted algorithm for small-angle X-ray spectroscopy.

An interesting novel extracorporeal device system for the accumulation of circulating tumor cells (CTCs) is currently under development. CTC devices consist of elements that are capable of binding to receptors on CTCs in peripheral blood. The quantification and characterization of CTCs enables the clinician to monitor disease progression and response to chemotherapy. The group of L. Terstappen, who significantly contributed to the development of the "Cell Search System," describes the diagnostic potential of the Cell Search System as the current standard in Chapter 12. However, the major limitation of the Cell Search System is the small number of CTCs that can be evaluated per volume blood.

Currently, an international consortium works on the development and clinical evaluation of a CTC apheresis system in order to enrich the CTCs from circulating blood. A higher number of CTCs is essential for improving the diagnosis of disease progression and treatment success. CTC apheresis may probably be the starting point for developing more specific and personalized anti-tumor strategies in the future.

From a technical point of view, following are the challenges in this setting: (a) the CTC high affinity trapping biomolecule has to be stably immobilized to the surface (e.g., on open porous polyurethane foams with optimized blood rheology) to prevent unappreciated systemic effects. (b) The high specificity of cell trapping has to be guaranteed even during a treatment period of about 1–2 h in extracorporeal blood circulation. (c) The trapped cells have to be eluted from the surface for further diagnostic procedures by using an adequate linker with a defined breaking point. To achieve these goals, large interdisciplinary efforts in the construction of the biofunctionalized CTC trapping surface will have to be done prior to clinical evaluation.

In the field of orthopedics, approaches to improve the healing and long-term stability of implants are several decades old. However, it has currently not been achieved to stably and efficiently couple bone morphogeneic proteins (BMP), an osteoconductive growth factor, on implant material so that the biofunctionalized end product can be terminally sterilized. Currently, the implant surface is mechanically coated with sterile BMP-2 within the operation room because the biomolecules are known to lose their functionality after gas sterilization, irradiation, or other procedures. In osteoblast cell culture models, BMP-2 retained the functional activity after irradiation when embedded by the nano-coating in a similar way as it is described in Chapters 2 and 7 for IgG and IgM antibodies, respectively.

For safety reasons, significant physical alterations such as aggregation or degradation of the biomolecules after thermal or irradiation stress are exclusion criteria for the approval of combination devices. Three-dimensional characteristics of reconstituted biomolecules on implant surfaces should not differ significantly from the native molecules. Reconstitution of an immobilized model IgM antibody after drying, irradiation, and reconstitution is described in detail in Chapter 7.

More stable molecules such as aptamers, nanofitins, and DARPins might be possible alternatives to large and fragile proteins for biofunctional surface engineering in the future. These biosimilars or biomimetics can be specifically designed by using existing databases for selecting desired sequences and by using systems such as phage display to produce large amounts of variants for further functional selecting steps. In this book, Avci-Adali et al., from the group of H. P. Wendel (Chapter 8), describe the progress of aptamers on the basis of high-affinity RNA or DNA oligonucleotides to be immobilized on the surface of vascular prostheses. In this example, the aptamers may directly bind to endothelial progenitor cells in the blood and promote the growth of endothelial cells on the artificial vascular wall.

The formation of biofilms is a significant issue in the field of implant medicine. Biofilms are a consequence of bacterial contamination and bacterial growth and may result in immediate reoperation. It is obvious that infection, biofilm formation, and reoperation are associated with extremely high costs and of course reduced life quality of the patient. In the chapters by K. Liefeith et al., (Chapter 5) who deal with surface characteristics and biofilms, and K.-D. Kühn (Chapter 6), who reviews the state of the art and current concepts of antimicrobial coatings, this important field for improvement of invasive biomaterials and medicine is intensively discussed. For example, Table 6.2 in the contribution of K.-D. Kühn (Chapter 6) summarizes the economic data of medical device infection in the US health care system. Possible savings by reducing the incidence of infections of specific medical implants are also calculated. Moreover, the value of arthroplasty registries to evaluate the long-term outcomes of total joint arthroplasty is discussed in Chapter 13 by A. Kontekakis et al. These registries seem to be extremely useful, e.g., to better define the need for alternative strategies such as the use of biofunctionalized medical devices.

Similarly, the need for anti-bacterial wound dressings is known for a long time. Currently, most companies offering wound dressings for advanced wound care include silver coatings to accelerate dermal wound healing processes. However, it has been reported that other factors play a role in delayed wound healing which are not addressed by silver. Moreover, as outlined by K.-D. Kühn in Chapter 6, silver has been shown to have unappreciated side effects and is discussed controversially.

Delayed wound healing is not only triggered by wound infection. There are rather other factors such as deregulated angiogenesis and thus insufficient oxygenation of the granulating tissue accounting for the development of chronic wounds. The orchestration and intercellular communication of different cell types within a wound may be disturbed in a highly complex manner. Therefore, more intelligent wound phase specific dressings are required in the future to relieve pain and suffering in the growing population of patients with chronic wounds, which are frequently observed in diabetic patients. A mini-review covering biofunctionalized wound dressings for advanced wound healing is provided in Chapter 11.

An interesting evolving technology related to biofunctional surface engineering is the vaccination with viral antigens immobilized on scaffolds such as microneedles. Microneedles are scaffolds for transdermal vaccination that carry the vaccine and avoid limited compliance (no syringe needed) of the patients. Moreover, the skin is an ideal tissue for antigen recognition and efficient antigen presentation by the Langerhans cells and dendritic cells that are present in a high density. The major requirements for vaccination with microneedles are high stability and sterility of the material that is introduced into the skin and the functionality of the antigens on the surface. The microneedle development, the challenges, and possible solutions to engineer these biofunctional surfaces are shortly introduced by the group of U. Protzer in Chapter 9.

Even the microarray technology used for diagnostic purposes is strongly associated with biofunctional surface engineering as it is described in Chapter 10 by Lueking et al. in the field of autoimmune diseases.

Regardless of the plausibility and proven efficacy of each single approach that involves biofunctionalized surfaces in the specific fields of medicine, every single approach has to consider commercial and regulatory aspects as early as possible.

There is no doubt that combination devices with biofunctionalized material surfaces will evolve to be an essential field of modern medicine in the near future. This book provides a comprehensive overview on the state of the art and the future of biofunctional surface engineering and will be of major interest for all those working in the fields of material sciences, medicine, and medical devices.

Martin Scholz
December 2013

Acknowledgment

This is to acknowledge the immense support by Simone Knappmann.

Chapter 1

Regulatory Requirements for Medical Devices, Including Combinations with Biological Products or Drugs as an Integral Part

Franziska Baumgarten
BSI Group Deutschland GmbH, Reindl 18A, D-82377 Penzberg, Germany
baumgartenfranziska@gmail.com

"One fits all" versus "tailor made," increasing competitive pressure, and substantial progress in technology have been drivers for the development of combinations of devices with drugs and biological products in recent years. This trend will continue and, as estimated, will even pick up speed. Two huge industry blocks are involved. European regulations and national laws are influenced and shaped by different requirements; regulations for medical devices follow the proportionality principle, while those for medicinal products follow the precautionary principle.

Many aspects have to be covered to accomplish the production of safe and effective products on the European market on the border of medical devices and drugs. People involved in the production and

Biofunctional Surface Engineering
Edited by Martin Scholz

ISBN 978-981-4411-60-8 (Hardcover), 978-981-4411-61-5 (eBook)
www.panstanford.com

marketing of these devices have to be knowledgeable about the state of the art of the regulations for both devices and drugs. Therefore, the interdisciplinary approach is the key.

This chapter gives an update on the regulatory facts to be considered for the approval of medical devices and combination products.

1.1 Definitions and Classification

Medical devices and combinations of medical devices with biological products or drugs are regulated in the EU by two major directives: the Medical Device Directive (MDD) 93/42/EEC[1] and the Active Implantable Medical Device Directive (AIMDD) 90/385/EEC. The MDD and AIMDD had to be transposed into law in the EU member states. In Germany, for example, the MDD and AIMDD requirements are implemented by the German "Medizinproduktegesetz."

The regulatory pathways and the relationships between directives and regulations that are relevant for the approval for a medical device in the EU are depicted schematically in Fig. 1.1.

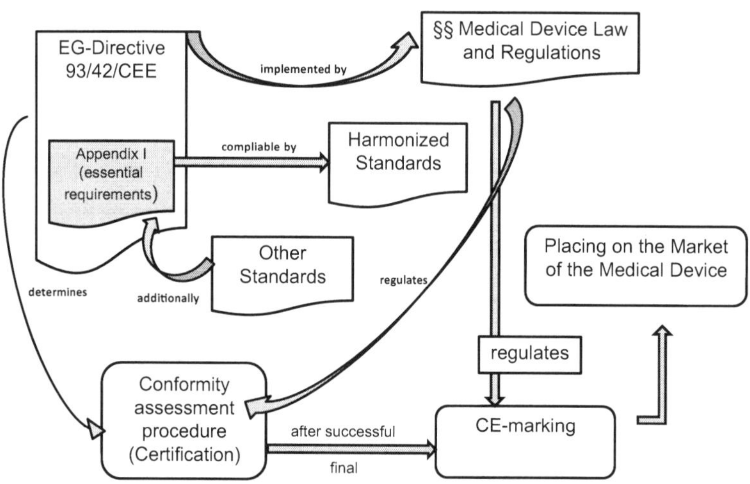

Figure 1.1 Regulatory relationships between directives and country regulations in the EU (for example, Germany). Only medical devices with a CE label can be commercially distributed.

[1]http://ec.europa.eu/health/medical-devices/index_en.htm.

Combinations of medical devices with drugs or biologic compounds are named "combi products" in this chapter. Advanced therapy medicinal products (ATMP), which are similar to combi products at the first sight, follow a different legal route and have been excluded here. Medical devices can be defined as used for

1. diagnosis, prevention, monitoring, treatment, or alleviation of diseases;
2. diagnosis, monitoring, treatment, alleviation of or compensation for an injury or handicap;
3. investigation, replacement, or modification of the anatomy or a physiological process; and
4. control of conception.

The demarcation between medical devices and medicinal products (regulated under Directive 2001/83/EC) is defined by the principal intended action. In general, the principal intended action of medical devices cannot be reached by pharmacological, immunological, or metabolic means. One of the core principles of medical device regulations is the risk-based approach, leading to the allocation of all medical devices into six different classes. The level of control corresponds to the level of potential hazard inherent in the type of device concerned. The manufacturer is responsible for device classification. The basis of classification are the claims made for the product and the method by which the principal intended action is achieved. The mode of action should be clear and should be evidenced with appropriate data. The following questions are relevant for proper classification:

- Is the medical device invasive?
- What is the nature and duration of the exposition?
- Does the device need energy supply and thus may be defined as an active medical device?

Depending on the answers, the devices may be judged as follows:

Class I: non-invasive medical devices

Class II (a, b): invasive devices, including those with energy supply, such as implants

Class III: medical devices that involve critical organs such as the heart and the brain, for example, implants made of absorbable material

1.2 Combi Products: Definitions and Classification

If the substances incorporated in medical devices are liable to act upon the body with action ancillary to that of the device, the regulation of the devices is governed by the MDD. These devices are in the highest risk class and fall under a separate classification rule (rule 13).

1.3 Evidence of Conformity to the Essential Requirements of the Directives

Medical devices placed on the European market should ensure a high level of protection for patients and users: A manufacturer states that their device conforms to the essential requirements as listed in Annex I of the MDD and the AIMDD; this is the "conformity declaration," CE, which the manufacturer affixes to their device. For Class Is, Im, IIa, IIb, and III devices, notified bodies have to check whether the declaration of conformity of the manufacturer is true and whether the essential requirements of the directives are met.

First, this is achieved by regular audits within the companies. The implementation of design, production, risk management, clinical evaluation, and post-market surveillance in the QM system is checked. Second, notified bodies assess the technical documentation—or the design dossier for Class III devices—in a structured and systematic way.

1.4 Specific Essential Requirements for Combi Products

If a device incorporates, as an integral part, a substance that, if used separately, may be considered a medicinal product as defined in Article 1 of Directive 2001/83/EC and that is liable to act upon the body with action ancillary to that of the device, then the following applies: The quality, safety, and usefulness of the substance must be verified by analogy with the methods specified in Annex I of Directive 2001/83/EC,[2] the directive for pharmaceutical products.

[2]Medical Device Directive 93/42/EEC essential requirement 7.4

This particular essential requirement requires data on quality and safety, which have to be verified by a competent drug authority of the EU member states or the European Medicines Agency (EMA). The notified body conducts a review of the usefulness of the ancillary substance and the device aspects. Additionally, the notified body has to consult the competent authority or the EMA for the quality and safety of the medicinal substance. If the ancillary substance is a human blood derivative, the consultation is between the notified body and the EMA. Figure 1.2 describes the steps of a consultation procedure in detail.

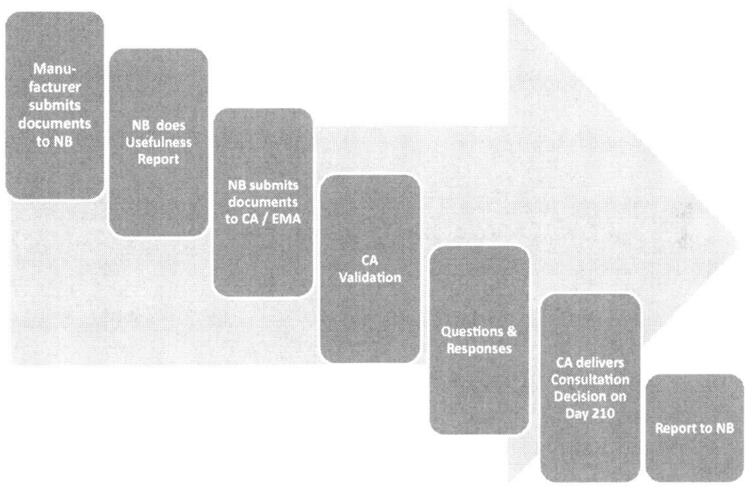

Figure 1.2 Stages in medicinal consultation and timelines. NB, notified body; CA, competent authority; EMA, European Medicines agency.

1.5 Use of Harmonized Standards: Presumption of Conformity

Member states and notified bodies shall presume compliance with the essential requirements of the directives when harmonized standards are used. All harmonized standards are published in the *Official Journal of the European Union* (OJEU). For combi products, which are in Class III by definition and are in most cases long-term invasive, three standards are important:

1. biocompatibility
2. bioburden
3. sterilization

The standard family of ISO 10993-(1-20) defines the requirements for the evaluation of the biocompatibility of a medical device prior to a clinical study. For example, the biocompatibility of each material that has contact with the patient tissue or blood, according to the intended use, will be evaluated. Related trials are cell culture testing and/or hemolysis assays.

The required bioburden testing procedures are described in ISO 11737-1:2006 "Sterilization of medical devices—Microbiological methods—Part 1: Determination of a population of microorganisms on products" and in ISO 11737-2:2009 "Sterilization of medical devices—Microbiological methods—Part 2: Tests of sterility performed in the definition, validation, and maintenance of a sterilization process."

The required sterilization procedures are defined in separate ISO standards: ISO 11137-1:2006 "Sterilization of health care products—Radiation—Part 1: Requirements for development, validation, and routine control of a sterilization process for medical devices" and ISO 11137-2:2012 "Sterilization of health care products—Radiation—Part 2: Establishing the sterilization dose."

The ISO standards 11137-1:2006 and 11137-2:2012 are described in more detail in Chapter 2. Figure 1.3 summarizes the required testing and documentation to apply for clinical evaluation of the device.

1.6 Clinical Evaluation

Before a device can be placed on the market and applied to patients, its safety and performance have to be approved. By definition, clinical evaluation is the assessment and analysis of the clinical data pertaining to a medical device to verify the clinical safety and performance of the device.[3] It is an ongoing process throughout the life cycle of the product, constantly being matched against post-market surveillance data and implemented in the QM system of the manufacturing company.

[3] MEDDEV. 2.7.1 Rev.3, p.4

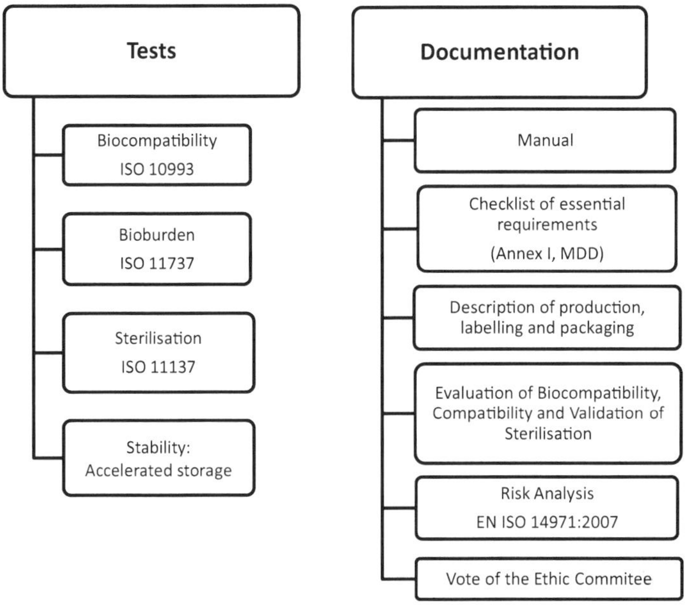

Figure 1.3 Annex VIII of the MDD requires testing and documentations as a prerequisite for starting a clinical trial.

Clinical evaluation always contains literature research. All medical devices have to undergo literature research, regardless of which class they belong to. Literature data are the basis for the decision whether a clinical investigation, or a clinical study, has to be performed. For a Class III medical device, clinical studies are mandatory.

EU member states have different approval routes before a clinical investigation can be started: Ethical commissions of the clinical testing sites have to approve the ethical conformity. The criteria are, for example, medical need, safety, additional risks for the patients, quality of the study design, and data safety.

Ethical evaluation is a central element for the start of clinical studies, which in turn are important for regulatory evaluation. After positive evaluation and approval of the ethical commissions and the state authorities, the study may begin. The clinical data have to be summarized in a final report, which is part of the clinical evaluation. It is important to note that the clinical data should be collected according to Annex X of the MDD, especially regarding the question whether the risk–benefit ratio is adequate, which in turn is defined in Annex I of the MDD.

A practical example for a risk–benefit consideration is presented here. It is a device for extracorporeal blood circulation and enrichment of circulating tumor cells (CTCs), which is currently in the development phase.

The classical method for collecting CTCs in a Cell Search System has been described by Coumans and Terstappen in Chapter 12. The Cell Search System allows the analysis of 7.5 mL blood containing only a few CTCs. The diagnostic potential of the Cell Search System is rather limited. It would be beneficial to have a new method available to be able to collect a significantly larger number of CTCs.

With the new approach under development—the "CTCtrap"—it is intended to achieve this. The CTCtrap is a plastic housing with open porous polyurethane foam that carries covalently immobilized biomolecules for trapping and enriching EpCAM+ tumor cells. The CTCtrap module will be interconnected into the circuit of an extracorporeal blood circulation system. After the termination of the apheresis, the housing is decoupled from the circuit and the trapped CTCs can be eluted for further diagnostic purposes.

The extracorporeal apheresis will last approximately 1–2 h, and it is very obvious that the risk for the patient is much higher when CTCs are collected with the CTCtrap method compared with the classical method, which means only collecting 7.5 mL blood from the patient with a syringe.

The potential benefit for the cancer patient could be much higher with the CTCtrap method, though. The larger amount of eluted cells could result in better diagnostics for further treatment.

Preclinical testing and the clinical evaluation, including the study plan, have to show that the trap is (1) safe to be used in humans (risk) and (2) that it can be expected that there is a diagnostic advantage over the classical method as a general outcome (benefit).

Ethical commissions and authorities have to approve the clinical study plan, taking into account this risk–benefit balance as an intrinsic part of their evaluation. After the clinical study has been finished successfully, it will be part of the technical documentation, which has to be reviewed for conformity according to EU requirements.

1.7 Outlook: New Regulation for Medical Devices in the EU

The two important directives for medical devices, AIMD and MDD, will be modified to become one single European regulation until 2016. This new regulation will become effective without transposition into country regulations of EU member states.

Chapter 2

Terminal Radiation Sterilization of Combination Products

Kristina Kemter
LEUKOCARE AG, Am Klopferspitz 19, 82152 Martinsried/Munich, Germany
kristina.kemter@leukocare.com

This review deals with the challenge of using radiation to terminally sterilize medical devices combined with biologic components. The market for these combination devices is rapidly growing and will determine the competition and the research and development activity of medical device and biopharmaceutical enterprises in the future. However, the conflict of the developers in this field is to achieve sterile products at the end of the production step and, at the same time, to enable sustained functionality of the biomolecule after sterilization. In the following, we give an overview of the regulatory issues that are relevant for sterilization and thus for the approval of combination devices. We also provide examples for technical solutions to achieve fully functional terminally sterilized biomolecules alone or immobilized on a scaffold. In conclusion, it can be said that innovative technologies enable terminal sterilization

Biofunctional Surface Engineering
Edited by Martin Scholz

ISBN 978-981-4411-60-8 (Hardcover), 978-981-4411-61-5 (eBook)
www.panstanford.com

of new combination products and catalyze the increasingly growing market at the interface between Medtech and Biotech.

2.1 Introduction

Radiation sterilization of medical devices has proved to be highly effective for more than 50 years (Fairand and Razem, 2010). The validation of a sterility assurance level (SAL) of 10^{-6} is possible for many different products, including heat-labile devices. Another advantage is the exact determination of absorbed dose of radiation by means of dosimetry. In general, a minimum dose of 25 kGy was considered sufficient to achieve a SAL of 10^{-6}. Today, different methods to establish the minimum sterilization dose are defined and embodied in ISO standards. An attractive method is the VD_{max}, which requires fewer test samples compared with the other methods. Therefore, the VD_{max} method is described here as a common method in more detail.

The VD_{max} method can be used for doses down to 15 kGy and requires the determination of bioburden and the performance of a verification dose experiment. The sterilization dose will change with the selection of different values for the maximum bioburden. For example, at a maximum bioburden of 1000 colony forming units (CFUs), the sterilization dose is 25 kGy, and for a maximum bioburden of 1.5 CFUs, the sterilization dose is 15 kGy. The verification dose experiment is performed at a SAL of 10^{-1}.

The validation protocol is specified in the ANSI/AAMI/ISO 11137-1:2006 document entitled "Sterilization of health care products—Radiation—Part 1: Requirements for development, validation, and routine control of a sterilization process for medical devices" and in the ANSI/AAMI/ISO 11137-2:2006 document entitled "Sterilization of health care products—Radiation—Part 2: Establishing the sterilization dose" (ISO11137-1:2006; ISO11137-2:2006).

In this review, some examples are provided that show the feasibility of terminal sterilization by irradiation. The underlying enabling technology is a coating layer that covers and protects the biomolecules in dry form until further use. The excipients within the amorphous layer substitute for the water molecules during drying and freezing and can be removed by water during reconstitution. The coating can be used for immobilized biomolecules, such as monoclonal antibodies, on any biocompatible scaffold material. The principle of the coating procedure and its proposed beneficial integration in various fields of Medtech are graphically shown in Fig. 2.1.

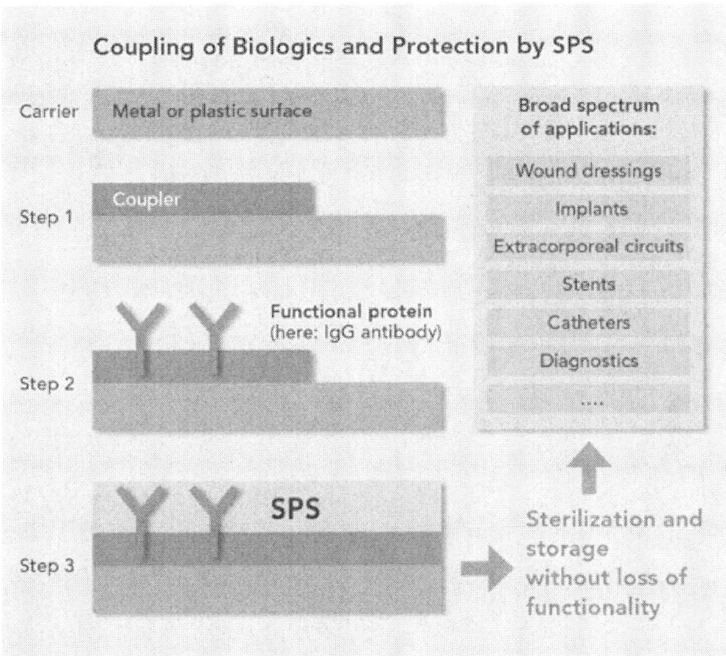

Figure 2.1 Principle design of the protecting layer as proposed for the use in different fields of Medtech and medicine. SPS: stabilizing and protecting solution.

2.2 Interaction of Radiation with Biomolecules

The radiation of biomolecules or drug products is associated with a high energy input (high energy electrons, for example, have energy in the 1–10 MeV range) and increases the risk for altered molecular and functional integrity (Fairand and Razem, 2010). For example, as outlined further below, the radiation-mediated protein misfolding in therapeutic drugs may result not only in biological dysfunction but also in unappreciated aggregation and subsequent immunogenic responses in the patient.

It is important to mention that the radiation-mediated damage of biomolecules cannot be easily predicted by the law of reciprocity (law of Bunsen–Roscoe) that can be applied for the sole physical modifications of materials. According to this law, the amount of radiation energy is reciprocal to the duration of radiation to achieve a certain physical effect. For biomolecules, such as proteins, this is not necessarily true because of intrinsic molecular repair mechanisms that have to be taken into account. On the other hand, the duration of irradiation is an important factor because of secondary damaging effects. Specifically, gamma ray irradiation takes longer than electron beam irradiation to achieve a defined dose on the product, and thus secondary reactions such as oxygen radical formation may accumulate over time and indirectly damage molecular structures. From this, it is evident that the amount of residual water content of the irradiated drug products is an important critical factor and should be carefully balanced. Radiation of water leads to ionizing of water (water hydrolysis) molecules and to the formation of aggressive oxidizing hydroxyl radicals and reactive oxygen intermediates (ROIs), which subsequently react with and damage the protein. It is well accepted that lyophilized drugs, therefore, better resist irradiation-mediated damage compared with wet samples (Fairand and Razem, 2010).

Of course, when biofunctional coatings of solid surfaces or devices for controlled drug release (CDR) are utilizing biopolymers, radiation-mediated chain scissions, cross-linking, and also formation of free radicals may occur. As a result, color, physical properties, and change in drug release characteristics might be the consequence.

In summary, radiation sterilization of combination devices or of biofunctionalized surfaces entails two biomolecule-damaging pathways, which have to be carefully considered: (a) toxic products elicited by radiated carrier material or CDR devices, and (b) chain reactions forced by oxygen radicals and ROIs in the residual water or in the biomolecule itself.

In the following paragraphs, examples of both, radiation sterilization of free lyophilized biomolecules and immobilized biomolecules, respectively, are described.

Radiation sterilization of lyophilized biomolecules

Aseptic filtration of biomolecules does not lead to a 10^{-6} SAL, leaves the risk of contamination during fill and finish (see also the online collection of recent FDA warning letters), and may also lead to significant economic loss (Rathore and Rajan, 2008; FDA warning letters; Shire, 2009). Furthermore, pharmaceutical guidelines recommend terminal sterilization methods (European Pharmacopoeia, 2005; EMEA, 2000; USP, 2000) so that the need for technologies and procedures that enable terminal sterilization of biomolecules, including proteins, increases along with cost pressure and safety concerns (Bhamra et al., 2000; Zbikowska et al., 2006). On the other hand, irradiation is currently not considered a standard and valid sterilization protocol for proteins and other biologics since it is associated with a high energy input and increased risk for chemical and physical modifications, misfolding, formation of aggregates, and fragmentation (Zbikowska et al., 2006; Garrison et al., 1962; Kapoor and Priyadarsini, 2001). Especially, aggregates may lead to modified immunogenicity of therapeutically applied biologics (De Groot and Scott, 2007).

Accordingly, new approaches to avoid sterilization-mediated damage of therapeutic biomolecules have been developed. Earlier studies showed that radiation-induced functional degradation of proteins was reduced by low irradiation temperatures and by certain excipients. For example, the addition of antioxidants in combination with low temperatures maintained the integrity of the protein even at high irradiation doses (Zbikowska et al., 2006). Therefore, the components of the protein formulation and the temperature should be carefully considered when radiation sterilization of drug products is the goal.

Recently, a novel stabilizing and protecting solution (SPS) has been reported that proved to stabilize biological macromolecules such as therapeutic antibodies and vaccines during sterilization by gamma or beta irradiation and ethylene oxide (Scholz and Altenhofer, 2011; Scholz and Lüking, 2012; Tscheliessnig et al., 2012). The specific composition of SPS consists of 5–7 different small molecule-type excipients, including a rigid amphiphilic molecule, and is void of commonly used stabilizers in pharmaceutical formulations, like sugars, proteins, and salts. These commonly used excipients are discussed controversially when lyophilization and sterilization procedures are involved (Wakankar and Borchardt, 2006; Han et al., 2007). For example, high concentrations of sugars often necessary for cryo- and lyoprotection are known to damage the biomolecule during freezing and thawing by crystallization (Han et al., 2007; Wang, 2000). The sugar-free SPS composition can be adjusted to the specific requirements of the biomolecule to be protected. SPS fulfills all safety and regulatory requirements for therapeutic use in patients.

Mechanistically, SPS works by replacing stabilizing interactions between the protein and water by similar interactions with less reactive small molecules. Upon removal of water, these molecules form an amorphous coat, which protects the substrate against physical and chemical destabilization during storage and against the destructive impact of different kinds of stress such as heat, oxidation, irradiation, or EtO gas sterilization. Proteins such as therapeutic antibodies and vaccines are certainly the major drug products that should be considered. Here, we give examples for both groups to allow a better view into the radiation-associated problems and possible solutions. All biomolecules can be utilized either as pharmacologically formulated free drugs or, when required, as effector molecules immobilized on scaffolds or in CDR biopolymers. An interesting example for immobilized vaccines is the recently propagated technology, designated "microneedles." Microneedles are vaccine carriers for transdermal application and require stable biomolecule coating with defined eluting kinetics. Microneedles are discussed in Chapter 9.

2.2.1 Example 1: Sterilization of Herceptin®

Therapeutic antibodies are certainly interesting proteins to study the protective effects of new formulations, particularly during terminal sterilization. Irradiation of a protein is associated with chemical and physical modifications. Chemical instability refers to oxidation, deamidation, reduction, and hydrolysis, and physical modifications are fragmentation, unfolding, dissociation, denaturation, aggregation, and precipitation. The degradation pathways are often synergistic, and a chemical event like oxidation can trigger a physical event like aggregation or fragmentation. The aggregate content as well as degradation products of therapeutically applied biologics should be as low as possible (e.g., below 2%) and are crucial parameter for regulatory compliance.

The molecular structures as well as the critical aggregation and fragmentation sites within these proteins are well known (Vlasak and Ionescu, 2011). The sites in the polypeptide chain susceptible to fragmentation are determined by a multitude of factors. Of course, the secondary, tertiary, and quaternary structures of the protein have a significant impact in modulating the distribution of the cleavage sites by altering local flexibility and accessibility to solvent or by bringing in close proximity side chains that are remote in sequence (Vlasak and Ionescu, 2011). Efforts to stabilize therapeutic monoclonal antibodies begin as early as during purification (Falconer et al., 2011).

By using trastuzumab (Herceptin®) as a model antibody (Jeyakumar and Younis, 2012), we studied the efficacy of an SPS provided by LEUKOCARE AG, Munich, in combination with a low temperature irradiation protocol (β- or γ-irradiation at −80°C) to prevent irradiation-mediated protein damage. For the lyophilization, a standard protocol was used, as shown in Table 2.1. Interestingly, β- or γ-irradiation with 25 and 40 kGy impaired functional HER2 binding of the original trastuzumab formulation and the negative control formulation in PBS only to a moderate degree, as shown by ELISA. This finding is remarkable in itself since irradiation at such elevated doses typically significantly decreases the activity of a protein. To better understand the nature of possible molecular modifications after irradiation, we applied nonreducing SDS-PAGE, fluorescence-based aggregation assay, size exclusion chromatography (SEC), and Fourier transform infrared spectroscopy (FTIR).

Table 2.1 A representative lyophilization protocol with an Epsilon 2-6D (Martin Christ; Osterode am Harz, Germany) was used for these experiments

Protocol step	Target (*T*) (°C)	Slope (*h*)	Hold (*h*)	Pressure (mbar)
Introduction	20	0	0	1000
Freezing	−50	1:30	2:30	1000
Sublimation	−50	0:15	0	0.045
	−15	1:30	30:00	0.045
Secondary drying	−15	0:15	0	0.009
	20	1:30	10:00	0.009

FTIR analysis confirmed the functional data that after reconstitution and refolding, the secondary structure, surprisingly of all irradiated and nonirradiated samples, was comparable to the original untreated antibody even in the negative control formulation in PBS.

However, the molecular integrity was markedly impaired particularly in terms of aggregate formation, as detected by nonreducing SDS-PAGE, fluorescence-based aggregation assay, and SEC.

By means of semiquantitative nonreducing SDS-PAGE and a fluorescence-based microplate assay, we observed substantial formation of aggregates and degradation products of Herceptin following both 25 and 40 kGy β- and γ-irradiation (not shown). When samples were lyophilized and irradiated in SPS, irradiation-mediated aggregates and degradation products were found to be markedly reduced. SEC analysis showed that either irradiation type induced severe aggregation and degradation of Herceptin in the original formulation but not in SPS-formulated samples, thus confirming the findings by SDS-PAGE and fluorescent aggregation tests. Interestingly, even at 40 kGy irradiation, the content of high molecular weight aggregates was around 2% or less when SPS-formulated samples were irradiated at −80°C. The lower temperature during irradiation itself showed an about 30% reduction of aggregates probably due to reduced thermal stress for the protein during the high irradiation-associated energy input (Garrison et al., 1962; Kapoor Priyadarsini, 2001). However, this modification in the irradiation protocol alone may not be sufficient to fulfill current production standards of therapeutic antibodies (< 2% aggregates). However, in our own experiments, the procedure involving a combination of low temperature irradiation with SPS-formulated biomolecules reached this goal (Altrichter et al., 2012).

Additionally, we found by the FTIR analysis of the freeze-dried samples that the secondary structure of the originally formulated, but not of SPS-formulated, Herceptin was significantly impaired in the lyophilized samples.

These results substantiate the hypothesis that the native conformation of the antigen-binding site of the antibody remains unimpaired upon irradiation even in the negative control formulation and that other parts of the antibody are chemically modified by exposure to irradiation leading to aggregation.

In summary, SPS formulation of trastuzumab almost fully prevented aggregation and fragmentation. Aggregate formation was further reduced when SPS-formulated samples were irradiated at −80°C. In addition, the secondary structure of trastuzumab was preserved by SPS but not by the original formulation during lyophilization. Moreover, SPS formulation alone or in combination with low temperature irradiation protocols enables terminal sterilization of trastuzumab by irradiation and thus may significantly reduce production costs and the risk of contamination in protein drugs.

The stabilizing and protecting effects of SPS have been shown in the past with several proteins, including IgM, IgG antibodies, enzymes, cytokines, etc. (Scholz and Altenhofer, 2011; Scholz and Lüking, 2012; Tscheliessnig et al., 2012). According to the concept of preferential exclusion and preferential binding (Shimizu and Smith, 2004; Auton et al., 2008), SPS generically elicits its protecting effects by forming a protecting layer around the proteins during drying. In addition, the amorphous character of SPS, combined with the lack of sugars, avoids crystallization-mediated protein damage during freezing and thawing (Han et al., 2007; Wang, 2000) and thus promotes refolding during reconstitution (Tscheliessnig et al., 2012). In addition to the stabilizing features, SPS formulations enable excellent cake formation with rapid reconstitution times. All components of the SPS are available in pharmaceutical grade and are already routinely applied in parenteral solutions.

In conclusion, terminal irradiation of therapeutic antibodies or other biomolecules is possible with innovative formulations alone or in conjunction with modified irradiation protocols, e.g., at low temperatures. Such protocols enable the maintenance of both the functionality and the molecular integrity and thus might be a novel benchmark for terminal sterilization of biomolecules on scaffolds.

2.2.2 Example 2: Sterilization of Immobilized Antibodies in Three-Dimensional Carrier Foams

A nano-coating (NC) formulation to maintain the functionality of proteins on biologic-device combination products was developed. As a proof of concept, NC preserved the structural and functional integrity of an otherwise highly fragile antibody immobilized on polyurethane during deleterious sterilizing irradiation (≥25 kGy). The NC procedure enabled straightforward terminal sterilization of biofunctionalized materials while preserving optimal conditioning of the bioactive surface.

The protecting efficacy of the NC procedure is assumed to be in accordance with the concepts of preferential exclusion and preferential binding (Arakawa et al., 2001, 2007; Auton et al., 2008; Shimizu and Smith, 2004; Timasheff, 1993, 2002). Biomolecules immobilized on a biocompatible carrier are embedded in the NC solution. After drying, the biofunctionalized material can be stressed, e.g., by irradiation without loss of molecular integrity. It is, therefore, appreciated that the stabilizing excipients support a preferentially hydrated, native protein conformation in the liquid phase. Upon drying of the bioactive surface, excipients should substitute for water molecules at the protein surface by forming hydrogen bonds between the protein and the functional groups of the co-solvent. A glassy molecular film of co-solvent established at the end of the drying process is considered to protect the functionality of the surface.

As proof of concept, the multimeric and fragile anti-Fas IgM antibody (IgM_{Fas}, 900 kD) was covalently coupled to open porous polyurethane (PU) for the use in a medical device for extracorporeal immunotherapy. The antibodies used here agonistically recognize and stimulate Fas (CD95) (Scholz and Cinatl, 2005) on circulating hyper-activated neutrophils (most abundant white blood cells in humans) from severely ill patients to limit systemic inflammation (Scholz and Cinatl, 2005; Fadeel et al.,1998; Peter et al., 2007).

To protect radiation-sensitive PU-IgM_{Fas} during sterilization of the support, we overlaid the biomolecules with the nano-coating formulation and determined (a.) physicochemical characteristics, (b.) molecular mechanisms of protein stabilization, and (c.) safety and efficacy.

The physicochemical characteristics of the nano-coating technology were shown to fulfill the requirements for effective three-dimensional stabilization of proteins during drying, sterilization, and reconstitution as it was shown by small angle X-ray scattering (SAXS) analysis. SAXS allows for monitoring of structural changes of the protein coupled to a solid carrier upon physical stress. The adaptation of SAXS for the structural analysis of coupled IgM to biocompatible scaffold materials is described in more detail in Chapter 7.

By means of functional in vitro and ex vivo read-out assays, we confirmed the efficacy and clinical relevance of nano-coating by showing the preservation of specific antigen/epitope binding of IgM_{Fas} during irradiation.

The validity of standard sterilization of PU-IgM_{Fas} was demonstrated in accordance with the ISO 11137 VD_{max} (ISO1137-1:2006; ISO1137-2:2006) method resulting in a SAL of 10^{-6}. An explanation of the guidelines on sterilization issues has been provided earlier in this chapter.

2.2.3 Example 3: Sterilization of Immobilized Viral Antigens on Vaccine Scaffolds

An attractive approach in vaccination strategy is the concept to immobilize viral antigens on microneedles or nanopatches. Microneedles or nanopatches are used for transdermal vaccination, avoiding the use of a syringe. A closer look at the microneedle technology is provided in Chapter 9. In the following paragraphs, it will be shown that immobilized viral antigens, for example on stainless steel scaffolds that may be used as microneedles, may be terminally sterilized without relevant loss of antigenicity.

2.2.3.1 Influenza A functionality assay showing maintenance of antigenicity

Inactivated Influenza A (H1N1) whole virus particles were formulated in a protecting solution. The stainless steel scaffolds were dipped into the vaccine-containing formulation and subsequently air dried. The dried protecting and stabilizing solution forms an amorphous layer around the vaccine antigens. A part of the scaffolds was sterilized with 25 kGy β-irradiation after the drying step. After reconstitution of the antigens by rinsing the scaffolds by means of an aqueous buffer solution, the functionality of the antigens was evaluated in the hemagglutination assay (HA). By contrast to the nonstabilized control, which showed a complete loss of antigenicity of Influenza A, the hemagglutination activity was almost fully maintained after treatment with protecting coating. These results clearly show the feasibility of terminally irradiated vaccine scaffolds such as microneedles, nanopatches, or others. The efficacy of the immobilized and dried vaccine may be further increased by adding an adjuvant to the protecting layer. For example, saponins such as glycyrrhizic acid, which are known to both stabilize proteins and may serve as an adjuvant, may be attractive candidates for improved vaccine formulations.

The ability to develop vaccine-bearing scaffolds with high stress resistance and prolonged shelf life opens the door for vaccine distributors to circumvent rapid loss of antigenicity, e.g., during transportation in countries where cool chains are not guaranteed.

2.2.3.2 Maintenance of antigenicity despite inactivation of virus upon irradiation

When considering the aforementioned protecting layers around the biomolecules during the production process to allow irradiation as sterilization, an important question has to be answered: Does the protecting layer also protect contaminating bacteria or viruses? The sterility regarding bacterial contamination has already been discussed and experimentally proven, as outlined earlier. The viral contamination might also be a problem during production.

To answer this question, virus inactivation studies were performed using immobilized human adenovirus type 5 (Ad5). Specifically, 50 μL of virus suspension was dried at 37°C on the bottom of sterile polystyrol tubes. The dried virus was then overlaid with 50 μL of the protecting solution and dried again at 37°C. After β-irradiation at 25 kGy or 40 kGy (controls were not irradiated), the virus/protecting solution bilayer was resuspended in 1 mL of MEM, and the titer of infectious virus was determined by means of end-point titration (Tscheliessnig et al., 2012).

We showed that β-irradiation led to quantitative inactivation of Ad5 (25 kGy, ≥99.9% reduction; 40 kGy, ≥99.999% reduction), while the functionality of an IgM antibody was maintained. These results demonstrate that the protecting solution selectively stabilizes and protects protein structures, such as antigenic envelope proteins, but does not prevent viral genome destruction and thus inactivation of the virus replication machinery (Tscheliessnig et al., 2012).

In summary, there is no increased risk of bacterial and viral activity after covering the biomolecule with the protecting layer before sterilization. Functionality and sterility of terminally irradiated biomolecules in the dry form are achieved by the protecting layer. For example, this may be specifically important for the production of vaccines, especially when viral antigens are intended to be immobilized on the surface of scaffolds according to the concept of microneedles or nanopatches (as outlined earlier and in Chapter 9).

References

Altrichter J, Altenhofen W, Kemter K, Scholz M. 2012. *Stabilization and Protection of the Therapeutic Antibody Herceptin During Irradiation by a Novel Formulation and Sterilization Protocol* (manuscript submitted).

Arakawa T., et al. 2001. Factors affecting short-term and long-term stabilities of proteins. *Adv Drug Deliv Rev* **46**(1-3): 307–326.

Arakawa T., et al. 2007. Biotechnology applications of amino acids in protein purification and formulations. *Amino Acids* **33**(4): 587–605.

Auton M, Bolen DW, Rosgen J. 2008. Structural thermodynamics of protein preferential solvation: osmolyte solvation of proteins, amino acids, and peptides. *Proteins* **73**: 802–813.

Bhamra K, Harrison P, Phillips J, Hale G. 2000. Aseptic vial filling. *Methods Mol Med.*40:313-317.

De Groot AS and Scott DW. 2007. Immunogenicity of protein therapeutics. *Trends in Immunol* **28**: 482–490.

European Pharmacopoeia. 2005. 5th ed. Council of Europe, Strasbourg, France.

European Agency for the Evaluation of Medicinal Products (EMEA). 2000. *Decision Trees for the Selection of Sterilization Methods (CPMP/QWP/054/98 corr)*, London.

Fadeel B., et al. 1998. A three-dimensional model of the Fas/Apo-1 molecule: Cross-reactivity of anti-Fas antibodies explained by structural mimicry of antigenic sites. *Int Immunol* **10**(2): 131–140.

Fairand BP and Razem D. 2010. Radiation sterilization. In *Pharmaceutical Dosage Forms: Parenteral Medications, 3rd ed, Volume 2: Facility Design, Sterilization and Processing* (Nema S and Ludwig JD, ed). New York: Informa Healthcare. pp. 268–294.

Falconer RJ, Chan C, Hughes K, Munro TP. 2011. Stabilization of a monoclonal antibody during purification and formulation by addition of basic amino acid excipients. *J Chem Technol Biotechnol* **86**: 942–948.

FDA warning letters: http://www.fda.gov/ICECI/EnforcementActions/WarningLetters/default.htm

Garrison WM, Jayko ME, Bennett W. 1962. Radiation-induced oxidation of protein in aqueous solution. *Radiat Res* **16**: 483–502.

Han Y, et al. 2007. Effects of sugar additives on protein stability of recombinant human serum albumin during lyophilization and storage. *Arch Pharm Res* **30**: 1124–1131.

ISO1137-1:2006

ISO1137-2:2006

Jeyakumar A and Younis T. 2012. Trastuzumab for HER2-positive metastatic breast cancer: Clinical and economic considerations. *Clin Med Insights Oncol* **6**: 179–187.

Kapoor S and Priyadarsini KI. 2001. Protection of radiation-induced protein damage by curcumin. *Biophys Chem* **92**: 119–126.

Peter ME, et al. 2007. The Cd95 receptor: Apoptosis revisited. *Cell* **129**(3): 447–450.

Rathore N and Rajan RS. 2008. Current perspectives on stability of protein drug products during formulation, fill and finish operations. *Biotechnol Prog* **24**: 504–514.

Scholz M and Altenhofer W. 2011. Stabilising biologics for vaccine production. *Manufacturing Chemist* **9**: 32–34.

Scholz M and Lüking A. 2012. A protein-stabilizing technology for enhanced antibody stability and antibody-binding profiles in a microchip array. *Biotechnol J.* doi: 10.1002/biot.201100494. [Epub ahead of print]

Scholz M and Cinatl J. 2005. Fas/Fasl interaction: A novel immune therapy approach with immobilized biologicals. *Med Res Rev* **25**(3): 331–342.

Shimizu S and Smith DJ. 2004. Preferential hydration and the exclusion of cosolvents from protein surfaces. *J Chem Phys* **121**: 1148–1154.

Shire SJ. 2009. Formulation and manufacturability of biologics. *Curr Opin Biotechnol* **20**: 708–714.

Timasheff SN. 1993. The control of protein stability and association by weak interactions with water: How do solvents affect these processes? *Annu Rev Biophys Biomol Struct* **22**: 67–97.

Timasheff SN. 2002. Protein-solvent preferential interactions, protein hydration, and the modulation of biochemical reactions by solvent components. *Proc Natl Acad Sci USA* **99**(15): 9721–9726.

Tscheliessnig R., et al. 2012. Nano-coating protects biofunctional materials. *Materials Today* **15**(9): 394–404.

United States Pharmacopoeia (USP). 2000. *National Formulary 24.* Rockville, Maryland: United States Pharmacopoeial Convention.

Vlasak J and Ionescu R. 2011. Fragmentation of monoclonal antibodies. *mAbs* **3**: 253–263.

Wang W. 2000. Lyophilization and development of solid protein pharmaceuticals. *Int. J. Pharm.* **203**: 1–60.

Wakankar AA and Borchardt RT. 2006. Formulation considerations for proteins susceptible to asparagine deamidation and aspartate isomerization. *J Pharm Sci* **95**: 2321–2336.

Zbikowska HM, Nowak P, Wachowicz B. 2006. Protein modification caused by a high dose of gamma irradiation in cryo-sterilized plasma: Protective effects of ascorbate. *Free Radical Biol Med* **40**: 536–542.

Chapter 3

Polyelectrolyte Multilayers as Functional Coatings for Controlled Biomolecular Interactions

Hanna Hartmann and Burkhard Schlosshauer
Natural and Medical Sciences Institute at the University of Tübingen, Markwiesenstraße 55, 72770 Reutlingen, Germany
schlosshauer@nmi.de

The surface properties of implants and biotechnological devices are of outstanding importance to direct and control interactions with living cells. Whereas biomimetic surfaces attempt to reproduce the organization of natural matrices, nonphysiological additives such as antimitotic drugs could help to manipulate cell responses in specific ways. Both aspects might be desirable aims for specific targets. A current approach to functionalize implants is based on nano-coating with polyelectrolyte multilayers (PEMs) in the layer-by-layer (LbL) method introduced by Decher et al. (1992, 1997). LbL coating is realized by alternate deposition of polyelectrolytes on charged surfaces in a self-assembling and self-organizing process.

Biofunctional Surface Engineering
Edited by Martin Scholz

ISBN 978-981-4411-60-8 (Hardcover), 978-981-4411-61-5 (eBook)
www.panstanford.com

3.1 Controlled Interactions of PEMs with Cells

Contact interactions of PEMs with living matter such as bacteria or eukaryotic cells are based on direct adhesion of microorganisms and cells or indirect attachment via the prior absorbance of molecular factors such as glycans and proteins. Adhesion of cells to a synthetic surface typically provokes cellular responses due to changes in membrane proteins, subsequent intracellular signaling, and rearrangements of the cytoskeleton. This might, in turn, affect cell morphology and migration or cell proliferation and differentiation, including the extension or retraction of cell processes. As a consequence, for example, the therapeutic outcome of biomedical applications such as tissue engineering and implant integration into the host is significantly influenced.

Besides the chemical composition of surfaces (charge, hydrophilicity, functional molecular domains, etc.), other relevant parameters include rigidity/fluidity, roughness, topography, and spatial patterns. These multi-parametric aspects do represent not only challenges but also chances to design PEMs with specific functional impacts. An example is dental implants at the aseptic/septic interface in the mouth where adhesion/nonadhesion specificity is desirable for regenerative host cells versus infectious bacteria.

3.1.1 Physical PEM Parameters and Cell Adhesion

When the fairly cell-nonpermissive polydimethylsiloxane, which is widely used in medical applications, is coated with PEMs, the adhesion of fibroblasts and primary hepatocytes can be significantly improved. Most interestingly, periodic micropatterning of the surface allows to regulate cell attachment and proliferation (Kidambi et al., 2007), suggesting that physicochemically designed topographies might be of relevance for tissue engineering applications.

For various PEM films, including poly-L-lysine (PLL)/hyaluronic acid (HA), chitosan/HA, PLL/polygalacturonic acid (PGA), and PLL/poly-L-glutamic acid (PGA) increased cell adhesion has been reported (Zhu et al., 2004). Furthermore, if the stiffness of PLL/HA films is increased more than 100-fold based on a water-based chemical cross-linking method with defined N-(3-dimethylaminopropyl)-N′-ethylcarbodiimide hydrochloride (EDC) concentrations, the surface properties of the corresponding PEM are switched from a nonpermissive to a highly permissive substrate, which in turn facilitates not only the adhesion but also the proliferation of chondrosarcoma cells (Francius et al., 2006). The same effect could be shown for placenta-derived mesenchymal stem cells (MSCs) grown on PLL/HA multilayers (Semenov et al., 2009). With increasing stiffness by cross-linking with EDC, MSCs show elevated adhesion and cell spreading (Fig. 3.1).

The change in adhesive PEM properties has similar impact on a wide variety of cells, including chondrocytes, osteoblasts, neurons, skeletal muscle cells, macrophages, stem and tumor cells (for review, see Boudou et al., 2009). Also the stiffness of poly(allylamine hydrochloride)/polyacrylamide (PAH/PAA) PEMs can be varied over several orders of magnitude depending on the pH being employed for the generation of the films without changing the chemical composition. Again, increasing the stiffness of PEM films correlates with increased adhesion of human microvascular endothelial cells (Thompson et al., 2005). The same is true for hepatocytes isolated from the rat liver. However, in this case, the enhanced cell adhesion is counterproductive for the maintenance of cell function, since albumin secretion as a marker for hepatocyte differentiation ceases with increasing substrate stiffness (Chen et al., 2009). Other laboratories investigated the impact of the surface roughness. When titanium with PEM layers consisting of PLL/PGA and interspersed calcium apatite crystals are coated with calcium phosphate, spreading of osteoblasts is found to be hampered by the surface roughness (Schade et al., 2011). In summary, rigidity as well as terminal layer coating and PEM composition appear to be instructive for differential attachment and function of many cells.

Cell-type specificity can be partially imposed onto material surfaces by various means. Elastomeric silicone sheets coated with PEMs composed of polyacrylic acid modified with phosphorylcholine and triethylene glycol groups are essentially antiadhesive under rest. With stretching of the substrate, the adhesion of fungi remains abrogated, whereas fibroblasts become capable of spreading on the surface (Reisch et al., 2010). A different approach was taken by using poly(diallyldimethylammonium chloride) (pDADMAC) and sulfonated polystyrene (SPS) to create microstructured planar surfaces by contact printing. When these polyions are printed in a patterned fashion, either pDADMAC onto SPS surfaces or vice versa, selective cell adhesion becomes evident: Primary hepatocytes attach only onto SPS, whereas fibroblasts settle on both, pDADMAC and SPS surfaces (Kidambi et al., 2007).

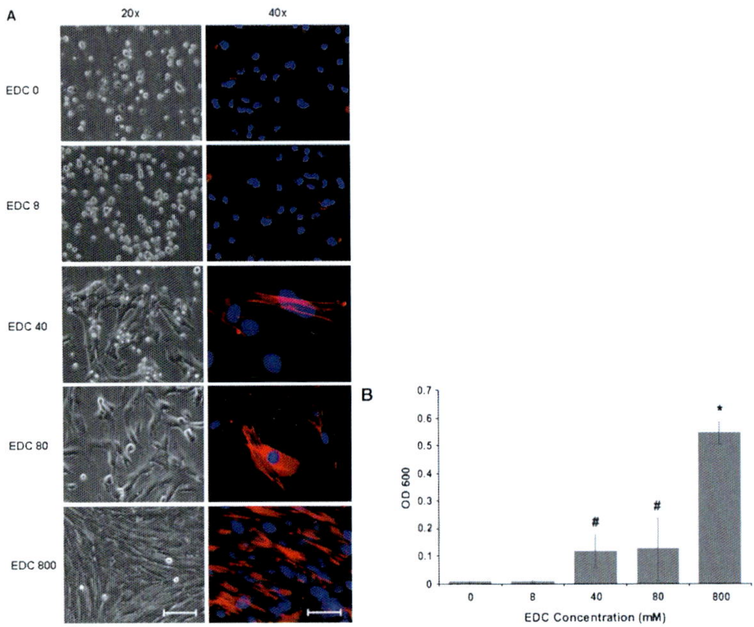

Figure 3.1 Stiffened multilayers for the promotion of MSC adhesion. (**A**) Images show PD-MSCs on PLL/HA multilayers that were stiffened to various degrees by cross-linking with increasing concentrations of N-(3-dimethylaminopropyl)-N′-ethylcarbodiimide hydrochloride (EDC) in combination with 100 mM N-hydroxysulfosuccinimide sodium salt. Images were taken 72 h after cell seeding. Phase microscopy (left column) and fluorescence microscopy (right column) of actin cytoskeleton (red color) show that stiffer coatings correlated with greater cell anchoring and spreading. Cell nuclei were stained with 4′,6-diamidino-2-phenylindole dihydrochloride (DAPI; blue color). (**B**) Determination of cell densities on native multilayers (EDC concentration 0 mM) or multilayers cross-linked with greater concentrations of EDC. The multilayer-bound MSCs were stained with crystal violet, and then the dye was eluted and quantified using colorimetry. * denotes $p<0.05$ versus EDC 40 and EDC 80 mM constructs; # denotes $p<0.05$ versus EDC 0 and EDC 8 mM constructs. Figure reproduced with permission from Mary Ann Liebert, Inc.

Another interesting aspect is the relation between topography and *cell differentiation*. In vivo, corneal epithelial cells are positioned on basement membranes that exhibit porosity on the nanoscale. PEMs that mimic the pore sizes of corneal membranes (100 nm to 600 nm) affect corneal epithelial cells since proliferation and migration speed are significantly higher on nanoporous PEMs, a phenomenon that is further supported by coating PEMs with fibronectin (Hajicharalambous et al., 2009).

3.1.2 Biofactor-Dotted PEMs and Biomimetic PEMs

PEMs can be further modified by the addition of extracellular matrix (ECM) proteins, nucleic acids, or low molecular weight components for directed growth, transfection, or guided cell differentiation.

Since heparin and chondroitin sulfate are prevalent noncollagen matrix molecules of vertebrates, heparin and chondroitin sulfate are employed to synthesize biomimetic coatings based on the LBL technique to support cell adhesion, spreading, proliferation, and maintenance of an osteoblast phenotype of osteosarcoma cells (Grohmann et al., 2011). The adhesion of L929 fibroblasts to poly(ε-caprolactone) (PCL) electrospun nanofibers can be improved via coating with self-assembled PEMs composed of four bilayers of pDADMAC and poly(sodium 4-styrene sulfonate) (PSS) when gelatin is incorporated. Gelatin represents partially hydrolyzed collagen, which is the most prominent ECM component in humans (Dubas et al., 2009). Similarly, PEMs made of PLL and dextran sulfate (DS) accelerate the spreading of human umbilical vein endothelial cells (HUVEC) if the films are pre-absorbed with fibronectin (Wittmer et al., 2007). Gelatin- and fibronectin-coated multilayer polyelectrolyte nanofilms are also advantageous for smooth muscle cell adhesion and growth, as shown in vitro with multilayers electrostatically constructed from PAH and poly(sodium 4-styrenesulfonate) (Li et al., 2005). In addition, repulsive surfaces can be generated: For example, heparin-terminated multilayers function as cell repellent, contrary to polyethyleneimine-terminated PEM, which promotes the adhesion of human dermal fibroblasts and growth on implants (Niepel et al., 2011).

As outlined in more detail below, nucleic-acid-modified PEMs provide promising tools to biofunctionalize medical implants. Introductory approaches proved the feasibility of this concept.

To generate transfection-competent implant surfaces, titanium substrates were polyplexed with deoxyribonucleic acid (DNA) as anionic polyelectrolyte and with poly-D-lysine (PDL) or PAH as cationic polyelectrolyte without adverse effects on mutagenesis, cell viability, and morphology in vitro (van den Beucken et al., 2006).

3.2 PEMs as Implant Coatings: Prerequisites for Applications

Prerequisites for medical applications include the compatibility of implant material and PEM processing as well as the maintenance of PEM stability and functionality during implantation procedure and exposure to the somehow corrosive physiological microenvironment.

Since the integration of orthopedic implants into the host bone still represents a major challenge in spinal fusion and joint arthroplasty, the functionalization of implant surfaces to improve this process is desirable. Hydrophilic protamine-based PEM films with a nanometer-scale roughness allow direct modulation of osteoblasts at the implant-bone interface and have been shown to facilitate increased deposition of calcified matrix in vitro (Samuel et al., 2011). The data suggest the compatibility of implant material and PEM processing. In a different context, dental titanium implants were coated with a polyethyleneimine (PEI) base layer and subsequent layers of PSS and PAH or of HA and PLL layers with or without cross-linking. The final architectures were: PEI-$(PSS/PAH)_{10}$, PEI-$(PSS/PAH)_{10}$-PSS, chemically cross-linked PEI-$(HA/PLL)_{10}$, and PEI-$(HA/PLL)_{10}$-HA. When exposed to human fibroblasts, PSS/PAH polyelectrolyte films coated with titanium display satisfactory biological performance and sufficient stability for a week in vitro (Brunot et al., 2008).

For tracheal implants, PEMs made of PLL and poly-L-glutamic acid (PGA) were functionalized by the covalent binding of a synthetic analogue of the anti-inflammatory peptide, α-melanocyte stimulating hormone, to PGA. Stable integrity and therapeutic efficacy of the films were evident in vivo as deduced from rats that had received implants for three months (Schultz et al., 2005). In another attempt, hyaluronan and chitosan on a polyethyleneimine primer layer were adsorbed onto metallic surfaces imitating endovascular stents. When PEM layers were dotted with the nitric-oxide-donor sodium nitroprusside to reduce the neointimal hyperplasia, it was found that in an ex vivo porcine aortic model, PEM coatings displayed sufficient stability to allow implantation (Thierry et al., 2003).

3.3 PEM as Biomaterial: Application Examples

3.3.1 Nucleic Acid Delivery

PEMs are an interesting tool for the development of local gene delivery systems for fundamental research; their application is also allowed for therapeutic gene delivery. The possibility to immobilize and release nucleic acid from surfaces offers the potential to gain localized delivery while maintaining an elevated concentration of nucleic acid within the cellular microenvironment. One can distinguish between direct integration of nucleic acid into PEMs (taking advantage of their negative charge), or integration as an aggregate, complexed with other agents that promote the internalization and processing in cells.

The simplest way is the *direct, layer-by-layer incorporation* of nucleic acid into degradable assemblies. Like this, PEMs can be efficient vectors for the delivery of plasmid DNA (pDNA). The group of David M. Lynn showed that naked pDNA encoding enhanced green fluorescent protein (EGFP) was released for up to four days from stent surfaces, taken up, and expressed in cells when integrated in hydrolytically degradable polyamine PEMs (Jewell et al., 2006; Zhang et al., 2004). The used polymer seems to facilitate uptake into adherent COS-7 cells (monkey kidney fibroblast cell line) and nuclear translocation of the DNA without the aid of additional transfection agents. Another group coated metal stents with dopamine-derivatized HA and subsequently deposited pDNA/polyethyleneimine nanoplexes. Under these conditions, pDNA is released over a period of 10 days with an enhanced gene transfection efficiency (Kim et al., 2010), implying that PEM layers might preserve their function over therapeutically relevant time periods. For the localized delivery of pDNA in vascular interventions, the above-mentioned hydrolytically degradable poly(β-amino ester) and pDNA coding for EGFP have also been immobilized by a LBL technique onto inflatable embolectomy catheter balloons. The successful labeling of injured carotid arteries in rats with film-coated balloons for 20 min demonstrates that PEM coating provides a means for acute gene delivery (Saurer et al., 2011). The positive outcome highlights that specific PEM compositions can meet the dual demands of stable film formation for surgical handling on the one hand and sufficiently rapid film disintegration on the other hand to guarantee instant plasmid delivery to vascular endothelial cells.

There is also increasing interest in the application of small interfering RNA (siRNA, used to specifically silence or knock down the expression of target proteins) as research tool and as potential therapeutic agent. Having similar characteristics as DNA (negative charge), siRNA internalization may be promoted by similar delivery systems. However, when the above-mentioned poly(β-amino ester) was used for the build-up of PEMs and integration of siRNA, no cellular transfection could be shown without supplement of an additional transfection agent (Flessner et al., 2011). In these studies, films with siRNA degraded quite fast within a few hours. However, the released siRNA was intact and functional when applied to HeLa cells. The authors attribute these differences in release profile and uptake at least in part to the large differences in size between siRNA and pDNA.

Cellular uptake can be facilitated by *complexation of nucleic acid* with other agents and integrating them as polyplexes or nanoparticles into or on the top of thin polymer films. This way, also small hairpin RNA (shRNA) can be complexed for cell transfection and gene silencing. Zhang et al. used triple shell calcium phosphate-shRNA nanoparticles consisting of a calcium phosphate core and further layers of shRNA, calcium phosphate, and shRNA (Zhang et al., 2010). These nanoparticles were incorporated into PEMs with PLL. Human osteoblasts cultured on the top of these layers showed inhibition of osteocalcin mRNA. This inhibition was even stronger than after application of the same nanoparticles in solution. An analysis of protein expression showed that osteopontin and osteocalcin were fully inhibited on $(PLL/NP)_6$ multilayered films (Fig. 3.2). The authors, therefore, suggest these films as a tool to control bone formation in the field of tissue engineering. Another approach of complexed siRNA delivery was described by Dimitrova et al. who incorporated PEI/siRNA nanoplexes into HA/chitosan PEMs to target hepatitis C virus infections (Dimitrova et al., 2008). Mehrotra et al. patterned similar PEI/siRNA nanoplexes on the top of pH-sensitive PEMs and showed that the resulting assemblies can be used to efficiently transfect HeLa cells with minimal cytotoxicity (Mehrotra et al., 2009).

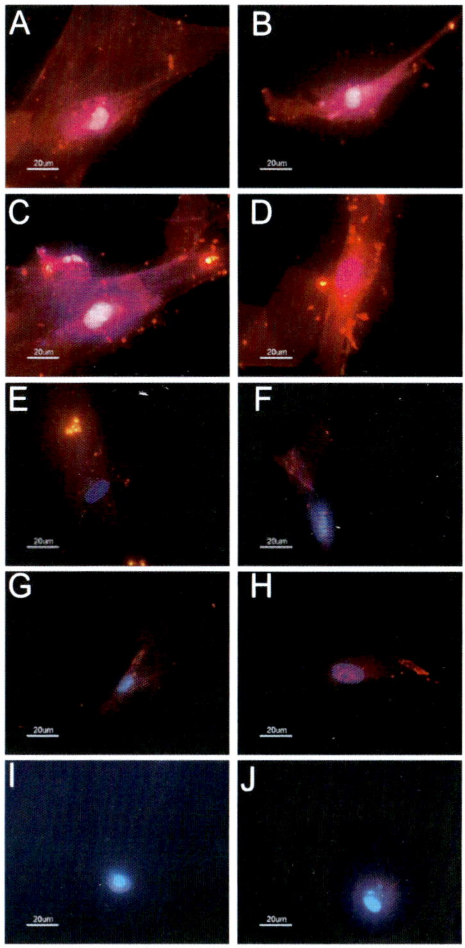

Figure 3.2 Osteopontin and osteocalcin in osteoblasts. Immunostaining was performed after 21 days with cells that were untreated (**A and B**), in the presence of free dissolved shRNA (**C and D**), in the presence of dispersed shRNA-functionalized nanoparticles (**E and F**), on (PLL-shRNA NP)$_1$ films (**G and H**), and on (PLL-shRNA NP)$_6$ films (**I and J**). The expression of osteopontin and osteocalcin was detected by using Cy3 immunostaining (red). Nuclei were visualized by Hoechst 33258 staining (blue). Figure reproduced with permission from Mary Ann Liebert, Inc.

DNA can be complexed in a similar way to facilitate cellular uptake. This method has, for example, been described by Meyer et al. who incorporated pDNA, precomplexed with PEI, into PEMs for local gene delivery. This method was showed to be efficient for transfection of the human hepato-cellular carcinoma cell line Huh-7 (Meyer et al., 2006). Lu et al. used a biodegradable polycationic poly(2-aminoethyl propylene phosphate) to build up layers with pDNA for long-term delivery over two months (Lu et al., 2008). Anionic DNA can be also complexed with cationic chitosan to facilitate cellular uptake. These complexes were shown to have good cytocompatibility and in vitro gene transfection ability when incorporated into PEMs with HA (Lin et al., 2009). As described for shRNA, efficient cell transfection can also be observed when DNA is co-precipitated with calcium phosphate and used for the build-up of fast degrading polymer films with cholic-acid-functionalized star poly(DL-lactide) (Zhang et al., 2009). HEK293, HeLa, and NIH 3T3 cells showed effective expression of a pGL3-Luc plasmid and no cytotoxicity in these transfection studies.

Further possibilities to enhance cell transfection have been examined, beyond complexing nucleic acids and applying them as nanoparticles or polyplexes. One possibility to enhance cell uptake is the use of a peptide analogue of the α-melanocyte stimulating hormone, which has been shown to enhance gene delivery in solution in a receptor-independent fashion due to its membrane-destabilizing properties (Chluba et al., 2001). Meyer et al. showed that this peptide grafted to PGA generates an efficient gene delivery for PEI precomplexed pDNA deposited on the top of PAH/ PSS multilayers (Meyer et al., 2008).

Cell-specific gene delivery could be shown by Cai et al., who built up multilayers incorporating galactosylated chitosan and pDNA (Cai et al., 2008). In this system, the galactose group serves as a specific ligand for hepatocyte binding. As a consequence, these films showed an increasing transfection rate specifically for the hepatoma cell line HepG2 but not for human embryonic kidney cells HEK293, which lack the necessary receptor.

If these promising studies can be confirmed in vivo, they have great potential for the development of gene-stimulating biomaterials, gene therapy, tissue engineering, and other biomedical applications.

3.4 PEMs with Antimicrobial Activity

Implant-associated infections can easily occur in conjunction with medical devices, ranging from minimally invasive contact lenses, to temporary urinary catheters, permanent cardiac valves, and orthopedic implants (Wu and Grainger, 2006). About half of the 2 million cases of nosocomial infections annually occurring in the United States are associated with indwelling devices (Darouiche, 2004). Biofilms can damage surrounding tissue and generate planktonic, nonattached bacterial cells that spread infections. The biofilm environment protects the bacteria from being easily targeted by normal therapeutic levels of antibiotics (Costerton et al., 1999; Hall-Stoodley et al., 2004). There are two general ways to prevent bacterial attachment and subsequent bacterial infections:

1. **Physical means**: Surface design that simply resists attachment of bacteria. This can be achieved without specific bactericidal characteristics but by special surface characteristics dependent on charge (Lichter and Rubner, 2009), surface hydrophobicity (Cistona et al., 2008), or roughness (Whitehead and Verran, 2006).
2. **Pharmacological means**: Surface design that kills bacteria before colonization by releasing antibacterial agents such as silver ions (Zan and Su, 2010), antibiotics (Wong et al., 2010; Chuang et al., 2008), or antimicrobial peptides (Shukla et al., 2010; Rudra et al., 2006).

Antimicrobial activity can be achieved by the "cationic killing effect" in which a cationic charged molecule is able to bind to the negatively charged bacterial membrane and permeabilize or lyse it, presumably by an ion-exchange mechanism (Murata et al., 2007; Kugler et al., 2005). For example, chitosan, a natural biocompatible cationic polysaccharide, is known to be biocidal because of its cationic charge. Therefore, chitosan has been incorporated into many PEMs for antimicrobial functionality (Feng et al., 2006; Elsabee et al., 2008). Like this, it could be shown that $(Ch/HA)_{10}$ films lead to about 80% decrease in bacterial adhesion of *Escherichia coli* compared to bare glass (Richert et al., 2004). Heparin can also prevent adhesion of bacteria. The antibacterial properties of films containing both polysaccharides, chitosan and heparin, were found to greatly decrease initial *E. coli* adhesion (Fu et al., 2005). The assembly pH was found to be an important parameter in the design of efficient antiadhesive and antibacterial films. Adjustment of assembly pH and postassembly conditions of polymers can be used to elevate cationic charge density, chain mobility, and contact-killing properties (Lichter et al., 2009). For this purpose, Lichter and Rubner created PEMs comprising PAH and PSS assembled at high pH and subsequently immersed in low pH solutions. Following the change in pH, this system undergoes a reversible swelling process, displaying accessible cationic charge. The viability of different bacterial strains of *Staphylococcus epidermidis* and *E. coli* was clearly reduced in this system.

As mentioned above, another approach to enhance antibacterial effects of multilayer films is the release of antibacterial substances. The most common biocidal material used in PEMs is *silver* (Cui et al., 2008; Yu et al., 2007; Fu et al., 2006; Podsiadlo et al., 2005; Grunlan et al., 2005). Silver ions act by binding to thiol groups on bacterial membranes, increasing cell membrane permeability, entering the cell, binding to DNA, and preventing bacterial replication (Feng et al., 2000). It is noteworthy that silver is effective against a broad spectrum of bacterial strains while minimally affecting human cells (Berger et al., 1976). This makes it a valuable tool for applications in the biomedical field where the incorporation of silver nanoparticles into PEMs renders implant surfaces antibacterial without significant side effects on mammalian cells (Fu et al., 2006). Zan and Su compared the incorporation of silver ions versus silver nanoparticles into PEMs. Their results show high antibacterial efficacy of the films against *E. coli* in both cases. However, short-term activity was observed for PEMs containing silver in the ionic form, whereas lower initial bactericidal effects, but prolonged activity, were evident for silver nanoparticles (Zan and Su, 2010). Another strategy is the loading of silver ions in liposomes, which can then be incorporated into PLL/HA films. In this case, also a strong bactericidal effect can be observed, attributed to the diffusion of silver ions out of the $AgNO_3$ coating, leading to a significant bactericidal concentration close to the membrane of the bacteria (Malcher et al., 2008).

The classical way to achieve antimicrobial activity is the *usage of antibiotics* released from devices to eradicate planktonic bacteria before biofilm formation. For example, incorporation of the antibiotic gentamycin was investigated in combination with the anti-inflammatory agent diclofenac incorporated into the top film of hydrolytically degradable PEMs (Kim et al., 2010). These PEMs could be shown to prevent bacterial attachment and to be biocompatible with A549 epithelial cancer cells and MC3T3-E1 osteoprogenitor cells. This underlines the potential application as coating of implantable devices to prevent the formation of biofilms. PEMs have also been described for controlled release of the antibiotic ciprofloxacin hydrochloride (Mao et al., 2005; Bhadra et al., 2004).

Another strategy relies on the incorporation of *antibacterial or antifungal peptides* into PEMs. For example, gramicidin A, a hydrophobic peptide, was found to perform antibacterial activity when complexed with nondenaturing anionic amphiphilic polysaccharide (hydrophobically modified carboxymethylpullulan). This negatively charged complex was used for the build-up of PEMs in combination with cationic PLL and was shown to inhibit the growth of the Gram-positive bacterium *Enterococcus faecalis* (Guyomard et al., 2008). Figure 3.3 shows that bacterial colonies are visible on all samples that did not incorporate gramicidin A. Samples with gramicidin A in the outer layer reveal total absence of bacteria, indicating that the peptide molecules get in close contact with the bacteria, penetrate their membrane, induce the formation of pores, and consequently cause bacterial lysis. In contrast, another PLL layer on the top of the gramicidin A layer seems to slightly promote cell adhesion but leads to swollen or lysed bacteria.

Other researchers described the incorporation of antifungal ß-peptides into PGA/PLL multilayers to gain antifungal activity and to inhibit the formation of biofilms (Karlsson et al., 2010). With this system, they could show the reduction of fungal growth, proliferation (measured by viability), metabolic activity, and hyphal elongation of *Candida albicans*. Therefore, this system could be helpful as coating for catheters, surgical instruments, and other devices. Shukla et al. incorporated the antimicrobial peptide ponericin G1 into hydrolytically degradable PEMs to inhibit biofilm formation and attachment of *Staphylococcus aureus* bacteria (Shukla et al., 2010). At the same time, the authors could show that these PEMs were biocompatible for wound-healing cells NIH 3T3 fibroblasts and endothelial HUVEC cell. Further on, the positively charged antimicrobial polypeptide hen egg white lysozyme was used in combination with negatively charged poly(lactic-co-glycolic acid) to build up PEMs, which were shown to inhibit growth of *Micrococcus luteus* (Rudra et al., 2006).

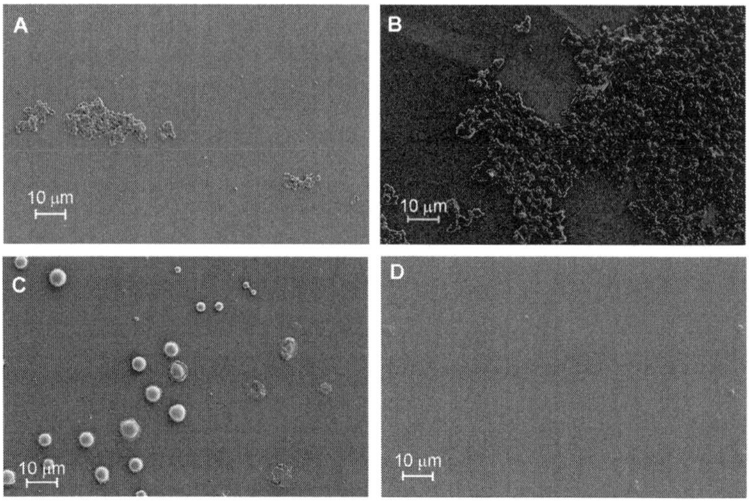

Figure 3.3 SEM images of LbL films. Films are ended by (**A**) (PLL/CMP$_L$-18C$_{10}$)$_3$-PLL, (**B**) (PLL/CMP$_L$-18C$_{10}$)$_3$, (**C**) (PLL/CMP$_L$-18C$_{10}$ _Gram A)$_3$-PLL, and (**D**) (PLL/ CMP$_L$-18C$_{10}$ _Gram A)$_3$. Subsequently, the films were exposed to *E. faecalis* suspension for 6 h. CMP$_L$: low-molar-mass carboxymethylpullulan. Figure reproduced with permission from John Wiley and Sons.

Taken together, the mentioned PEMs can be employed to optimize material surfaces, including those of medical devices, and to gain a large variety of surface characteristics. Modifications can be imprinted by physical means such as nanotopography or by chemical means such as the composition of PEMs. Additional modifications are already realized by the addition of diverse pharmacologically active components.

References

Berger TJ, Spadaro JA, Chapin SE, Becker RO. 1976. Electrically generated silver ions: Quantitative effects on bacterial and mammalian cells. *Antimicrob Agents Chemother* **9**(2): 357–358.

Bhadra D, Gupta G, Bhadra S, Umamaheshwari RB, Jain N. 2004. Multicomposite ultrathin capsules for sustained ocular delivery of ciprofloxacin hydrochloride. *J Pharm Pharm Sci* **7**(2): 241–251.

Boudou T, Crouzier T, Ren K, Blin G, Picart C. 2009. Multiple functionalities of polyelectrolyte multilayer films: New biomedical applications. *Adv Mater* **22**(4): 441–467.

Brunot C, Grosgogeat B, Picart C, Lagneau C, Jaffrezic-Renault N, Ponsonnet L. 2008. Response of fibroblast activity and polyelectrolyte multilayer films coating titanium. *Dent Mater* **24**(8): 1025–1035.

Cai K, Hu Y, Luo Z, Kong T, Lai M, Sui X, et al. 2008. Cell-specific gene transfection from a gene-functionalized poly(d,l-lactic acid) substrate fabricated by the layer-by-layer assembly technique. *Angew Chem Int Ed Engl* **47**(39): 7479–7481.

Chen AA, Khetani SR, Lee S, Bhatia SN, Van Vliet KJ. 2009. Modulation of hepatocyte phenotype in vitro via chemomechanical tuning of polyelectrolyte multilayers. *Biomaterials* **30**(6): 1113–1120.

Chluba J, Lima de Souza D, Frisch B, Schuber F. 2001. Enhancement of gene delivery by an analogue of alpha-MSH in a receptor-independent fashion. *Biochim Biophys Acta* **1510**(1–2): 198–208.

Chuang HF, Smith RC, Hammond PT. 2008. Polyelectrolyte multilayers for tunable release of antibiotics. *Biomacromolecules* **9**(6): 1660–1668.

Cistona S, Lueptowb RM, Gray KA. 2008. Bacterial attachment on reactive ceramic ultrafiltration membranes. *J Membrane Sci* **320**(1–2): 101–107.

Costerton JW, Stewart PS, Greenberg EP. 1999. Bacterial biofilms: A common cause of persistent infections. *Science* **284**(5418): 1318–1322.

Cui X, Li CM, Bao H, Zheng X, Lu Z. 2008. In situ fabrication of silver nanoarrays in hyaluronan/PDDA layer-by-layer assembled structure. *J Colloid Interf Sci* **327**(2): 459–465.

Darouiche RO. 2004. Treatment of infections associated with surgical implants. *N Engl J Med* **350**(14): 1422–1429.

Decher G, Hong JD, Schmitt J. 1992. Buildup of ultrathin multilayer films by a self-assembly process: III. Consecutively alternating adsorption of anionic and cationic polyelectrolytes on charged surfaces. *Thin Solid Films* **210–211**(Part 2): 831–835.

Decher G. 1997. Fuzzy nanoassemblies: Toward layered polymeric multicomposites. *Science* **277**(5330): 1232–1237.

Dimitrova M, Affolter C, Meyer F, Nguyen I, Richard DG, Schuster C, et al. 2008. Sustained delivery of siRNAs targeting viral infection by cell-degradable multilayered polyelectrolyte films. *Proc Natl Acad Sci USA* **105**(42): 16320–16325.

Dubas ST, Kittitheeranun P, Rangkupan R, Sanchavanakit N, Potiyaraj P. 2009. Coating of polyelectrolyte multilayer thin films on nanofibrous scaffolds to improve cell adhesion. *J Appl Polym Sci* **114**(3): 1574–1579.

Elsabee MZ, Abdou ES, Nagy KSA, Eweis M. 2008. Surface modification of polypropylene films by chitosan and chitosan/pectin multilayer carbohydrate polymers **71**(2): 187–195.

Feng YH, Han ZG, Peng J, Lu J, Xue B, Li L, et al. 2006. Fabrication and characterization of multilayer films based on Keggin-type polyoxometalate and chitosan. *Mater Lett* **60**(13–14): 1588–1593.

Feng QL, Wu J, Chen GQ, Cui FZ, Kim TN, Kim JO. 2000. A mechanistic study of the antibacterial effect of silver ions on *Escherichia coli* and *Staphylococcus aureus*. *J Biomed Mater Res A* **52**(4): 662–668.

Flessner RM, Jewell CM, Anderson DG, Lynn DM. 2011. Degradable polyelectrolyte multilayers that promote the release of siRNA. *Langmuir* **27**(12): 7868–7876.

Francius G, Hemmerle J, Ohayon J, Schaaf P, Voegel JC, Picart C, et al. 2006. Effect of cross-linking on the elasticity of polyelectrolyte multilayer films measured by colloidal probe AFM. *Microsc Res Tech* **69**(2): 84–92.

Fu J, Ji J, Fan D, Shen J. 2006. Construction of antibacterial multilayer films containing nanosilver via layer-by-layer assembly of heparin and chitosan-silver ions complex. *J Biomed Mater Res A* **79**(3): 665–674.

Fu J, Ji J, Yuan W, Shen J. 2005. Construction of anti-adhesive and antibacterial multilayer films via layer-by-layer assembly of heparin and chitosan. *Biomaterials* **26**(33): 6684–6692.

Grohmann S, Rothe H, Frant M, Liefeith K. 2011. Colloidal force spectroscopy and cell biological investigations on biomimetic polyelectrolyte multilayer coatings composed of chondroitin sulfate and heparin. *Biomacromolecules* **12**(6): 1987–1997.

Grunlan JC, Choi JK, Lin A. 2005. Antimicrobial behavior of polyelectrolyte multilayer films containing cetrimide and silver. *Biomacromolecules* **6**(2): 1149–1153.

Guyomard A, Dé E, Jouenne T, Malandain J-J, Muller G, Glinel K. 2008. Incorporation of a hydrophobic antibacterial peptide into amphiphilic polyelectrolyte multilayers: A bioinspired approach to prepare biocidal thin coatings. Adv Functional Mater **18**(5): 758–765.

Hajicharalambous CS, Lichter J, Hix WT, Swierczewska M, Rubner MF, Rajagopalan P. 2009. Nano- and sub-micron porous polyelectrolyte multilayer assemblies: Biomimetic surfaces for human corneal epithelial cells. *Biomaterials* **30**(23–24): 4029–4036.

Hall-Stoodley L, Costerton JW, Stoodley P. 2004. Bacterial biofilms: From the natural environment to infectious diseases. *Nat Rev Microbiol* **2**(2): 95–108.

Jewell CM, Zhang J, Fredin NJ, Wolff MR, Hacker TA, Lynn DM. 2006. Release of plasmid DNA from intravascular stents coated with ultrathin multilayered polyelectrolyte films. *Biomacromolecules* **7**(9): 2483–2491.

Karlsson AJ, Flessner RM, Gellman SH, Lynn DM, Palecek SP. 2010. Polyelectrolyte multilayers fabricated from antifungal beta-peptides: Design of surfaces that exhibit antifungal activity against *Candida albicans*. *Biomacromolecules* **11**(9): 2321–2328.

Kidambi S, Udpa N, Schroeder SA, Findlan R, Lee I, Chan C. 2007. Cell adhesion on polyelectrolyte multilayer coated polydimethylsiloxane surfaces with varying topographies. *Tissue Eng* **13**(8): 2105–2117.

Kidambi S, Sheng L, Yarmush ML, Toner M, Lee I, Chan C. 2007. Patterned co-culture of primary hepatocytes and fibroblasts using polyelectrolyte multilayer templates. *Macromol Biosci* **7**(3): 344–353.

Kim TG, Lee Y, Park TG. 2010. Controlled gene-eluting metal stent fabricated by bio-inspired surface modification with hyaluronic acid and deposition of DNA/PEI polyplexes. *Int J Pharm* **384**(1–2): 181–188.

Kugler R, Bouloussa O, Rondelez F. 2005. Evidence of a charge-density threshold for optimum efficiency of biocidal cationic surfaces. *Microbiology* **151**(Pt 5): 1341–1348.

Li M, Mills DK, Cui T, McShane MJ. 2005. Cellular response to gelatin- and fibronectin-coated multilayer polyelectrolyte nanofilms. *IEEE Trans Nanobioscience* **4**(2): 170–179.

Lichter JA, Rubner MF. 2009. Polyelectrolyte multilayers with intrinsic antimicrobial functionality: The importance of mobile polycations. *Langmuir* **25**(13): 7686–7694.

Lin QK, Ren KF, Ji J. 2009. Hyaluronic acid and chitosan-DNA complex multilayered thin film as surface-mediated nonviral gene delivery system. *Colloids Surf B Biointerfaces* **74**(1): 298–303.

Lu ZZ, Wu J, Sun TM, Ji J, Yan LF, Wang J. 2008. Biodegradable polycation and plasmid DNA multilayer film for prolonged gene delivery to mouse osteoblasts. *Biomaterials* **29**(6): 733–741.

Malcher M, Volodkin D, Heurtault B, Andre P, Schaaf P, Mohwald H, et al. 2008. Embedded silver ions-containing liposomes in polyelectrolyte multilayers: Cargos films for antibacterial agents. *Langmuir* **24**(18): 10209–10215.

Mao Z, Ma L, Gao C, Shen J. 2005. Preformed microcapsules for loading and sustained release of ciprofloxacin hydrochloride. *J Control Release* **104**(1): 193–202.

Mehrotra S, Lee I, Chan C. 2009. Multilayer mediated forward and patterned siRNA transfection using linear-PEI at extended N/P ratios. *Acta Biomater* **5**(5): 1474–1488.

Meyer F, Ball V, Schaaf P, Voegel JC, Ogier J. 2006. Polyplex-embedding in polyelectrolyte multilayers for gene delivery. *Biochim Biophys Acta* **1758**(3): 419–422.

Meyer F, Dimitrova M, Jedrzejenska J, Arntz Y, Schaaf P, Frisch B, et al. 2008. Relevance of bi-functionalized polyelectrolyte multilayers for cell transfection. *Biomaterials* **29**(5): 618–624.

Murata H, Koepsel RR, Matyjaszewski K, Russell AJ. 2007. Permanent, non-leaching antibacterial surface--2: How high density cationic surfaces kill bacterial cells. *Biomaterials* **28**(32): 4870–4879.

Niepel MS, Peschel D, Groth T. 2011. Controlling fibroblast adhesion with pH modified polyelectrolyte multilayers. *Int J Artif Organs* **34**(2): 185–191.

Podsiadlo P, Paternel S, Rouillard JM, Zhang Z, Lee J, Lee JW, et al. 2005. Layer-by-layer assembly of nacre-like nanostructured composites with antimicrobial properties. *Langmuir* **21**(25): 11915–11921.

Reisch A, Hemmerle J, Chassepot A, Lefort M, Benkirane-Jessel N, Candolfi E, et al. 2010. Anti-fouling phosphorylcholine bearing polyelectrolyte multilayers: Cell adhesion resistance at rest and under stretching. *Soft Matter* **6**(7): 1503–1512.

Richert L, Lavalle P, Payan E, Shu XZ, Prestwich GD, Stoltz JF, et al. 2004. Layer by layer buildup of polysaccharide films: Physical chemistry and cellular adhesion aspects. *Langmuir* **20**(2): 448–458.

Rudra JS, Dave K, Haynie DT. 2006. Antimicrobial polypeptide multilayer nanocoatings. *J Biomater Sci Polym Ed* **17**(11): 1301–1315.

Samuel RE, Shukla A, Paik DH, Wang MX, Fang JC, Schmidt DJ, et al. 2011. Osteoconductive protamine-based polyelectrolyte multilayer functionalized surfaces. *Biomaterials* **32**(30): 7491–7502.

Saurer EM, Yamanouchi D, Liu B, Lynn DM. 2011. Delivery of plasmid DNA to vascular tissue in vivo using catheter balloons coated with polyelectrolyte multilayers. *Biomaterials* **32**(2): 610–618.

Schade R, Dutour Sikiric M, Liefeith K, Fueredi-Milhofer H. 2011. Interaction of cells with organic-inorganic nanocomposite coatings for titanium implants. *Bioceramics Development and Applications* doi:10.4303/bda/D110159

Schultz P, Vautier D, Richert L, Jessel N, Haikel Y, Schaaf P, et al. 2005. Polyelectrolyte multilayers functionalized by a synthetic analogue of an anti-inflammatory peptide, alpha-MSH, for coating a tracheal prosthesis. *Biomaterials* **26**(15): 2621–2630.

Semenov OV, Malek A, Bittermann AG, Voros J, Zisch AH. 2009. Engineered polyelectrolyte multilayer substrates for adhesion, proliferation, and differentiation of human mesenchymal stem cells. *Tissue Eng Part A* **15**(10): 2977–2990.

Shukla A, Fleming KE, Chuang HF, Chau TM, Loose CR, Stephanopoulos GN, et al. 2010. Controlling the release of peptide antimicrobial agents from surfaces. *Biomaterials* **31**(8): 2348–2357.

Thierry B, Winnik FM, Merhi Y, Silver J, Tabrizian M. 2003. Bioactive coatings of endovascular stents based on polyelectrolyte multilayers. *Biomacromolecules* **4**(6): 1564–1571.

Thompson MT, Berg MC, Tobias IS, Rubner MF, Van Vliet KJ. 2005. Tuning compliance of nanoscale polyelectrolyte multilayers to modulate cell adhesion. *Biomaterials* **26**(34): 6836–6845.

van den Beucken JJ, Vos MR, Thune PC, Hayakawa T, Fukushima T, Okahata Y, et al. 2006. Fabrication, characterization, and biological assessment of multilayered DNA-coatings for biomaterial purposes. *Biomaterials* **27**(5): 691–701.

Whitehead KA, Verran J. 2006. The effect of surface topography on the retention of microorganisms: A review. *Food Bioproducts Processing* **84**: 253–259.

Wittmer CR, Phelps JA, Saltzman WM, Van Tassel PR. 2007. Fibronectin terminated multilayer films: Protein adsorption and cell attachment studies. *Biomaterials* **28**(5): 851–860.

Wong SY, Moskowitz JS, Veselinovic J, Rosario RA, Timachova K, Blaisse MR, et al. 2010. Dual functional polyelectrolyte multilayer coatings for implants: permanent microbicidal base with controlled release of therapeutic agents. *J Am Chem Soc* **132**(50): 17840–17848.

Wu P, Grainger DW. 2006. Drug/device combinations for local drug therapies and infection prophylaxis. *Biomaterials* **27**(11): 2450–2467.

Yu DG, Lin WC, Yang MC. 2007. Surface modification of poly(L-lactic acid) membrane via layer-by-layer assembly of silver nanoparticle-embedded polyelectrolyte multilayer. *Bioconjug Chem* **18**(5): 1521–1529.

Zan X, Su Z. 2010. Polyelectrolyte multilayer films containing silver as antibacterial coatings. *Thin Solid Films* **518**(19): 5478–5482.

Zhang J, Chua LS, Lynn DM. 2004. Multilayered thin films that sustain the release of functional DNA under physiological conditions. *Langmuir* **20**(19): 8015–8021.

Zhang X, Kovtun A, Mendoza-Palomares C, Oulad-Abdelghani M, Fioretti F, Rinckenbach S, et al. 2010. SiRNA-loaded multi-shell nanoparticles incorporated into a multilayered film as a reservoir for gene silencing. *Biomaterials* **31**(23): 6013–6018.

Zhang Q, Zhao D, Zhang XZ, Cheng SX, Zhuo RX. 2009. Calcium phosphate/DNA co-precipitates encapsulated fast-degrading polymer films for substrate-mediated gene delivery. *J Biomed Mater Res B Appl Biomater* **91**(1): 172–180.

Zhu H, Ji J, Shen J. 2004. Construction of multilayer coating onto poly-(dl-lactide) to promote cytocompatibility. *Biomaterials* **25**(1): 109–117; Yamanlar S, Sant S, Boudou T, Picart C, Khademhosseini A. 2011. Surface functionalization of hyaluronic acid hydrogels by polyelectrolyte multilayer films. *Biomaterials* **32**(24): 5590–5599.

Chapter 4

Polyelectrolyte Multilayers as Functional Coatings for Controlled Biomolecular Interactions

Xin Xiong, Susanne Hossfeld, Simona Margutti, and Rumen Krastev
NMI Natural and Medical Sciences Institute at the University of Tübingen, Markwiesenstraße 55, 72770 Reutlingen, Germany
xin.xiong@nmi.de

This review gives a short overview of the physical processes involved in the formation of the polyelectrolyte multilayers (PEMs) and their destruction. These two processes are vital for the formation of PEMs with desired physical and chemical structures, and for loading them with active substances and their spatial controlled release. It includes a survey of the physical and chemical properties that are key points for controlling film nanostructure in relation to biological processes and different possibilities for controlling cell behavior by means of film composition, bioactivity, mechanical properties, and three-dimensional organization.

Biofunctional Surface Engineering
Edited by Martin Scholz

ISBN 978-981-4411-60-8 (Hardcover), 978-981-4411-61-5 (eBook)
www.panstanford.com

4.1 Introduction

The demand for different implants—biomaterials such as orthopedic, cardiovascular, ocular, and dental implants and different medical devices—is growing continuously. The bulk properties—such as mechanical stability, sufficient tensile strength, yield strength, fatigue and corrosion resistance, elastic modulus, surface finish and hardness, durability, and integrity—of the materials used as biomaterials are well recognized as important for the overall properties and performance of the implants. In case of vascular graft, for example, the material should be flexible and should have the same mechanical properties as the normal artery. Differently, biomaterials for orthopedic implants should have high mechanical strength and deformation resistance, and biomaterials for tissue engineering should dissolve at the same rate as the regeneration of tissue.

For a long time, the biological activities of the biomaterials, together with their surface properties, were not considered important for their performance. The first-generation biomaterials in fact included inert materials, which did not interact with the body. These materials were designed to be low toxic and to cause a minimal biological response. The second-generation biomaterials included bioactive materials that were designed to interact with the surrounding tissues to promote surface bonding. They also included bioabsorbable materials, which had the ability to degrade while the tissue regenerates and heals. The up-to-date biomaterials appeared a decade ago, which were bioactive as well as biodegradable.

Biomaterials are usually three-dimensional materials such as scaffolds or implants. They can also be used as coatings for implants for triggering the properties of nonviable materials to that of the vital biological tissue. In fact, considerable efforts are currently devoted toward the functionalization of the surfaces of the materials commonly used in biomedical applications, such as metals, polymers, ceramics, and composites. Surface modifications can strongly influence many biological events, which include protein adsorption, cell adhesion and proliferation, and inflammatory response (Cowin, 2004; McEver and Zhu, 2010; Albanese et al., 2012; Berthiaume et al., 2011). All these processes affect the behavior of biomolecules at solid–liquid interfaces and consequently play a crucial role for the remodeling of the contact between the biological tissue and the surface of the implants.

In this respect, the development of switchable surfaces, which alter their physical–chemical properties in response to their environment, is a key enabling advancement for biomedical applications, including biomaterials and tissue engineering. Switch ability, in essence, enables temporal control, adding another dimension to controlled biomolecular manipulation. Examples are implants coatings for the delivery of therapeutic molecules wherefore hydrogels are typically used as drug-delivery vehicles because of their capability to change their shape in response to a change in the tissue environment, such as increase or decrease in metabolites. Besides this so-called "smart drug-delivery systems," such devices can be found in biosensing, bioelectronics, and tissue engineering. In case of nongel polymeric systems, the release process could be controlled by the degradation of the coating or by the controlled diffusion of the active substances through it or by the change of their hydrophobicity.

Different types of stimuli can be applied to modulate the "switch" of the surfaces, e.g., UV, temperature, ultrasound, chemicals, and biochemicals. Thermosensitive or light-responsive surfaces or surfaces that can be modified by changing pH or ionic strength may find great applicability as temporary scaffolds for topical delivery of drugs or cells. Systems that recognize independently or simultaneously more than one stimulus are also interesting for the development of new biomedical devices. Besides the typical response to temperature and pH, recent developments on materials that react to biochemical stimuli, including specific enzymes, antibodies, or cells, may be used for new medicinal applications.

Different coating deposition methods are developed, extensively studied, and widely used. These include the following: dipping the object in a liquid and its removal to create a thin surface film; spray coating to deposit a thin film; surface polymerization to create a film from a monomer vapor; physical vapor deposition to transfer a solid source to a surface film; ink jet placement of coating via impingement of tiny droplets; chemical vapor deposition for a surface reaction to create film; electrostatic self-assembly; freeze condensation of vapor to create a thin film of frozen liquid; and surface condensation to create a film of liquid. The choice of the deposition method is driven mainly by the object geometry, used liquid precursor, and coating-formation mechanism.

Concerning the type of materials used as biocoatings, porous metal and ceramic coatings deposited on implants facilitate implant fixation and bone in-growth. Implant surfaces modified by ion implantation or physical vapor deposition exhibit superior hardness and wear resistance. Polymeric coatings are used to enhance biocompatibility, biostability, hemocompatibility, antimicrobial action, dielectric strength, and lubricity; to make medical devices used within the body more visible to ultrasound; and to deliver drugs (Davis, 2003).

One of the most popular coating materials is based on polylactic acid or its blends. Designing coatings with nanometer-scale control and with preserved activity of embedded molecules with fine controlled delivery is a challenge, in particular when the delivery must be performed under physiological conditions (certain pH range, defined ionic strength, and existence of physiological fluids). Several techniques have been developed to design thin films at the molecular level, including Langmuir–Blodgett and self-assembled monolayers (Ulman, 1991; Magnussen et al., 1996; Ariga et al., 2006; Girard-Egrot, 2005). A technique that allows the formation of nanometer-scale coatings for medical implants and allows fulfilling the above-listed requirements is the layer-by-layer (LbL) method introduced by Decher, Möhwald, and Lvov (Lvov et al., 1993; Decher et al., 1992, 1994; Sukhorukov et al., 1996). It consists of alternate deposition of polyelectrolytes on charged surfaces. This is a self-assembled and self-organized process on the surfaces of the materials, leading to the formation of polyelectrolyte multilayer (PEM) films with a precisely defined thickness, which can be tuned down to only a few nanometers (Antipov and Sukhorukov, 2004; Yoo et al., 2008). The procedure is versatile and comparatively simple. It is applicable to many different kinds of substrate, which include complex geometrical structures, different areas, and even closed volumes. A large variety of polyelectrolytes was tested, which show the formation of excellent coatings for different applications. All deposition processes are performed from water-based solutions, which makes the process extremely environment friendly. On the other hand, this guarantees the stability of different biologically active molecules ("biologicals"), such as polypeptides, RNA, DNA, enzymes, and antibodies, during the deposition process and thereafter. Incorporation of various kinds of nanoparticles and nanosystems (clay platelets, carbon nanotubes, etc.) in PEM coatings was also reported (Nepal et al., 2008; Ai et al.,

2003; Baek et al., 2012; Richert et al., 2003). These functional layers were used for the preparation of coatings with different applications from electroconductivity via chemical and biological sensing to coatings with antiflammable or antibacterial properties.

The behavior of cells on the surfaces of implants is an important issue, which is crucial for the interaction between the biomaterial and the biological tissue. The process of cell deposition on PEMs has been explored since 2000. This was related to the discovery of different mechanisms of film growth (exponential and linear), which allowed for the formation of PEMs with different mechanical properties combined with reservoir capacities (Boudou et al., 2010). Possibilities for the control of cell immobilization and growth on PEM have been defined and the first in vivo studies have been performed (Boura et al., 2003). The opportunity for using a wide range of polyelectrolytes and nanoobjects combined with spatial confinement and controlled localized delivery enriches the biological applications for PEM films.

Several reviews on the properties of PEM have been published in the last years. They concern either the internal structure of the films or the applications of PEM films at the nanoscale, but they also include issues concerning the application of PEMs as coatings with biomedical purposes. These applications can be for controlled erosion, protein-inspired nanofilms, polyelectrolyte blends, and biomedical applications, including drug delivery, biosensors, biomimesis, and tissue engineering (Boura et al., 2003; Berg et al., 2004; Mansouri et al., 2011; Mhanna et al., 2011; Picart et al., 2005; Picart, 2008; Reisch et al., 2010; Rengaraj, 2011; Szarpak et al., 2010; Zhao et al., 2011).

In this review, we focus on the design of PEM films for biomaterial surface coatings and tissue engineering. The review gives a short overview on the physical processes involved in the formation of PEMs and their destruction. These two processes are vital for the formation of PEMs with desired physical and chemical structures, and for loading them with active substances and their spatial controlled release. It includes a survey of the physical and chemical properties that are key points for controlling film nanostructure in relation to biological processes and different possibilities for controlling cell behavior by means of film composition, bioactivity, mechanical properties, and three-dimensional organization.

4.2 Layer-by-Layer Technology and Preparation of PEMs

Polyelectrolyte multilayers are prepared by the sequential deposition of positive and negative polyelectrolytes on charged surfaces. The deposition is based on the electrostatic interaction between the polyelectrolytes and the surfaces. The stability of the coatings is guaranteed by the increased entropy of the whole system in this process. PEMs consist of polyelectrolyte couples that define the properties of the whole PEM coating.

4.2.1 Polyelectrolytes

The properties of polyelectrolytes are responsive for the properties of the whole PEMs after the LbL preparation; therefore, the basic knowledge about the properties of a single polyelectrolyte and their control is important for the choice of suitable components for the formation of PEMs.

Polyelectrolytes are macromolecules that dissociate when placed in a suitable ionizing solvent. The dissociation leads to the formation of charged polyions and usually small oppositely charged ions, which neutralize the repeating charges on the polymer molecule. The polyelectrolytes can be divided into two types: "weak" and "strong". "Strong" polyelectrolytes are those that dissociate completely in contrast to "weak" polyelectrolytes, which are only partially dissociated at intermediate pH. Thus they are not fully charged in solution, and their charge can be modified by changing the pH of the solution, or ionic strength.

The static properties of the polyelectrolytes, mostly related to their conformation in solutions, are different from those of their electrically neutral counterparts. This is a result of the specific electrostatic interaction between the charges in the molecules and their screening in the presence of small counter ions (Verwey, 1947; Derjaguin and Landau, 1993). The conformation of any polymer in solution depends on the polymer architecture and the solvent affinity. In case of polyelectrolytes, charge and charge density have a vital effect. Usually, an uncharged linear polymer possesses random conformation in solution. The charges on a linear polyelectrolyte chain repel each other, and thus the chain takes more expanded, rod-like conformation. At higher salt concentration, the charges of the polyelectrolyte chains are screened and consequently the chains collapse to a random conformation similar to that of a neutral chain (Liu et al., 1998; Decher, 2003). This behavior of the polyelectrolytes allows their "form" to be precisely controlled via changes in the ionic strength of the solution (Huddleston et al., 2001; Stuart et al., 2010).

Polyelectrolytes can also bear both cationic and anionic repeat groups. These polyelectrolytes are called polyampholytes. These polymers usually dissolve only when a sufficient amount of salt is added. Typical examples of polyampholytes are many proteins where some amino acids tend to be acidic while others are basic.

Polyelectrolytes can also be divided into different groups according to their origin. Usually, these are two large groups of synthetic and natural polyelectrolytes. The natural polyelectrolytes play an important role in biology and biochemistry. These include, for instance, polypeptides, proteins, nucleic acids, and polysaccharides prepared from natural sources (e.g., chitosan, alginate, and hyaluronic acid) and have excellent biocompatibility. The synthetic polymers are obtained as result of chemical synthesis. These polyelectrolytes usually have better defined structure and are used in many technical applications. However, because of their strong adhesion and formation of stable PEM coatings, these polyelectrolytes also can find applications as coatings for biomaterials. Blends of natural and synthetic polyelectrolytes may be used in different applications as one can control very precisely the properties of the PEM by varying the amount and type of both types of polyelectrolytes used in the formation of PEMs. Table 4.1 summarizes the most used polyelectrolytes as coatings and their possible applications as biomaterials.

4.2.2 Formation of LbL Coatings

The formation of PEMs is based on the LbL deposition technique, which exploits the fact that polyelectrolytes adsorb onto surfaces of opposite charge and that the surface charge density is reversed by this process. Therefore, a multilayer can be built up by alternating the adsorption of positively and negatively charged polyelectrolytes. The thickness of such multilayers can be controlled down to molecular dimensions and varied by the number of adsorption cycles, salt concentration of the polyelectrolyte solutions, and with the fine-tuning of the adsorption conditions (Antipov and Shukhorukov, 2004; Decher, 2003; Decher, 1997; Anzai et al., 1998). The multilayer formation and the final internal structure are the result of the balance between different interactions. These include electrostatic as well as nonelectrostatic interactions, e.g., hydrophobic interaction, hydrogen bonds, van der Waals forces, charge transfer halogen interactions, and possibly covalent bonds (Schönhoff, 2003; Steitz et al., 2000). The intrinsic properties of the polyelectrolytes (structure of the polyelectrolyte, charge density, and chain stiffness) and the physical and chemical properties of the suspending medium (type and concentration of salt, pH) are key parameters for the buildup process.

Table 4.1 Examples of polyelectrolytes with applications as coatings for biomaterials

Polyelectrolyte	Application	Reference
PSS/pDNA	Delivery of plasmid DNA	Jewell et al., 2006
(Collagen-polylactid glycolid) + DNA	Delivery of DNA	Perlstein et al., 2003
Heparin/pDNA	Delivery of DNA	Walter et al., 2004
Chitosan/Heparin	Stent coating	Meng et al., 2009
Hyaluronan/PEI-DNA	Delivery of DNA	Kim et al., 2010
Heparin/Collagen	Antithrombosis	Lin et al., 2011
Heparin/Collagen	Stent coating	Lin et al., 2010

The charge inversion after each deposition step is believed to be a precondition for multilayer formation. It is assumed that electrostatic interactions are the main driving forces for the formation of PEMs. This opinion is supported by the fact that after each deposition step, the ζ-potential changes its sign. However, some recent experiments (Lundström-Hämälä et al., 2010; Johansson et al., 2009) showed that a change in sign of the surface potential is not the necessary condition for the formation of a stable PEM. This gives a hint that electrostatic attraction between the adsorbing polyelectrolytes and the surface is not the only reason for multilayer formation.

The charge density of the polyelectrolytes is important for the formation of PEMs. A minimum charge density is required for the formation of multilayers. Below this charge limit, the charge reversal is not sufficient. In case of strong polyelectrolytes, the charge density is varied by modifying the chemical structure. The charge density of the weak polyelectrolytes can be controlled by the pH of the solution used for the preparation of PEMs. The charge density controls also the film thickness. A sharp maximum in film thickness is observed at the intermediate charge density. A reason for the maximum is that in case of weak polyelectrolytes, the polyanion is charged in the basic regime and uncharged in the acidic regime. For the polycation, the opposite is valid. The distribution of the charges along the chains plays an important role in building up multilayers, e.g., by the deposition of block-copolymers.

The thickness of PEMs can be controlled by adding salt to the aqueous polyion solutions. Due to the screening of the charges along the polyelectrolyte chains, the polymer molecules are more coiled with increasing salt concentration, which results in a larger thickness and a stronger roughness of the adsorbed layers. The increase in thickness is proportional to the ionic strength. This effect varies for different polyanion–polycation combinations. Besides the segment–segment repulsion, the attraction between the polyelectrolyte and the oppositely charged interface is also screened at high salt concentration. Therefore, one would expect a decrease in the adsorbed amount at high ionic strength.

The type of used polyelectrolyte also affects the total thickness of PEMs. The intrinsic persistence length of the polymers related to their chain stiffness is one reason for the differences in multilayer thickness (v. Klitzing, 2006). Another reason is the balance between the hydrophilicity and hydrophobicity of the polyelectrolytes, which plays an important role for their thickness. The solvent of the polyelectrolyte solution affects the interactions between the counter ions and the respective polyelectrolyte. Methanol and ethanol have a poorer solvating effect on the ions than water, which leads to a stronger ion–polyelectrolyte association, i.e., a stronger screening (respectively coiling) of the polyelectrolyte chains, which leads to increasing multilayer thickness with increasing ethanol concentration.

It is proved that the driving force for multilayer formation is not only of electrostatic origin, but also the gain in entropy due to the release of a large amount of counter ions during the deposition process. This explains the fact that PEMs cannot be formed from polyelectrolytes below certain threshold charge density. The entropic origin of the forces responsible for the formation of PEMs explains also the stability of the layers even in a medium with a high concentration of salts.

4.2.3 Methods for Deposition and Anchoring of PEMs

Polyelectrolyte multilayers are prepared by the sequential adsorption of polyions. Various depositing methods have already been proposed for LbL buildup, including dip coating, spin coating, and spraying. The most common is probably the dip coating technique. A substrate is immersed into an aqueous solution of polyion 1. After a specific time needed for polyelectrolyte adsorption and the formation of a layer on the substrate, the sample is rinsed to remove weakly bounded polyion molecules to avoid their bulk reaction with polyion 2, which could happen during the following adsorption step. The procedure is repeated until the required number of layers is obtained, and rinsing is applied after every single deposition step. Because of the long deposition time of single-layer deposition, the procedure is time consuming and difficult for routine sample preparation.

For future use and industrial applications of LbL films, the total time required for film preparation and the anchorage of the layer to the underlying substrate are important constraints. Therefore, particularly rapid methods such as spraying were also developed. In this case, the polyion solutions and rinsing solutions are supplied by enforced spraying. The procedure requires two spraying steps per single layer with waiting time in between. This waiting time is to allow for the solution drainage. Spraying with rinsing solution is needed after a complete layer is formed. Spray depositing is effective even under conditions for which dipping failed to produce homogeneous films (e.g., extremely short contact times). The main advantage of spraying is the meaningful reduction of time needed for multilayer formation.

Adherence of the PEM to the underlying substrate is an important topic. In many applications, this is assured by the use of polyethyleneimine (PEI) with different chain lengths. It was shown that branched PEI used as a first layer acts as a uniform anchoring network for the formation of consecutive layers; therefore, uniform layer growth can be observed and the resulting PEM film should be more homogeneous. The use of PEI as anchoring layer is not a universal solution. It works very well on charged surfaces. Some results also confirm that PEI activation layer could be used also on hydrophobic surfaces. Recent publications open the way to better anchoring of the film and could be applied in the case of hydrophobic surfaces such as poly(tetrafluoroethylene) (PTFE) and poly(ethylene) (Lan et al., 2011; Rofaiel et al., 2012; Rinckenbach et al., 2008). This is based on the use of mussel-adhesive-inspired polymers containing catechol and amine functional groups. They can be grafted to various polyelectrolytes and allow the adsorption of polyelectrolytes and LbL buildup on various polymeric surfaces. These catecholamine-containing polymers could thus be used as universal surface primers for facilitating LbL assembly on metal, oxide, and polymer substrates (Boudou et al., 2010). Overall, the numerous possibilities for depositing methods, as well as the recent development of polyelectrolyte/surface anchoring, strengthen the concept that PEM films can be efficiently and reproducibly coated onto any kind of substrate.

4.3 Structure of PEM and Its Relation to the Basic Components and Preparation Conditions

4.3.1 Film Stability

The temporal control of film stability and its degradability is an important issue concerning the use of PEMs in biomedical applications, e.g., in drug delivery. The different stimulus pathways used to control the deconstruction or dissolution of PEM deposit on solid substrates or organized in capsules is already summarized (Tang et al., 2006; Lynn, 2007; de Geest et al., 2007). Usually, the degradation process is based on hydrolytically degradable polymers (Lynn, 2007), weakening of the interactions between the polymer chains at a certain pH or ionic strength, or use of natural polyelectrolytes, which are enzymatically degraded. New strategies rely on the preparation of films with adjustable biodegradability, depending on the enantiomer ratio, e.g., D- over L-lysine in the polyelectrolyte solution (Benkirane-Jessel et al., 2005), where the degradation is controlled by THP-1 macrophages produced TNF-α. The production of TNF-α starts after adjustable induction time and depends on the composition of the PEM and the embedding depth of the microorganisms.

4.3.2 Exponential Versus Linear Growth

An important feature of the formation of PEMs is their growth mode (Schönhoff, 2003; Steitz et al., 2000; Picart et al., 2002). There are two limiting aspects: linear growing versus exponential growing layers. The thickness of polystyrene sulfonate (PSS) and poly(allylamine hydrochloride) (PAH) multilayers, for instance, increases linearly with the number of deposition cycles, while the thickness of PSS/poly(diallyldimethylammonium chloride) (pDADMAC) multilayers increases linearly or nonlinearly depending on the charge density of pDADMAC. In general, the linear growth leads to thinner films than exponential growth does. The linear increase is due to the charge overcompensation, which is required for the multilayer formation. The roughness and the surface potential remain the same after a full deposition cycle, and the increment per deposition cycle is constant. Much more complex is the nonlinear growth. A transition between both types of growth can be observed, depending on the combination of polyelectrolytes and preparation conditions.

Most of the biologically relevant polyelectrolytes such as polypeptides and polysaccharides show a nonlinear growth. This regime is characterized by film thickness and the amount of adsorbed polyelectrolytes, which increase more rapidly than linearly with the number of deposited layers.

Not only biologically relevant polyelectrolytes lead to an exponential increase in adsorbed amount. For many synthetic polyelectrolytes, a transition from linear to exponential growth can be tuned by preparation conditions. A transition from linear to exponential growth requires an increase in the vertical mobility of polyelectrolyte chains. This can be achieved by an increase in the flexibility of the polyelectrolyte chains, leading to a better protrusion through the voids formed by the matrix of polyelectrolytes and the formation of fewer complexes between the chains. Usually, the growth becomes nonlinear with increasing salt concentration and the amount of adsorbed polymer increases more rapidly than linearly with the number of deposition cycles. A change from a linear to exponential buildup is also observed when the temperature of the preparation increases.

4.3.3 Polyelectrolyte Blends

Controlling the chemical composition of PEMs makes possible to tailor their physical properties. Constructing PEMs using polyelectrolyte blends offers new possibilities for the modulation of film thickness, film morphology, secondary structure, degradation rates, protein adsorption, or even mechanical properties. Multicomponent polymer blends can yield numerous advantages over single-component polymers. Blends may allow the tailoring of the bulk material behavior, increasing its applications and process ability. Blending of polymers can be used to create films with tailored interfacial properties for controlling drug release (Cui et al., 2011). Polyelectrolyte blends can be applied for producing highly functional films and coatings with nanoscale dimensions and tailored interfacial properties assembled from aqueous solutions. In 2008, a review by Caruso and coworkers (Quinn et al., 2008) stressed on the advantages of these new types of films. Examples of applications in the fields of biology or nanoporous thin film preparation were demonstrated. The properties of the polyelectrolyte blends are given by the balance that dictates PEM formation. The details of polyelectrolyte arrangement within blend films are still unresolved and difficult to investigate. Obviously, the particular molecular organization of the polyelectrolytes within the films plays the most important role. The control of the chemical composition of the film is of high importance, as it is the origin of the desired, tailored properties of the film.

An example of the application of polyelectrolyte blends formed by hyaluronan and chitosan was recently demonstrated. These polyelectrolytes are biocompatible, but alone they are known to be rather soft and strongly viscoelastic. Salomäki and Kankare (Salomäki and Kankare, 2009) have shown that incorporating synthetic nonsaccharide polyelectrolytes such as PAH and poly(acrylic acid) (PAA) in various proportions into the hyaluronan/chitosan layers forms diffusion barriers when deposited between the layers. If its proportion is higher, the film growth adopts a linear buildup in the LbL process. Polyacrylic acid forms a kind of scaffold inside the film, giving the natively soft hyaluronan/chitosan film more mechanical strength.

4.3.4 Cross-Linking of Polyelectrolytes in PEMs

Chemical cross-linking of the polyelectrolytes in PEMs can control the stability of PEMs against chemical or biological degradation. It also plays an important role by changing the mechanical properties of PEMs, which is an important condition for the immobilization and proliferation of cells on the PEM-coated surfaces. Two types of cross-linking are mostly used: chemical and photochemical, depending on the factors that activate the cross-linking process.

It is known that temperature higher than 130°C can induce the formation of amide or imide bonds within films (Dai et al., 2001). Richert et al. (2004) and Schuetz et al. (2003) have proposed protocols based on the carbodiimide chemistry for cross-linking carboxyl groups with amine groups. The carbodiimide used [1-ethyl-3-(3-dimethylaminopropyl)carbodiimide] does not require additional molecule to be inserted into the film. The cross-linking process is due to the transformation of ionic cross-links into covalent cross-links.

Cross-linking has major consequences on film structure and mechanical properties. The result of cross-linking is considerable stiffening of PLL/hyaluronan and chitosan/hyaluronan when compared to the native (uncross-linked) films (Richert et al., 2004; Schneider et al., 2006). Cross-linking improves also the resistance of PEMs to biodegradation (Picart et al., 2005; Etienne et al., 2005). Li and Haynie (2004) used another strategy for the cross-linking and stabilization of polypeptide PEMs by the formation of disulfide bonds. These bonds are involved in the structural stabilization of proteins. Disulfide cross-linking could be particularly useful for decreasing the rate of film disintegration or for modulating the mechanical properties of a PEM (Haynie et al., 2005). Photo-cross-linking techniques were also used to adjust the mechanical properties of PEMs. Yang and Rubner (2002) demonstrated the proofs of concept for this type of cross-linking. Recently, they synthesized a photo-cross-linkable weak polyanion poly(acrylic acid-ran-vinylbenzyl acrylate) (PAArVBA) and associated it with PAH to make films. Native and photo-cross-linked films were found to exhibit similar thickness, but the swelling of the cross-linked films is much limited.

4.3.5 Mechanical Properties of PEMs

Many applications in chemistry, physics, and biology require the formation of PEMs with adjustable mechanical properties. The stiffness of PEMs can be modulated from a few kPa to several GPa by the proper choice of polyelectrolytes, and the degree of cross-linking inside the film affected mostly by pH and ionic strength as well as covalent cross-links. The stiffness of a PEM film is also related to the buildup regime in the LbL process. Exponentially growing films are generally considered to be softer than those with a linear buildup (Collin et al., 2004). The mechanical properties of the films can be modulated by using polyelectrolytes with different conformations. Schönhoff and colleagues characterized the stiffness of PEMs containing PAH as the polycation and two different anionic sulfated polysaccharides: i-carrageenan, which forms helical structures, and λ-carrageenan, which has a random coil conformation (Schönhoff, 2003). It was found that films prepared with λ-carrageenan were about three times stiffer than those with i-carrageenan. This proves the strong influence of polyelectrolyte structures on the rigidity of PEMs (Podsiadlo et al., 2007). Phospholipid-grafted sugar molecules (Schneider et al., 2006) also significantly influence the stiffness of the films. Another strategy for adjusting the mechanical properties of PEMs is to incorporate nanoparticles into the films. The formation of multilayer films containing cationic polyelectrolytes and anionic nanoparticles such as carbon nanotubes (Tang et al., 2003), montmorillonite (Podsiadlo et al., 2007), or metallic nanoparticles (Park et al., 2005; Kolasinska et al., 2009) has already been reported. The Young's modulus of these films could be up to two orders of magnitude higher than that of the pure PEMs. The use of blends of strong and weak polyelectrolytes also leads to the formation of films with high rigidity, for instance, by inserting "stiff" PSS/PAH layers on the top of a "soft" PLL/hyaluronan film (Francius et al., 2007) or between the layers of chitosan/hyaluronan (Salomäki and Kankare, 2009). Films prepared from weak polyelectrolytes, which are only partially charged at moderate pH, are strongly influenced by pH and ionic strength (Pavoor et al., 2004). Usually, an increase in the salt concentration reduces intermolecular interactions in the films and makes them softer. Increased ionic strength was also used for the enhancement of drug delivery through salt-induced structural changes and the formation of nanopores (Fery et al., 2001; Dubas and Schlenhoff, 2001; Heuvingh et al., 2005).

4.4 Summary and Outlook

Contemporary medicine is looking continuously for new biomaterials that combine the excellent mechanical and physical properties of inorganic materials with the requirements of living tissues. Sometimes, it is impossible to combine the requirements in one single material. Then the modification on the surfaces of the implants where the biological tissues meet nonbiological materials is necessary. The PEM prepared by the LbL technology is an excellent candidate to meet these requirements. They can be prepared using well-known and biocompatible natural polyelectrolytes whose properties can be tuned very precisely according to the specific applications. This is based on the huge variety of deposition conditions, which may change the properties of the coatings dramatically. Even though the PEM coatings offer many opportunities for surface modification, these layers are still not widely used in the manufacturing of specific products. One of the main obstacles in that way is the comparatively slow coating/deposition process. Although there is already a variety of improved deposition techniques, their optimization and application in the near future will still be one of the main challenges for the scientists and in particular for the engineers working in this field.

Many efforts are necessary to understand better the contact between the PEMs and the biological tissues and cells. Two main challenges should be mentioned. One is the influence of the physical properties of the layers (e.g., thickness, roughness, and viscosity) on cellular behavior such as adhesion and proliferation of different types of cells in contact with the modified surfaces. Another challenge is the preparation of coatings that are able to reduce drastically the undesired immunological response of the tissues that are in contact with the implants. First results in these areas are already obtained, but further work among chemists, material scientists, and biologists is required.

The PEMs have high potential to become standard coating technology in many applications, including that of medical devices. The extreme efforts in the last years to understand their structure and control it on molecular level will give new insight into different applications.

References

Ai, H., Jones, S., and Lvov, Y. 2003. Biomedical applications of electrostatic layer-by-layer nano-assembly of polymers, enzymes, and nanoparticles. *Cell Biochem. Biophys.* **39**(1): 23–43.

Albanese, A., Tang, P.S., and Chan, W.C.W. 2012. The effect of nanoparticle size, shape, and surface chemistry on biological systems. *Annu. Rev. Biomed. Eng.* **14**(1): 1–16.

Antipov, A.A., and Sukhorukov, G.B. 2004. Polyelectrolyte multilayer capsules as vehicles with tunable permeability. *Adv. Colloid Interface Sci.* **111**(1–2): 49–61.

Anzai, J.-I., Kobayashi, Y., Nakamura, N., Nishimura, M., and Hoshi, T. 1998. Layer-by-layer construction of multilayer thin films composed of avidin and biotin-labeled poly(amine)s. *Langmuir* **15**(1): 221–226.

Ariga, K., Nakanishi, T., and Michinobu, T. 2006. Immobilization of biomaterials to nano-assembled films (self-assembled monolayers, Langmuir–Blodgett films, and layer-by-layer assemblies) and their related functions. *J. Nanosci. Nanotechnol.* **6**(8): 2278–2301.

Baek, H., Lee, C., Park, J., Kim, Y., Koo, B., et al. 2012. Layer-by-layer assembled enzyme multilayers with adjustable memory performance and low power consumption via molecular-level control. *J. Mater. Chem.* **22**(11): 4645–4651.

Benkirane-Jessel, N., Lavalle, P., Hübsch, E., Holl, V., Senger, B., et al. 2005. Short-time tuning of the biological activity of functionalized polyelectrolyte multilayers. *Adv. Funct. Mater.* **15**(4): 648–654.

Berg, M.C., Yang, S.Y., Hammond, P.T., and Rubner, M.F. 2004. Controlling mammalian cell interactions on patterned polyelectrolyte multilayer surfaces. *Langmuir* **20**(4): 1362–1368.

Berthiaume, F.O., Maguire, T.J., and Yarmush, M.L. 2011. Tissue engineering and regenerative medicine: History, progress, and challenges. *Annu. Rev. Chem. Biomol. Eng.* **2**(1): 403–430.

Boudou, T., Crouzier, T., Ren, K., Blin, G., and Picart, C. 2010. Multiple functionalities of polyelectrolyte multilayer films: New biomedical applications. *Adv. Mater.* **22**(4): 441–467.

Boura, C., Menu, P., Payan, E., Picart, C., Voegel, J.C., et al. 2003. Endothelial cells grown on thin polyelectrolyte mutlilayered films: An evaluation of a new versatile surface modification. *Biomaterials* **24**(20): 3521–3530.

Collin, D., Lavalle, P., Garza, J.M.N., Voegel, J.-C., Schaaf, P., et al. 2004. Mechanical properties of cross-linked hyaluronic acid/poly-(l-lysine) multilayer films. *Macromolecules* **37**(26): 10195–10198.

Cowin, S.C. 2004. Tissue growth and remodeling. *Annu. Rev. Biomed. Eng.* **6**: 77–107.

Cui, D., Jing, J., Boudou, T., Pignot-Paintrand, I., de Koker, S., et al. 2011. Hydrophobic shell loading of biopolyelectrolyte capsules. *Adv. Mater.* **23**(24): H200–204.

Dai, J., Jensen, A.W., Mohanty, D.K., Erndt, J., and Bruening, M.L. 2001. Controlling the permeability of multilayered polyelectrolyte films through derivatization, cross-linking, and hydrolysis. *Langmuir* **17**(3): 931–937.

Davis, J.R. (ed). 2003. *Handbook of Materials for Medical Devices.* Ohio: ASM International.

de Geest, B.G., Sanders, N.N., Sukhorukov, G.B., Demeester, J., and de Smedt, S.C. 2007. Release mechanisms for polyelectrolyte capsules. *Chem. Soc. Rev.* **36**(4): 636–649.

Decher, G. 1997. Fuzzy nanoassemblies: Toward layered polymeric multicomposites. *Science* **277**(5330): 1232–1237.

Decher, G. 2003. Polyelectrolyte multilayers, an overview. In *Multilayer Thin Films: Sequential Assembly of Nanocomposite Materials* (Decher, G., and Schlenoff, J. B. ed). Weinheim, FRG: Wiley-VCH Verlag GmbH & Co. KGaA. pp. 1–46.

Decher, G., Hong, J.D., and Schmitt, J. 1992. Buildup of ultrathin multilayer films by a self-assembly process: III. Consecutively alternating adsorption of anionic and cationic polyelectrolytes on charged surfaces. *Thin Solid Films* **210–211, Part 2**: 831–835.

Decher, G., Lvov, Y., and Schmitt, J. 1994. Proof of multilayer structural organization in self-assembled polycation-polyanion molecular films. *Thin Solid Films* **244**(1–2): 772–777.

Derjaguin, B. and Landau, L. 1993. Theory of the stability of strongly charged lyophobic sols and of the adhesion of strongly charged particles in solutions of electrolytes. *Prog. Surface Sci.* **43**(1–4): 30–59.

Dubas, S.T., and Schlenoff, J.B. 2001. Swelling and smoothing of polyelectrolyte multilayers by salt. *Langmuir* **17**(25): 7725–7727.

Etienne, O., Schneider, A., Taddei, C., Richert, L., Schaaf, P., et al. 2005. Degradability of polysaccharides multilayer films in the oral environment: an in vitro and in vivo study. *Biomacromolecules* **6**(2): 726–733.

Fery, A., Schöler, B., Cassagneau, T., and Caruso, F. 2001. Nanoporous thin films formed by salt-induced structural changes in multilayers of poly(acrylic acid) and poly(allylamine). *Langmuir* **17**(13): 3779–3783.

Francius, G., Hemmerlé, J., Ball, V., Lavalle, P., Picart, C., et al. 2007. Stiffening of soft polyelectrolyte architectures by multilayer capping evidenced by viscoelastic analysis of AFM indentation measurements. *J. Phys. Chem. C* **111**(23): 8299–8306.

Girard-Egrot, A.S.P., Godoy, S.P., and Blum, L.C.J. 2005. Enzyme association with lipidic Langmuir–Blodgett films: Interests and applications in nanobioscience. *Adv. Colloid Interface Sci.* **116**(1–3): 205–225.

Haynie, D.T., Zhang, L., Rudra, J.S., Zhao, W., Zhong, Y., et al. 2005. Polypeptide multilayer films. *Biomacromolecules* **6**(6): 2895–2913.

Heuvingh, J., Zappa, M., and Fery, A. 2005. Salt softening of polyelectrolyte multilayer capsules. *Langmuir* **21**(7): 3165–3171.

Huddleston, J.G., Visser, A.E., Reichert, W.M., Willauer, H.D., Broker, G.A., et al. 2001. Characterization and comparison of hydrophilic and hydrophobic room temperature ionic liquids incorporating the imidazolium cation. *Green Chemistry* **3**(4): 156–164.

Jewell, C.M., Zhang, J., Fredin, N.J., Wolff, M.R., Hacker, T.A., et al. 2006. Release of plasmid DNA from intravascular stents coated with ultrathin multilayered polyelectrolyte films. *Biomacromolecules* **7**(9): 2483–2491.

Johansson, E., Lundström, L., Norgren, M., and Wågberg, L. 2009. Adsorption behavior and adhesive properties of biopolyelectrolyte multilayers formed from cationic and anionic starch. *Biomacromolecules* **10**(7): 1768–1776.

Kim, T.G., Lee, Y., and Park, T.G. 2010. Controlled gene-eluting metal stent fabricated by bio-inspired surface modification with hyaluronic acid and deposition of DNA/PEI polyplexes. *Int. J. Pharm.* **384**(1–2): 181–188.

Kolasinska, M., Gutberlet, T., and Krastev, R. 2009. Ordering of Fe_3O_4 nanoparticles in polyelectrolyte multilayer films. *Langmuir* **25**(17): 10292–10297.

Lan, Y., Cheng, C., Zhang, S., Ni, G., Chen, L., et al. 2011. Plasma-induced styrene grafting onto the surface of polytetrafluoroethylene powder for proton exchange membrane application. *Plasma Sci. Tech.* **13**(5): 604.

Li, B., and Haynie, D.T. 2004. Multilayer biomimetics: Reversible covalent stabilization of a nanostructured biofilm. *Biomacromolecules* **5**(5): 1667–1670.

Lin, Q., Ding, X., Qiu, F., Song, X., Fu, G., et al. 2010. In situ endothelialization of intravascular stents coated with an anti-CD34 antibody functionalized heparin-collagen multilayer. *Biomaterials* **31**(14): 4017–4025.

Lin, Q., Yan, J., Qiu, F., Song, X., Fu, G., et al. 2011. Heparin/collagen multilayer as a thromboresistant and endothelial favorable coating for intravascular stent. *J. Biomed. Mater. Res. Part A* **96A**(1): 132–141.

Liu, H., Skibinska, L., Gapinski, J., Patkowski, A., Fischer, E.W., et al. 1998. Effect of electrostatic interactions on the structure and dynamics of a model polyelectrolyte. I. Diffusion. *J. Chem. Phys.* **109**(17): 7556–7566.

Lundström-Hämälä, L., Johansson, E., and Wågberg, L. 2010. Polyelectrolyte multilayers from cationic and anionic starch: Influence of charge density and salt concentration on the properties of the adsorbed layers. *Starch-Stärke* **62**(2): 102–114.

Lvov, Y., Decher, G., and Moehwald, H. 1993. Assembly, structural characterization, and thermal behavior of layer-by-layer deposited ultrathin films of poly(vinyl sulfate) and poly(allylamine). *Langmuir* **9**(2): 481–486.

Lynn, D.M. 2007. Peeling back the layers: Controlled erosion and triggered disassembly of multilayered polyelectrolyte thin films. *Adv. Mater.* **19**(23): 4118–4130.

Magnussen, O.M., Ocko, B.M., Deutsch, M., Regan, M.J., Pershan, P.S., et al. 1996. Self-assembly of organic films on a liquid metal. *Nature* **384**(6606): 250–252.

Mansouri, S., Merhi, Y., Winnik, F.O.M., and Tabrizian, M. 2011. Investigation of layer-by-layer assembly of polyelectrolytes on fully functional human red blood cells in suspension for attenuated immune response. *Biomacromolecules* **12**(3): 585–592.

McEver, R.P., and Zhu, C. 2010. Rolling cell adhesion. *Annu. Rev. Cell Dev. Biol.* **26**: 363–396.

Meng, S., Liu, Z., Shen, L., Guo, Z., Chou, L.L., et al. 2009. The effect of a layer-by-layer chitosan-heparin coating on the endothelialization and coagulation properties of a coronary stent system. *Biomaterials* **30**(12): 2276–2283.

Mhanna, R.F., Vörös, J., and Zenobi-Wong, M. 2011. Layer-by-layer films made from extracellular matrix macromolecules on silicone substrates. *Biomacromolecules* **12**(3): 609–616.

Nepal, D., Balasubramanian, S., Simonian, A.L., and Davis, V.A. 2008. Strong antimicrobial coatings: Single-walled carbon nanotubes armored with biopolymers. *Nano Lett.* **8**(7): 1896–1901.

Park, J., Fouché, L.D., and Hammond, P.T. 2005. Multicomponent patterning of layer-by-layer assembled polyelectrolyte/nanoparticle composite thin films with controlled alignment. *Adv. Mater.* **17**(21): 2575–2579.

Pavoor, P.V., Bellare, A., Strom, A., Yang, D., and Cohen, R.E. 2004. Mechanical characterization of polyelectrolyte multilayers using quasi-static nanoindentation. *Macromolecules* **37**(13): 4865–4871.

Perlstein, I., Connolly, J.M., Cui, X., Song, C., Li, Q., et al. 2003. DNA delivery from an intravascular stent with a denatured collagen-polylactic-polyglycolic acid-controlled release coating: Mechanisms of enhanced transfection. *Gene Ther.* **10**(17): 1420–1428.

Picart, C. 2008. Polyelectrolyte multilayer films: From physico-chemical properties to the control of cellular processes. *Curr. Med. Chem.* **15**(7): 685–697.

Picart, C., Elkaim, R., Richert, L., Audoin, F., Arntz, Y., et al. 2005. Primary cell adhesion on RGD-functionalized and covalently crosslinked thin polyelectrolyte multilayer films. *Adv. Funct. Mater.* **15**(1): 83–94.

Picart, C., Mutterer, J., Richert, L., Luo, Y., Prestwich, G.D., et al. 2002. Molecular basis for the explanation of the exponential growth of polyelectrolyte multilayers. *Proc. Nat. Acad. Sci. USA* **99**(20): 12531–12535.

Picart, C., Schneider, A., Etienne, O., Mutterer, J., Schaaf, P., et al. 2005. Controlled degradability of polysaccharide multilayer films in vitro and in vivo. *Adv. Funct. Mater.* **15**(11): 1771–1780.

Podsiadlo, P., Tang, Z., Shim, B.S., and Kotov, N.A. 2007. Counterintuitive effect of molecular strength and role of molecular rigidity on mechanical properties of layer-by-layer assembled nanocomposites. *Nano Lett.* **7**(5): 1224–1231.

Quinn, A., Such, G.K., Quinn, J.F., and Caruso, F. 2008. Polyelectrolyte blend multilayers: A versatile route to engineering interfaces and films. *Adv. Funct. Mater.* **18**(1): 17–26.

Reisch, A., Hemmerle, J., Chassepot, A., Lefort, M., Benkirane-Jessel, N., et al. 2010. Anti-fouling phosphorylcholine bearing polyelectrolyte multilayers: Cell adhesion resistance at rest and under stretching. *Soft Matter* **6**(7): 1503–1512.

Rengaraj, S., Mani, V., Kavanagh, P., Rusling, J., and Leech, D. 2011. A membrane-less enzymatic fuel cell with layer-by-layer assembly of redox polymer and enzyme over graphite electrodes. *Chem. Commun.* **47**(43): 11861–11863.

Richert, L., Boulmedais, F., Lavalle, P., Mutterer, J.R.M., Ferreux, E., et al. 2004. Improvement of stability and cell adhesion properties of polyelectrolyte multilayer films by chemical cross-linking. *Biomacromolecules* **5**(2): 284–294.

Richert, L., Engler, A.J., Discher, D.E., and Picart, C. 2004. Elasticity of native and cross-linked polyelectrolyte multilayer films. *Biomacromolecules* **5**(5): 1908–1916.

Richert, L., Lavalle, P., Payan, E., Shu, X.Z., Prestwich, G.D., et al. 2003. Layer by layer buildup of polysaccharide films: Physical chemistry and cellular adhesion aspects. *Langmuir* **20**(2): 448–458.

Rinckenbach, S., Hemmerlé, J., Dieval, F., Arntz, Y., Kretz, J.-G., et al. 2008. Characterization of polyelectrolyte multilayer films on polyethylene terephtalate vascular prostheses under mechanical stretching. *J. Biomed. Mater. Res. Part A* **84A**(3): 576–588.

Rofaiel, A., Ellis, J.S., Challa, P.R., and Bazylak, A. 2012. Heterogeneous through-plane distributions of polytetrafluoroethylene in polymer electrolyte membrane fuel cell gas diffusion layers. *J. Power Sources* **201**: 219–225.

Salomäki, M., and Kankare, J. 2009. Influence of synthetic polyelectrolytes on the growth and properties of hyaluronan-chitosan multilayers. *Biomacromolecules* **10**(2): 294–301.

Schneider, A., Vodouhê, C., Richert, L., Francius, G., Le Guen, E., et al. 2006. Multifunctional polyelectrolyte multilayer films: Combining mechanical resistance, biodegradability, and bioactivity. *Biomacromolecules* **8**(1): 139–145.

Schönhoff, M. 2003. Layered polyelectrolyte complexes: Physics of formation and molecular properties. *J. Phys.: Condens. Matter* **15**(49): R1781.

Schuetz, P., and Caruso, F. 2003. Copper-assisted weak polyelectrolyte multilayer formation on microspheres and subsequent film crosslinking. *Adv. Funct. Mater.* **13**(12): 929–937.

Steitz, R., Leiner, V., Siebrecht, R., and v. Klitzing, R. 2000. Influence of the ionic strength on the structure of polyelectrolyte films at the solid/liquid interface. *Colloids Surf. A.* **163**(1): 63–70.

Stuart, M.A.C., Huck, W.T.S., Genzer, J., Muller, M., Ober, C., et al. 2010. Emerging applications of stimuli-responsive polymer materials. *Nat. Mater* **9**(2): 101–113.

Sukhorukov, G.B., Möhwald, H., Decher, G., and Lvov, Y.M. 1996. Assembly of polyelectrolyte multilayer films by consecutively alternating adsorption of polynucleotides and polycations. *Thin Solid Films* **284–285**: 220–223.

Szarpak, A., Cui, D., Dubreuil, F.d.R., de Geest, B.G., de Cock, L.J., et al. 2010. Designing hyaluronic acid-based layer-by-layer capsules as a carrier for intracellular drug delivery. *Biomacromolecules* **11**(3): 713–720.

Tang, Z., Kotov, N.A., Magonov, S., and Ozturk, B. 2003. Nanostructured artificial nacre. *Nat. Mater* **2**(6): 413–418.

Tang, Z., Wang, Y., Podsiadlo, P., and Kotov, N.A. 2006. Biomedical applications of layer-by-layer assembly: From biomimetics to tissue engineering. *Adv. Mater.* **18**(24): 3203–3224.

Ulman, A. 1991. *An Introduction to Ultrathin Organic Films: From Langmuir Blodgett to Self-Assembly*. California: Academic Press.

V. Klitzing, R. 2006. Internal structure of polyelectrolyte multilayer assemblies. *Phys. Chem. Chem. Phys.* **8**(43): 5012–5033.

Verwey, E.J.W. 1947. Theory of the stability of lyophobic colloids. *J. Phys. Colloid Chem.* **51**(3): 631–636.

Walter, D.H., Cejna, M., Diaz-Sandoval, L., Willis, S., Kirkwood, L., et al. 2004. Local gene transfer of phVEGF-2 plasmid by gene-eluting stents. *Circulation* **110**(1): 36–45.

Yang, S.Y., and Rubner, M.F. 2002. Micropatterning of polymer thin films with pH-sensitive and cross-linkable hydrogen-bonded polyelectrolyte multilayers. *J. Am. Chem. Soc.* **124**(10): 2100–2101.

Yoo, P.J., Nam, K.T., Belcher, A.M., and Hammond, P.T. 2008. Solvent-assisted patterning of polyelectrolyte multilayers and selective deposition of virus assemblies. *Nano Lett.* **8**(4): 1081–1089.

Zhao, Q., Li, H., and Li, B. 2011. Nanoencapsulating living biological cells using electrostatic layer-by-layer self-assembly: Platelets as a model. *J. Mater. Res.* **26**(02): 347–351.

Chapter 5

Surface Characteristics and Biofilms

Klaus Liefeith, Holger Rothe, Marion Frant, and Ronald Schade
Department of Biomaterials, Institute for Bioprocessing and Analytical Measurement Techniques eV (iba), Rosenhof, 37308, Heilbad Heiligenstadt, Germany
klaus.liefeith@iba-heiligenstadt.de

In this chapter, an overview of the current understanding of noncovalent interfacial forces in relevant biological aqueous media is given, followed by a more in-depth discussion of initial bacterial adhesion and biofilm formation as a consequence of those interfacial forces. Particular emphasis is given to provide an overview of the existing active and passive antifouling strategies, especially in the light of the tremendous self-association potential of vicinal water. Corresponding test strategies based on the application of mixed bacterial cultures and bioreactors as microbiological test platform to establish a suitable culture environment are presented.

Biofunctional Surface Engineering
Edited by Martin Scholz

ISBN 978-981-4411-60-8 (Hardcover), 978-981-4411-61-5 (eBook)
www.panstanford.com

5.1 Introduction

Research on bacterial adhesion phenomena and biofilm formation is, as previously, a major topic especially for biomaterials scientists. With this background, it can be stated that the central point is, even after decades of worldwide research, the development of protein-resistant surfaces or contamination-preventing strategies to reduce the risk of implant-associated infections caused by pathogens.

While the development of protein-resistant surfaces builds the basis for the manufacturing of blood-compatible surfaces, since often the amount of adsorbed fibrinogen has been correlated with the reaction of blood cells and hemocompatibility approaches (Ratner, 2007), the nature of a proper biomaterial from a physicochemical point of view remains unclear. Promising approaches were published based on both hydrophilic polymers such as poly(ethylene glycol) (PEG) or zwitterionic phosphorylcholine (Cao et al., 2007; Ishihara et al., 1994) and hydrophobic polymers such as Teflon or silicone (Hanson et al., 1980).

However, it can be summarized that our lack of understanding the complex basic biology and physicochemistry of the interaction between blood proteins and cells on the one hand and artificial materials on the other hand is the reason for using basically still the same materials in the clinic for more than 50 years.

Furthermore, it is acknowledged that today's biomaterials science suffers from some analytical and conceptual barriers that can be summarized briefly as follows:

a. Analytical barriers are still existent due to the fact that biomaterials or, more precisely, biomaterial surfaces should be evaluated in a manner that the resulting data reflect the complex biological milieu of the target tissue or, generally spoken, the aqueous environment of the end use, which is typical especially for biological entities.
b. Conceptual barriers are of special importance and comprise all efforts to interpret the terms biocompatibility and biofunctionality by means of material or surface properties with practical relevance.

According to the detailed and ground-breaking studies of Vogler (Vogler, 1993) and Della-Volpe (Morra, 2000), it is widely accepted that only the uppermost layers of an arbitrary biomaterial are in direct physicochemical contact with the surrounding biological system independently of the nature of the real contact situation. The interaction of a material with the biological environment occurs at the so-called biointerface, a liquid or, generally spoken, an aqueous interface extended over some atomic bond-length distances. Vogler's proposal that biocompatibility cannot be interpreted on the basis of microscopic and spectroscopic data alone because these approaches are often based on dry-state chemistry represents a pioneering work from a biomaterials point of view. Taking into consideration that this aqueous milieu is not a neutral carrier of biosystems such as proteins or cells, but builds up a narrow zone of vicinal water that interacts actively with the biological environment via acid–base reactions, ion exchange, and hydrogen bonding, it is not unusual to accept that surfaces possess a tremendous potential to reorganize in an aqueous environment and to influence the intensity of protein adsorption or to induce surface-associated changes of the secondary structure of proteins.

Having this in mind, it is quite understandable that tensiometric methods experience a renaissance in biomaterials surface science. Wetting experiments show an extremely high surface sensitivity in the subnanometer region and are basically focused to detect the fundamental energetics between biosystems and biomaterials.

It can be assumed that this theoretical framework will provide enough information in future research to identify the fundamental parameters that drive the biological response to artificial materials, e.g., in the field of biofilm formation and biofilm monitoring.

5.2 Interfacial Energy at Biointerfaces

In the past decades, a large number of in vitro models have been developed to investigate bacterial adhesion and/or biofilm formation. They can be classified roughly as follows:

a. Static test systems (Petri dishes, tissue culture plates, etc.) or
b. Dynamic test systems (parallel-plate flow chamber, radial flow chamber, rotating disc apparatus, Robbins device, etc.)

As a rule the sample surface can be fixed at the bottom of the culture device or inside the flow-through chamber system, e.g., as a part of the perfusion system. Many of the designed adhesion test setups allow a microscopic control to observe the kinetic of bacterial adhesion. The recorded kinetics for the initial adhesion may be described by Eq. 5.1.

$$q(t) = q_{\max} \cdot (1 - e^{-\beta \cdot t}) \tag{5.1}$$

The maximum cell loading ($q_{\max}$) and the exponential accumulation factor (β) were obtained from the exponential fit of the adhesion kinetics as published by Montag et al. (2012). The microorganisms must be selected carefully to meet the clinical situation as accurately as possible. In many cases multispecies biofilms are formed under physiological conditions, and therefore it is common practice to use defined mixed cultures consisting of up to five microorganisms to achieve optimum results. It is of value to point out that any such adhesion experiments require a long-term stable, sterile, and reproducible cultivation process. To guarantee corresponding cultivation conditions, bioreactor-based test systems were designed in association with flow-through chamber systems, which offer a lot of analytical possibilities to allow a continuous biofilm monitoring, e.g., in dependence of the physicochemical nature of the substrate surface.

As previously, colloid-chemical approaches are used to predict or to interpret bacterial attachment data in terms of noncovalent interaction forces acting under aqueous conditions. Recently, bacterial adhesion has been interpreted in terms of surface free energy comprising electrodynamic Lifshitz van der Waals interaction forces, and increasingly in terms of electrostatic interactions. The combination of both surface energy components is generally known as the DLVO approach (after Derjaguin, Landau, Verway, and Overbeek) (Derjaguin and Landau, 1941; Verwey and Overbeek, 1948). It can be expected that electrostatic interactions are long-range interactions becoming especially important at charged surfaces.

However, if the assumption of Vogler (Vogler, 1998) is true, there is an enormous difference in the self-association of water molecules between vicinal water and bulk-phase water based on the tetraether structure of water and the electron-acceptor and electron-donor capabilities of water molecules. Consequently, this leads to a situation where at hydrophobic surfaces, dominated by completely apolar electrodynamic Lifshitz van der Waals interaction forces, another structure and reactivity of vicinal water were observed than at hydrophilic surfaces, associated essentially with polar electron-acceptor and electron-donor sites or Lewis acid–base sites and the corresponding Lewis acid–base interaction forces.

That is the reason why advanced theoretical approaches explain the initial bacterial adhesion processes as interplay between DLVO energies and non-DLVO energies. Furthermore, it is widely accepted that the most important contribution is caused by polar Lewis acid–base interaction forces often resulting from hydrogen bonds or water molecules with their excellent proton-donor and proton-acceptor capabilities.

Although a considerable amount of debate remains, it is clear that some of the basic assumptions that have guided biomaterials research during the last decades seem to be imprecise, because they neglect the basic role of structured water at biointerfaces and the herewith related reactivity between water and the biological environment. On this background, we follow a proposition of Vogler (Vogler, 1998) that (i) the free energy of biomaterial surfaces determines the structure and the reactivity of water at the biointerface, including the solvent properties within the vicinal water zone and (ii) the biological response is controlled by the solvent properties within the vicinal water zone and therefore only indirectly related to the free surface energy of the biomaterial itself.

The noncovalent interaction forces that dominate the reactivity at aqueous biointerfaces were summarized by van Oss (van Oss, 1994) as follows:

a. Apolar electrodynamic, or Lifshitz van der Waals interactions
b. Polar, electron-donor–electron-acceptor, or Lewis acid–base interactions
c. Electrostatic interactions
d. Brownian movement

This theoretical concept leads, without any further assumption, to the conclusion that hydrophobic surfaces induce a biological response of Type I and hydrophilic surfaces induce a biological response of Type II (Vogler, 1999) as confirmed by own investigations concerning the initial adhesion of a bacterial mixed culture containing *Staphylococcus aureus* and *Staphylococcus epidermidis* in a mixing ratio of 1:1. Noteworthy that the limit between Type I and Type II responses was observed at a water contact angle close to the BECB limit, which is given with 65° (Berg, 1994; Vogler, 1999).

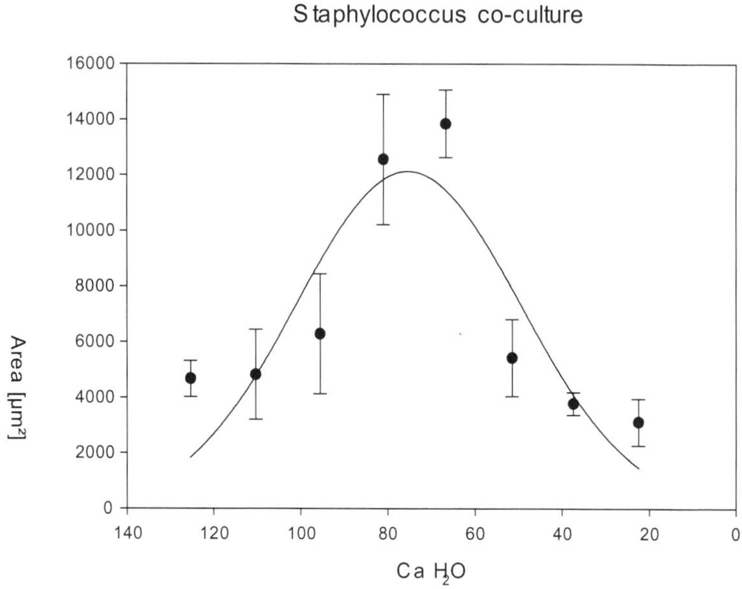

Figure 5.1 Biofilm formation on material surfaces chemically modified by means of thiols coupled with hydroxyl groups and methyl groups of different mixing ratios to get surfaces with a stepwise varied hydrophobicity. Shown is the area colonized with bacteria in dependence of the surface hydrophobicity (Ca H_2O – water contact angle).

5.3 Biofilm Formation

The majority of bacteria in all ecosystems is organized in aggregates or biofilms. This kind of survival strategy facilitates the microorganisms to respond and adapt to physiologically limited and strongly versatile environments and can protect them against antimicrobial strategies of competitive organisms or the host organism. Biofilms can be considered multicellular organisms involving mechanisms of physiological interactions, communication, signaling, mutualistic and antagonistic strategies similar to higher forms of life (Costerton et al., 1999). Bacterial adhesion with subsequent growth and propagation results in a steady state characterized by complex interactions between the microorganisms that enable the microhabitat community to withstand surrounding influences and protect themselves to attacks of the host defense system. Depending on their appearance and functions, biofilms are classified as "negative" or "positive" biofilms according to their effects on the human society (Karunakaran et al., 2011). The complex physiological pathways within biofilms contribute to convert waste materials into less dangerous intermediate products or carbon dioxide and water. Bioremediation processes in waste water management benefit from microbiological metabolism and are one of the best known applications of "positive" biofilms. Conversely, biofilms often negatively affect substrates, hosts or technical systems. Substrate-degrading effects, failures of technical devices such as flow inhibition, e.g., in heat exchangers, or biofouling, e.g., on optical sensor surfaces, and especially infection-associated bacterial populations in biomedicine can cause drastic damages and high costs. The enhanced knowledge about biofilms, their formation, and the involved interactions accumulated over the last decades led to a more detailed approach to monitor and control biofilms. So it is of great importance to understand which aspects are the key to understand the complex scenario of biofilm accumulation. Here some selected aspects of biofilm formation, structural aspects, and factors involved in cell–surface and cell–cell interactions are briefly discussed. Over the years, significant work has been done and the readers are referred to actual reviews published recently by Karunakaran et al., Lopez et al., and Hojo et al. (Karunakaran et al., 2011; Lopez et al., 2010; Hojo et al., 2009).

According to Karunakaran et al. *(*Karunakaran et al., 2011*)*, biofilm research has to be handled as a multidisciplinary study involving microbiology, biochemistry, medicine, infection biology as well as material science and physics. They introduced the term "biofilmology" to point out the high complexity of biofilms and related interactions. In other words, biofilm research has to merge investigations and data concerning the surface characteristics from both the material and the microorganism, the external environment (biofilm matrix, host conditions), and the intracellular processes (gene activities, signaling, proteomics) (Filoche et al., 2010). Each of these biofilm characteristics can differ in an unexpected large scale. This is expressed in a wide range of different biofilm communities. For instance, natural biofilms can show an enormous complexity of involved bacterial strains, matrix structures, and physiological pathways. In contrast, infectious biofilms often are characterized by a dominance of a few or a single bacterial strain (Burmolle et al., 2010) due to the ecological interactions of the microorganism population with the host and it's specific defense mechanisms. But there are some common basic processes in biofilm formation and propagation. According to a meanwhile widely accepted scheme, the biofilm genesis is passing several phases starting from surface modifications by media components, the settlement and initial adhesion of early biofilm colonizers with subsequent formation of microcolonies by cell–cell adhesion coupled with the activation of interbacterial signaling, gene transfer, and changes of gene activities to the formation of stable matured biofilm in a steady state (Costerton et al., 1999; Lopez et al., 2010; Hojo et al., 2009; Filoche et al., 2010). In this phase, the biofilms serve as a well-organized microenvironment only disturbed by active and/or passive detachment of more or less biofilm communities and their further spreading on the substrate surface (Fig. 5.2).

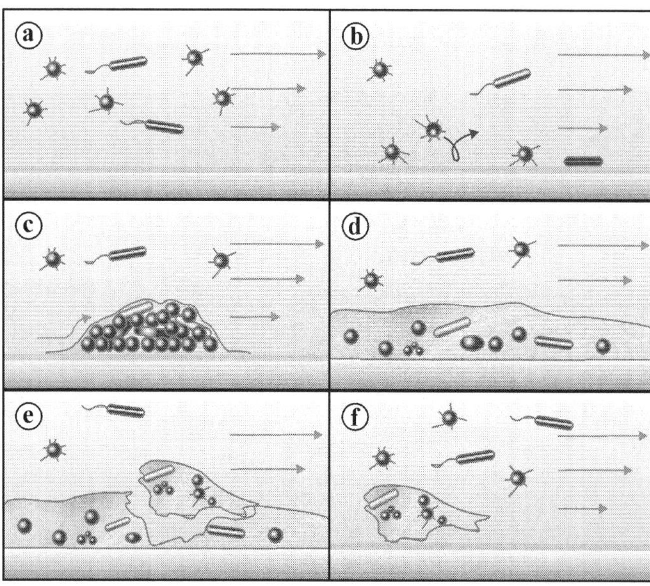

Figure 5.2 Biofilm formation on material surfaces. (a) Biofilm formation in aqueous systems starts with the adsorption of a "conditioning" layer on the material surface; (b) transportation of microorganisms to the surface by turbulent flow, reversible and irreversible adhesion; (c) formation of microcolonies; (d) formation of a stable matured biofilm; (e) active and passive detachment of biofilm components; (f) further spreading of the biofilm and attachment.

Especially in the early phase of initial adhesion, surface-associated interactions play a crucial role whether, and if so, how the biofilm formation is initialized. A common approach to understand this process has been to apply colloid-chemical concepts based on the surface or interface energies of the respective substrates and the attaching microorganisms in an aqueous milieu as described in the chapter before. Surface modifications by the adsorption of different patterns of media components such as ions and proteins within a few seconds and minutes can affect the surface properties of the substrate and change the local physiological environment, such as pH value and fluid structure in terms of proton-acceptor and proton-donor capacities. A well-known example is the acquired pellicle as a thin layer of salivary proteins on tooth and restorative materials, which can modulate the initial adhesion of dental bacteria (Dawes et al., 1963; van Dijk et al., 1988; Rosentritt et al., 2008). The adhesion of early colonizers is determined by surface-associated interactions such as hydrogen bonds, charge interactions, and specific bindings of cell wall molecules and cell adhesins. It is not surprising that the diversity of surface modifications by the adsorption processes of media components leads to a diversity of cell–material interactions in the early phase of biofilm formation. The ability of certain bacteria to bind to proteins of the surface layers favors these bacteria as early colonizers. For instance, the dental pellicle is characterized by salivary proteins such as alpha-amylase, immunoglobulin A, proline-rich proteins, and glycoproteins, which interact with many oral streptococci (Kolenbrander et al., 2002). Bacteria-to-surface and bacteria-to-host/tissue contacts are mediated by adhesins such as pili, Type I fimbriae (*Escherichia coli*), glycosyltransferase (*Streptococcus mutans*), protein F (*Streptococcus pyogenes*), lipoteichoic acid (*Streptococcus salivarius*), and cell-bound protein (*Staphylococcus aureus*) (Lopez et al., 2010; Todar). The predominant cell–material interactions in the first phase of biofilm formation are increasingly replaced by interbacterial interactions characterized by the changes of the intracellular activities and the associated protein and gene expression pattern, which lead to the formation of microcolonies and biofilm growth. In *S. aureus* biofilms, cell-wall-anchored adhesive proteins (Bap) interact with neighboring bacteria as a kind of "glue molecules." This type of cell-to-cell interactions seems to be independent on the common production of extracellular polymeric substances (EPS) (Cucarella et al., 2004).

Furthermore, lectin-binding proteins are involved in *Pseudomonas aeruginosa* biofilms (Tielker et al., 2005) and play an important role in coaggregation between early and late colonizers of dental plaque biofilms mediated by *Fusobacterium nucleatum* (Kolenbrander et al., 2002). Amyloid-like proteins in *Bacillus subtilis* biofilms (TasA) are required to form biofilms despite the fact that the bacteria still produce EPS (Branda et al., 2006). It was found that TasA forms extracellular filaments (Romero et al., 2010). Such filaments as well as extracellular DNA found in many biofilms contribute to the final structure and architecture of biofilms (Lopez et al., 2010).

It is of value to point out that the change of the gene expression pattern is typical for the conversion from the suspended to the sessile form of bacteria. A well-known example is the change of the phenotype of *Ps. aeruginosa* from nonmucoid free-floating populations to mucoid bacteria populations within the biofilm in human lung epithelia, causing cystic fibrosis (Gill et al., 1987). It was also found that changes in lipopolysaccharide structure of *Azospirillum brasilense* correlate with the activation of biofilm formation (Sheludko et al., 2008). One of the most important processes in biofilm formation is the activation of signaling patterns coupled with changes in gene activities. The so-called quorum sensing is a density-dependent form of cell-to-cell communication by small-molecule signals (Decho et al., 2010). This chemical communication involves several types of molecules depending on the kind of interacting bacteria. One of the best-described systems is the LuxR/LuxI system of Gram-negative proteobacteria using bacterial acyl homoserine lactones, their interactions with the Lux-proteins, and the subsequent induction of transcription of several quorum sensing genes in the *up* operon resulting in a wide range of bacterial activities such as production of EPS, virulence induction, toxin production, motility, and plasmid transfer (Waters and Bassler, 2005; Hanzelka and Greenberg, 1995). Gram-positive bacteria produce oligopeptides as signal molecules (Miller and Bassler, 2001). Furthermore, autoinducers play an important role in intra- and interspecies cell-to-cell communication and initiation of biofilm growth processes (Costerton et al., 1999). Their concentration can be correlated with the population density (Lopez et al., 2010), implying an autocatalytic effect of biofilm formation. An overview about the bacterial interactions and the quorum sensing processes is given by Decho et al. (Decho, 2010). With this background, it is surprising that low-dose antibiotics can induce biofilm formation (Hoffman et al., 2005; Kaplan, 2011). The mechanisms are not fully understood yet, but the antibiotics produced within bacterial micropopulations can be not only weapons against competitors but can also contribute to the interbacterial communication and the triggering of changes in gene expression (Yim et al., 2007).

However, specific global patterns that are characteristic for biofilm formation could not be identified. Obviously, the high diversity of biofilms is coupled with a high diversity of underlying intrabacterial processes. This situation is similar to the high diversity of microenvironments in different biofilms. A characteristic feature of all biofilms is the extracellular matrix containing EPS. Key components of the EPS matrix are polysaccharides, proteins, DNA, enzymes, lectines, inorganic elements, divalent cations, and water. The composition depends on the biofilm communities, the age of biofilms, the environment and influences, and the properties of the mature biofilms. The EPS is crucial for the formation of biofilm, imposition of stability, protection against xenobiotics, and serving as a nutritional reservoir (Flemming and Wingender, 2010). From the point of view of metabolic pathways, EPS represents secondary metabolites (Lopez et al., 2010). Their production is controlled at the genetic level. The involved expression patterns are complex and specifically for biofilm colonizers. The EPS production by biofilm colonizers can be considered a structural tool to adapt to the natural site conditions and to guarantee a functional microhabitat in a steady state, including as well mutualistic physiological interactions as antagonism in close proximity. It is not surprising that bacterial populations organized within an EPS biofilm community are protected against disinfectants or the host immunological defense 500–1,000 fold more effective than their planctonic counterparts due to the slow growth within biofilms and the associated less sensitivity to growth-dependent killing and drug-inactivating enzymes (Hojo et al., 2009).

It is interesting that there are differences between natural and infectious biofilms in terms of kind and composition of bacteria. Natural or commensal biofilms, e.g., in water ecosystems, human intestine, and oral cavity or industrial systems, normally are characterized by multispecies displaying an adapted survival strategy and a pronounced mutualism. In contrast, infectious biofilms often include only one or a few bacterial strains due to changes in the selection pressure at the infection place (Burmolle et al., 2010). Furthermore, changing environmental conditions can trigger the switch from commensal to infectious biofilms. One of the well-described examples is the dental plaque. Marsh and colleagues (Marsh, 1994) have introduced the ecological plaque hypothesis. The balance between natural mouth microorganisms on teeth and gingival tissues can shift to a prevalence of as well acidogenic and acidotolerant microorganisms as anaerobic Gram-negative organisms, resulting in dental caries and periodontal diseases. The shift to the infectious dental plaque is linked with the formation of anaerobic microenvironments within EPS-covered dental biofilms, changes of the bacterial composition, release of endotoxins followed by tissue and periodontal damages, and metalloprotein-triggered binding of metal ions contributing to an increased corrosion rate of metallic dental biomaterials (Neu and Lawrence, 2009).

In principle, the structure, organization, and interactions within biofilms are comparable basically to the structural organization and the economical interactions of a human mega city covering many orders of magnitude from the macro down to the micro and the nano range.

5.4 Antifouling Strategies

In general, medical-device-associated infections caused by biofilm formation represent one of the most important problems in medicine (Donlan, 2002). Especially fatal is the fact that most of the coagulase bacteria are resistant to antibiotics and therefore represent a hazardous germ reservoir (Bridier et al., 2011). Early biofilms are defined as matrix-enclosed bacterial population adherent to each other and/or to surfaces or interfaces (Costerton et al., 1995). The biofilm formation is a complex, heterogeneous process, which will be affected by the organisms, the surfaces, the liquid media as well as the temperature and hydrodynamic conditions (Donlan, 2002). Protein fouling on medical implants reduces their efficacy and may result in harmful effects such as thrombosis (Werner et al., 2007). Accordingly to the kinetic of an initial bioadhesion process and the different growth phases of biofilm formation, key strategies for establishing antifouling surfaces should be based on the molecular mechanisms and the time sequence of these processes (Banerjee et al., 2011). Consequently, antifouling concepts or contamination-preventing strategies can be subdivided according to the following classification:

- **Passive Concepts**: Development of antiadhesive surfaces by means of modification strategies based on physicochemical and topographic surface parameters to control the free energy of interaction at the interface between substrate and microorganism (e.g., PEG coatings/hydrogels). Corresponding surfaces inhibit the adherence of microorganisms without interfering with the proliferation or the metabolism of the microorganisms.
- **Active Concepts**: Development of antimicrobial surfaces by means of the direct inactivation of adherent organisms and biofilms via leaching systems that contain toxic substances (e.g., antibiotics) or superficial integration of specific molecules that could prevent signal exchange, influence gene expression, or effect membrane integrity (e.g., antimicrobial peptides). Corresponding surfaces interfere with the proliferation process or the microbial metabolism.

A combination of several strategies to suppress initial adhesion and to increase antimicrobial activity probably represents the most promising antifouling concept from today's point of view, in particular if based on a biomimetic surface (Banerjee et al., 2011; Frant, 2008). Numerous processes to control and prevent biofilms at surfaces have been patented, and they provide a basis for future applications. Interested readers are referred to the excellent review of de Carvalho (de Carvalho, 2007) who concluded that a mixture of biocidal agents and disinfectants seems to be the most efficient way to destroy biofilms.

5.5 Passive Concepts That Do Not Interfere with the Adhering Microorganisms

Surface characteristics such as topography and roughness, chemistry, surface energy, and surface charge play a key role in initial bioadhesion processes and the subsequent cell response triggered hereby (Zhao et al., 2009). Development of multiple scales in topography in response to variation of shape and size of fouling organisms (proteins: few nm;

bacteria: 1 μm; diatoms and spores: 3–15 μm) results in biomimetic microtextured surfaces (Marechal and Hellio, 2009). The chemical modification of medical-grade titanium represents another approach to establish nonfouling surfaces. Using the photocatalytic activity of anatase surfaces, ultraviolet light irradiation leads to a significant increase in wettability on titanium dioxide (Gallardo-Moreno et al., 2009). In other words, changing the crystalline structure of the surface oxide layer can also reduce bacterial adhesion due to the photocatalytic effect (Gopal et al., 2004). More then 30 years ago, the first antifouling concepts were published with the aim to reduce the attractive forces between bacteria and biomaterial surfaces by optimizing physicochemical surface properties. Meanwhile, there have been discussions about the relevance of the different nonspecific interaction forces. Theories assume that generally ideal colloidal particles with homogeneous surface properties and consequently any such approaches are limited when applied to living systems. Nonetheless, these models provide a useful conceptual framework to understand bioadhesion, detachment, and biofilm formation (Dickinson et al., 2000; Busscher et al., 1992; Abu-Lail and Camesano, 2006). One of the first correlation studies between surface hydrophilicity and bacterial adhesion was published by Glantz (Glantz, 1971). About 23 years later, Quirynen and Bollen came again to the statement that high-energy hydrophilic surfaces collect plaque, improve customer retention, and favor specific bacteria (Quirenen and Bollen, 1995). Steinberg et al. found with increasing hydrophilicity a decrease in the adsorption of proteins (Steinberg et al., 1995). Ferreiros et al. summarized the microbial adhesion of 29 *Staphylococcus epidermidis* strains on polymers with different hydrophilicity and showed an optimum adhesion in the range where the hydrophilic properties of the bacterium and of the material were comparable (Ferreiros et al., 1989). In contrast to this, some results described an increased biofilm formation on the more hydrophobic polymer surface (Pedri, 2004). Chaudhury et al. showed the effect of a gradient of hydrophobicity to an increasingly denser hydrophobic algae adhesion (Chaudhury et al., 2006). Contact angle hysteresis as an additional parameter of the hydrophilicity was used by Schmidt et al. to demonstrate an improved antifouling with modified copolymers showing a small hysteresis (Schmidt et al., 2004). However, it can be stated that numerous model studies covering surface wettability and attachment/detachment of bacteria led obviously to different and partly inconsistent relations (Vogler, 1999). Further, the explicit reference to energetic surface parameters such as surface tension and polarity is part of numerous studies of initial bioadhesion. In 1993 and 2004, interesting results were published by Boulange-Petermann et al. focusing on biofouling of stainless steel surfaces. The authors found a direct correlation between the polarity of the steel surface and bacterial adhesion (Boulange-Petermann et al., 1993, 2004). Furthermore, Allion et al. described an increase in dead microorganisms on metallic surfaces of higher polarity (Allion et al., 2006). Polar components of surface tension comprise essentially acid–base interactions of the Lewis type. In aqueous media, interfacial Lewis acid–base interactions comprise mainly the interplay between hydrogen-donor entities and hydrogen-acceptor entities or more generally between electron-acceptor and electron-donor entities.

In addition to apolar interaction forces of the Lifshitz van der Waals type and polar interaction forces of the Lewis acid-base type, electrostatic or Coulomb interaction forces are discussed for decades as a third type of noncovalent interaction forces. Taking into consideration the laws of physical chemistry, it seems to be clear that a microbial adhesion process leads to an overlap of the electrical double layer and following that to an electrostatic interaction. As a pioneer in this field, Mozes et al. published already in 1987 a study on the interplay of electrostatic and nonelectrostatic interactions (Mozes et al., 1987). From that time, the key role of electrostatic interactions on protein adsorption controlled by the surface potential of material surfaces, the isoelectric point (IEP) of the protein, and the ionic strength of aqueous media is considered accepted. Brandes et al. confirmed this correlation by the analysis of ubiquitous proteins such as albumin. They presented a maximum of protein adsorption, exactly when the medium assumes a pH value, which corresponds to the IEP of the protein (Brandes et al., 2004). Gross et al. specified the role of charged cell wall polymers (teichoic acid) of bacteria and showed that, in particular, the initial bioadhesion is controlled electrostatically (Gross et al., 2001). A similar hypothesis regarding the initial bacterial adhesion was presented by Gottenbos et al. and van Merode et al. (Gottenbos et al., 2003; van Merode et al., 2006).

As can be seen from the above-cited literature, the published results concerning the correlation between different physicochemical surface parameters and bacterial adhesion and/or biofilm formation are often inconsistent and questionable. One reason for this situation is based on misleading assumptions with regard to the basic role of structured water at biointerfaces and the herewith related reactivity between water and the biological environment. A direct consequence is the application of the well-known DLVO approach even though non-DLVO interaction forces are acting. Keeping in mind that wetting behavior becomes sensitive to induce bioactivity as described above, it can be concluded that the extended DLVO theory (Ista et al., 2010; Xu and Siedlecki, 2007; Yang et al., 2010; Boulange-Petermann et al., 1993, 2004; Allion et al., 2006; Mozes et al., 1987) possesses the potential to quantify interfacial forces and energies in an aqueous environment adequately.

Another problem usually consists in the derivation of a myriad of variables and parameters to describe the wetting behavior of biomaterial surfaces. Most of these parameters are not directly measurable or disregard the interaction of the surface with liquid phases containing proteins. From that point of view, it is quite understandable that such surface energy parameters cannot be correlated with the biological response to a biomaterial surface. Furthermore, we have to accept that interfacial tensions cannot be measured using contact angle or tensiometric methods.

Nonetheless, a lot of biomaterial practitioners started to develop polymer-based hydrophilic coatings due to their capacity to act as protein-resistant coatings. Often these approaches were found by way of trial and error and not as a logical consequence of the self-association properties of vicinal water.

Without the pretense to follow a predictive theoretical framework, biomimetic approaches were introduced to mimic the antiadhesive properties of the hydrated physiological environment. Basically, a biomimetic design process is defined as the study of structure and function of biological systems and processes as inspiration for engineering of materials and machines (Salta et al., 2010). One of the most commonly used approaches to provide protein resistance based on immobilized PEG (Wagner et al., 2004; Tziampazis et al., 2000; Emoto et al., 2000; Mehne et al.,2008; Halperin et al., 2007; Tosatti et al., 2003) was employed to establish a hydration-controlled antifouling. Similar strategies were used to introduce anti-infective coatings (Wang et al., 2011; Saldarriaga-Fernandez et al.,2007;

Roosjen et al., 2006; Park et al., 1998) and antiadhesive surfaces (Lee et al., 2000; Sharma et al., 2004; Ostuni et al., 2001). If we recognize the fundamental role of water self-association and the related electron-donor–electron-acceptor or Lewis acid-base interactions, it can be concluded that the ability to form stable hydrogen bonds with water and the extraordinary conformational flexibility belong to the most important properties of PEG in the light of antifouling. In this context, Ksrko and Libera have described a specific coupling strategy of PEG to achieve antiadhesive properties at biomaterial surfaces. The efficiency of this approach was discussed with respect to several theoretical ideas: (i) increase in volume by swelling, (ii) repulsive osmotic pressure, (iii) high molecular mobility, and (iv) availability of only a few binding sites (Krsko and Libera, 2005). Nearly all attempts to explain these properties in relation to different structural parameters of the PEG molecule (chain length, linkage density, type of coupling) are discussed controversially as commented by J. Israelachvili (Israelachvili, 1997). Klee et al. reported dependence between the bioadhesion on the one hand and the chain length of PEG on the other hand. PEG molecules with chain length of 5,000 led to a reduction in protein adsorption and bacterial adhesion, while PEG 30,000 led obviously to the opposite result (Klee et al., 2003). Roosjen et al. confirmed this classification using an antiadhesive PEG 9,600 in comparison to a more or less ineffective PEG with a chain length of 526 (Roosjen et al., 2006). In an actual study published by Wang et al., the role of hydrophilic chain length in perfluoropolyether/PEG networks was investigated. In contrast to shorter PEG macromonomers, an enhanced antifouling performance could be determined by means of PEG 1,100 (Wang et al., 2011). Feng et al. analyzed PEG coupling densities between 0.06 and 0.39 molecules/nm^2 in relation to the adsorption of fibrinogen. As a result, a more pronounced effect was obtained by a density variation of the polymer in comparison to a variation of the chain length (Feng et al., 2006). Vacheethasanee et al. (Vacheethasanee and Marchant, 2000) and Tiller et al. (Tiller et al., 2001) coupled PEG 2,000 and PEG 5,000 on surfaces using different concentrations. According to the authors, the variation of the PEG concentration led to a reinforcement of steric repulsion of bacteria, while the cells were only slightly affected. Mehne et al. published various arrangements of different immobilized PEG chains. The short PEG chains (2,000/3,000) form a uniform polymer brush, whereas the longer chains (6,000) tend to entangle or collapse on the surface. For the mixed polymers, a more three-dimensional surface morphology was expected. The results showed that the medium-sized PEG offers the best properties (Mehne et al., 2008).

Based on the hydration approach of PEG, alternative biomimetic molecules and membrane-analogous concepts were reported that reduce bacterial adhesion. Zwitterionic surfaces based on phosphorylcholine have also been prominent to form a hydration layer that inhibits protein adsorption and cell adhesion effectively (Chen et al., 2005; Rose et al., 2004; Lewis et al., 2003). Recently it was reported that polyoxazolines (POX) possess a certain potential to show antifouling properties due to their extreme high water affinity. Polyoxazolines are amphiphilic and nontoxic, and they show a high self-assembling capacity (Adams and Schubert, 2007). Due to the possibility to create dense packed superficial water films via brush-like grafted polymers or dendritic structures, a good protein resistance and an effective antifouling were reached (Giardi et al., 2009; Pidhatika et al., 2008). Waschinski et al. optimized the antibacterial efficacy by the terminal coupling of positively charged functional groups on POX (Waschinski et al., 2005).

Natural models were taken as a basis for the design of biomimetic antifouling surfaces. In this context, covalently fixed biomimetic structures could be developed by a combination of hydrophilic dextran oligosaccharides with hexanol groups (Ruegsegger et al., 2001). The glycocalyx-like layers show a significantly reduced protein adsorption (Holland et al., 1998) and platelet adhesion (Gupta et al., 2006) as well as a reduced adhesion of *S. epidermidis* (Vacheethasanee and Marchant, 2000). The antifouling effect is probably based on the formation of hydrated brush-like structures in connection with a specific contact activation process, which allows a targeted antibacterial effect. Moreover, the antibacterial effectiveness of chitosan is commonly accepted, but the basic principle of the underlying effect and the in vivo performance are not yet well known as published recently (Zhao et al., 2009; Martinez et al., 2010). Yang et al. immobilized (hydroxyethyl)methacrylate (HEMA) brushes on stainless steel. The hydroxyl groups of HEMA were converted to carboxyl groups for coupling of chitosan. As a consequence, a reduced albumin adsorption and bacterial adhesion could be demonstrated (Yang et al., 2011).

5.6 Active Concepts That Interfere with the Adhering Microorganisms

The integration of toxic agents in the surface near layers with defined release kinetics is a widely accepted antifouling concept that has been used for several years (Vasilev et al., 2009). The essential advantage of leaching systems is the controlled release of antibacterial agents triggered by various polymer modifications, which lead to specific adapted designs. As a rule, a local delivery in high doses without exceeding a toxic level is possible. A disadvantage may be the exhaustion of antimicrobial substances after a short time. Consequently, long-term effective antifouling concepts are more desirable. An essential requirement for coatings loaded with antimicrobial agents is that these substances should not affect the desired reactions of eukaryotic cells, e.g. tissue integration and cell adhesion (Zhao et al., 2009). Biofilm deterrence by leaching biocidal agents is often patented, e.g., by the use of peroxides, halogens, quaternary ammonium compounds (QACs), phenols, and terpenes (de Carvalho, 2007). Using the example of medical titanium, antibacterial coatings were divided into (i) antibiotics, (ii) nonantibiotic organic agents, and (iii) inorganic agents. The former group includes especially vancomycin and gentamicin incorporated in calcium phosphate coatings or polyelectrolyte films (Zhao et al., 2009; Jang et al., 2010; Neut et al., 2003). Chlorhexidine and poly(hexamethylenebiguanide) are representative as nonantibiotic organic agents (Mohammadi and Abbott, 2009; Jeon et al., 2011). Silver appears to be the broadest spectrum antibiotic available and does not appear to induce resistance (Zhao et al., 2009: Vasilev et al., 2009). Silver ions are effective against various bacteria in vitro. They bind strongly to the electron-donor groups present in biological molecules containing sulfur, oxygen, or nitrogen. The level of clinical effectiveness is discussed controversial. The best approaches are reported by silver impregnation in degradable polymer coatings because directly coated silver components can be inactivated by physiological media. Stobie et al. presented the reduction of initial bioadhesion of four infective strains and a biofilm inhibition of *S. epidermidis* by silver-doped perfluoropolyether-urethane coatings (Stobie et al., 2009). Besides silver impregnated in hydroxyapatite films or coupled in silver zeolite complexes, recent studies show the efficient antimicrobial property of silver nanoparticle due to their large surface area and their strong binding to electron-donor groups present in biological molecules containing sulfur, oxygen, or nitrogen (Juan et al., 2010). In addition to silver and silver-containing compounds are numerous other toxins in antifouling applications. For example, Domenico et al. discussed the activity of bismuth thiols, which had been shown to have a 1,000 times stronger antibacterial effect compared with currently used bismuth salts (Domenico et al., 2001). Various antibiotics have been loaded into polymers for biomedical applications. Kohnen et al. present catheter surfaces (silicone) impregnated with a combination of rifampin and sparfloxacin (Kohnen et al., 2003). Especially for use in urethral catheters, Park et al. and Hubner et al. developed antibiotic-loaded polymers; used antibiotics are norfloxacin, chlorhexidine, and polyhexanide (Park et al., 2003; Hubner et al., 2010).

One of the recent problems of antibiotic leaching systems concerns the necessary selection of new antibiotics due to the enhanced antimicrobial resistance and high dose of antibiotics. Bacteria protected in biofilms can require 1,000-times the dose necessary to bacteria in suspension (Vasilev et al., 2009). Bridier et al. reviewed the resistance of biofilms against antibiotics and disinfectants and related it to the three-dimensional structure of biofilms, the heterogeneity, and the multifactorial accumulation (Bridier et al., 2011).

Besides slow-releasing systems and release-on-command systems, nonleaching systems have also been developed based on the covalent immobilization of antibacterial molecules. The basic principle can be subdivided into two phases: first, there are interactions between the covalently bonded molecule and the surface of microorganisms; subsequently, channels are formed in biological membranes, thus destroying the microorganism. The advantage—the suppression of the release of excess toxic substances and the high chemical and physical resistance to environmental conditions—is contrary to the factor that the contact-coupled effect requires the adhesion of bacteria, and thus dead organisms must be removed, which may be the basis for a renewed biofilm formation. The application of furanones (bromine compound) as a toxic substance is the subject of other studies (Baveja et al., 2004; Hume et al., 2004). As a result, a reduction in bacterial adhesion, which was correlated with the reduced formation of slime, could be observed. However, a cytotoxic effect was reported. Taylor et al.

(Taylor et al., 2004) describe a mechanism of furanones to affect quorum sensing and so disrupting the cell–cell communication within a biofilm. Further, antimicrobial surfaces were developed by the addition of enzymes to surfaces. Bacterial protection can be the result of production of inhibitors, reduction of oxygen, secretion of antimicrobial proteins, or degradation of biofilm matrix (de Carvalo, 2007). Lactones are also known to influence quorum sensing. Tiller et al. provide the basis for antifouling surfaces modified with QACs (Tiller et al., 2001). Until today, it could be shown that QACs act against all bacteria (Gram-positive and Gram-negative). However, to understand the antibacterial mechanism, two approaches do exist: (i) cell membrane penetration due to cationic polymer chains of molecules and (ii) ion exchange caused by highly charging (Murata et al., 2007). Generally, surfaces functionalized with antimicrobial peptides (AMPs) represent new strategy to develop biocidal materials because AMPs have been shown a broad antimicrobial activity at low concentrations (Banerjee et al., 2011; Som et al., 2008; Zasloff, 2002; Zhang et al.,2001; Friedrich et al., 2001).

Friedrich et al. compared several AMPs of different amino acid sequences and chain lengths in terms of their impact on clinical isolates and infectious germs. The authors pointed to the cytocidal effect due to the depolarization of the membrane (Friedrich et al., 2001). The peptides substitute divalent cations, which are important for the outer membrane integrity, and lead to permeabilization. Besides the use of natural peptides, first synthesis of antimicrobial active peptides succeeded (Som et al., 2008).

Another important class of protein-resistant surfaces is based on kosmotropicity, which means the ability of molecules to function as osmolytes (Banerjee et al., 2011). Kosmotropes such as taurin, betain, or Trimethylamine N-oxide are preferentially excluded from the protein surfaces in water (Kane, 2003). Coupled on implant surface, they offer the possibility to establish new anti-infective surfaces.

Recently published approaches present a certain potential to benefit from the excellent properties of carbon nanotubes and nanocomposites in preventing biofouling, as discussed by Upadhyayula et al. (Upadhyayula and Gadhamshetty, 2010). This new class of surface modification leads to promising biocidal and protein-resistant properties, but unfortunately they are often associated with human health risk caused by manufacturing processes.

5.7 Conclusion and Future Prospects

Microbial colonization of a biomaterial surface proceeds in different stages. It is necessary to understand how a biofilm is formed and which mechanisms are involved in adhesion and colonization (Marechal and Hellio, 2009).

Vasilev et al. reviewed a number of antifouling strategies and published some general key issues for the design of a future anti-infective biomaterial (Vasilev et al., 2009):

- cytotoxicity of antibacterial coatings
- duration over which antibiotic release is needed
- close collaboration between clinicians and material scientists
- design of smart coatings
- antimicrobial resistance against pathogens

In the previous section, numerous antifouling concepts were presented and described with respect to their antiadhesive and antimicrobial effect commonly known as passive and active strategies to reduce bacterial adhesion and biofilm formation (Fig. 5.3).

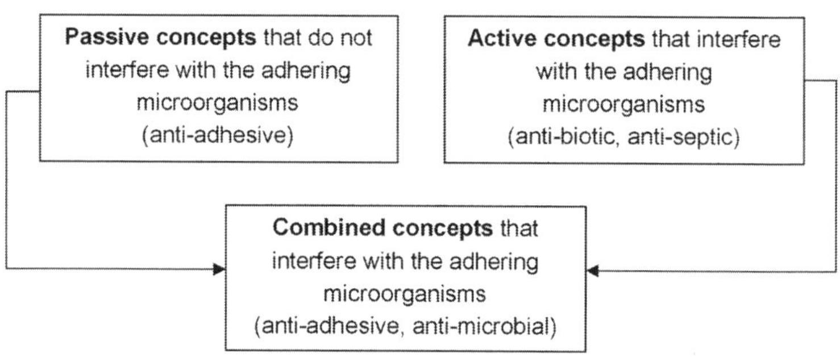

Figure 5.3 Classification of antifouling concepts.

The perfect antifouling concept has not been found, but the best solution would certainly be a combination of different technologies. In this way, Haamann et al. presented an antibacterial coating by the incorporation of silver nanoparticles and peptides in a hydrogel layer based on PEG (Haamann et al., 2010). Salta et al. published a further excellent review about designing biomimetic antifouling surfaces, which include a bioinspired coating derived from natural membranes, a tailor-made surface to achieve superhydrophobic properties ("lotus leaf effect") or alternatively hydrophilic properties produced by grafted polymers such as PEG (Salta et al., 2010). Additional natural antimicrobial agents such as zosteric acid were included. Another example describes Subramanyan et al. as a combination of the antimicrobial activity of silver halogens and the membrane-dissolving action of polyhexamethylbiguanid (Subramanyan et al., 2000). Dalsin et al. have shown the protective effect of PEG-bound water combined with the effect of bactericide shellfish proteins (Dalsin et al., 2003).

Based on the statement that the development of antifouling strategies for biomaterial surfaces seems to be something like a "never-ending story", Morra (Morra, 2000) formulated a very pragmatic approach, which enables an elegant correlation between material surface chemistry, interfacial properties, and biological response. Taking into consideration the above-mentioned effects related to hydrogen bonding and self-association of vicinal water, Morra suggests a new approach in contrast to the previous view of existing ideas. Correspondingly, the molecular basis of antifouling can be explained by interfacial interactions between surfaces or suspended phases and water. With regard to the electron-donor (oxygen) and the electron-acceptor (hydrogen) sites of water molecules, this interfacial interaction is controlled by Lewis acid–base interaction forces. By means of this conception, it is easy to explain the well-known effect of PEG by a synergistic effect of the molecular structure of the polymer chain and the polar structure of water molecules.

From the authors' point of view, this concept has the potential to be a quantum jump forward if realized chemically by means of an adapted polymer structure with a specific number and a spatial arrangement of electron-donor and electron-acceptor sites.

5.8 Biofilm Testing

Most frequently used systems for in vitro biofilm testing represent microtiter plate-based systems in various designs. These approaches are often applied for screening the purposes of effects on biofilm formation. However, the design as static system without shear stress and the batch cultivation of bacterial cultures characterized by changing the culture conditions without regulation limit the microtiter plate-based approaches (Busscher and van der Mei, 2006).

In consideration of the complex interactions under natural conditions, flow systems provide a much better approach for testing biofilm formation (Andersen and Rasmussen, 2009). Although the design of individual flow systems is very versatile, the flow-chamber-based principle of the Modified Robbins Device (MRD) became one of the most applied biofilm test setups. The principle of an MRD is a linear array of samples along a channel of rectangular cross section in a flow chamber. Jim Robbins developed the device at the beginning of the 1980s at the University of Calgary (McCoy et al., 1981), and many research groups now apply the MRD or the homemade variations of the MRD principle. The flexibility of the MRD principle, for instance, coupling with a bioreactor (chemostat), the self-contained design, and the application of different bacterial models from single-strain cultures to more complex mixed cultures made this principle a standard tool for the dynamic investigation of biofilm formation and the testing of antibiotic substances or surface effects of (bio)materials. The authors have developed a series of variations of water-bath-heated flow chambers in terms of the number, shape, and size of samples, the design of the cross-flow section, the possible addition of in situ measurement devices such as optical windows for microscopic investigations on transparent and opaque biomaterials, fluorescence-based probes, and corrosion probes to enable the investigation of biofilm accumulation under the influence of metallic corrosion. The principle of a possible setup is given in Fig. 5.4. Lately, modifications of flow chamber systems as microfluidic devices are used to improve single-cell detection and to allow high-throughput screening (Benoit et al., 2010).

Other dynamic systems represent chemostat-based designs with sample holders directly placed in the reactor vessel. Here the constraints in respect of flow rates within flow-chamber-based setups can be overcome (Teodioso et al., 2011) by applying flow rates for in vitro simulation of biofilm processes in ecosystems with extremely high flow rates (such as water management and industrial systems) compared to common biomedical implantation sites, e.g., in the oral cavity, the blood circulation system where catheters are applied, or around implants where biomaterial-associated infections can occur. Examples of such setups are the CDC-biofilm reactor (Donlan, 2004), the rotating disc reactor (Buckingham-Meyer et al.,

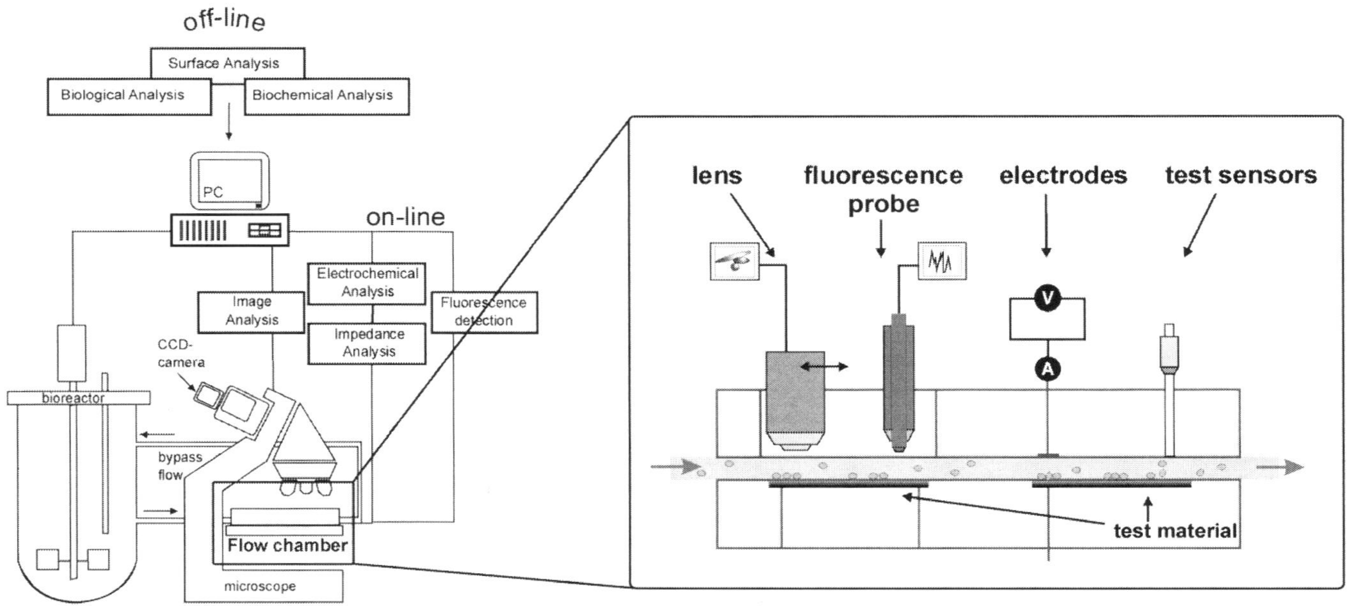

Figure 5.4 Flow-through chamber-based in vitro biofilm simulation with integrated online analysis.

2003; Lawrence et al., 2000), and the constant depth film fermenter (Peters and Wimpenny, 1988).

It is of importance to note that the so-called artificial mouth is specifically focused on the complex situation in plaque biofilms. Based on the aim of this approach, the substrate materials, as well the bacterial flora, are designed to reflect the natural conditions of plaque formation in the oral cavity and to simulate multi-laque conditions (microcosm). The system allows the long-term investigation of the biodiversity and functional interactions in mature plaque layers. Further, biofilm-testing models include eukaryotic cell models in combination with bacterial biofilms and in vivo approaches to study the interactions of biofilms with tissues in different body tracts. Surveys of the different techniques for biofilm simulation and testing are published by Coenye (Coenye and Nelis, 2010) and Sissons (Sissons, 1997).

Obviously, each of the biofilm models possesses advantages and disadvantages, and the selection of a suitable model should be made on the basis of the respective biofilm problem and the questions being addressed, especially during the development and testing of new biomaterials or medical products. The conceptual design of biofilm investigations must involve all essential parameters, which are of crucial importance for the initial adhesion of microorganisms and biofilm formation on biomaterial surfaces under natural conditions, e.g., at the infection site. This includes not only controlled growth conditions, incubation times, and shear forces, but also adequate bacterial culture models in terms of the type and the number of strains, their importance in sequential biofilm formation phases, and their physiological interactions with the host organism. Clearly, the conceptual design of any such experiments includes also the establishment of continuous and reproducible biofilm monitoring. There is no doubt that offline measurements performed after the removal of attached microorganisms, such as the determination of the cell number by counting, FISH-based fluorescence techniques, and the analysis of EPS components (staining, chemical proofs), possess a tremendous potential to provide additional important data for the validation of biomaterials in general or possible antimicrobial effects associated with biomaterials or drug-release systems. Consequently, such investigations will not lose their importance for the evaluation of the initial adhesion of bacteria and the biofilm propagation. Suitable techniques include the confocal laser scanning microscopy

(CLSM), bioluminescence measurements, Raman and Fourier transform infrared spectroscopy/microscopy in combination with the evaluation of biofilm data with material surface parameters such as topography, free surface energy, surface charge, and the role of surface-active groups.

It must be stressed that the evaluation of the complex biofilm-formation process implies in many cases that the different phases of biofilm formation, like in the initial phase of adhesion and the phase of biofilm propagation, must be isolated from each other. This is not surprising because the affecting parameters are quite different. It is widely accepted that the phase of initial adhesion as starting point for biofilm growth on biomaterials is influenced by physicochemical interactions between microorganisms and the substrate surface. As already mentioned, the free surface energy, surface charges, and surface topography are of supreme importance influenced by the nature of the culture medium. The later phases of biofilm growth become more and more independent of the nature of the material surface and will be affected by intensifying bacterial interactions such as signaling, gene transfer, surface–surface contacts, and physiological relations. These interactions can be characterized as mutualistic as well as antagonistic. So it can be concluded that a comprehensive investigation of biofilms has to include three main aspects (Karunakaran et al., 2011):

- The characterization of surface properties of both the material and the microbial surface, including the noncovalent interaction forces and energies typical for an aqueous environment.
- The characterization of the external environment (extracellular matrix) and possible changes during biofilm maturation and propagation.
- The characterization of intracellular processes such as gene expression, signaling (quorum sensing), protein content, and phenotype changes.

However, common approaches for biofilm testing focus often on the detection and analysis of the partial aspects of the complex interactions in biofilm formation and maturation. Considering especially the point of data interpretation, experimental requirements, and laboratory resources, these experimental setups are very effective and scientifically accepted due to their practical relevance and their potential to solve specific problems. As a result, the key question in biofilm testing is basically to decide which biofilm model is needed for solving the actual biofilm problem. Commonly, the following aspects must be taken into consideration to select a proper biofilm model:

- simple cultures (monocultures) versus complex cultures (mixed bacterial strains)
- short-term tests versus long-term tests
- focus on microorganisms versus focus on EPS components
- adhesion and biofilm formation versus detachment of the biofilm components
- experimental studies versus theoretical modeling, simulation

Donlan et al. summarized more than 20 methods for biofilm testing in static and dynamic mode and on that basis a comparison of various methods for the quantification of biofilm properties was performed. Although they favored particular test designs for specific biofilm investigations, a reasonable combination of monitoring techniques in dependence of the questions being addressed seems to be the best way to gain acceptable data (Donlan, 2001; Goeres et al., 2005). With regard to the complex situation within a matured biofilm matrix, the determined data show as a rule a more or less strong dependence from the applied biofilm model, the test conditions, and the established experimental approach. It is, therefore, common practice to evaluate this data in terms of three aspects:

1. Reproducibility of the data provided by single methods
2. Validation of new methods by established methods (standardization)
3. Complementarity of the data provided by several methods (correlation)

It is of value to point out that the majority of in vitro methods often does not accurately mimic the in situ or the in vivo situation. Often the absence of control strategies to acquire the experimental conditions leads to some difficulties to compare the observed results.

Therefore, it is no surprise that a discrepancy exists between biofilm-testing models using bacterial monocultures or mixed cultures even if the mixed culture consists of the same bacterial species than the bacterial monocultures. Own data of biofilm tests in the field of water management confirm these discrepancies. For this purpose, three model systems (mixed cultures) were established to represent the microbiological situation in drinking water, river water, and waste water. Each model system consists of five bacterial strains with a proven potential to form biofilms on solid substrates. Static biofilm tests on uncoated (hydrophilic) and lipid-coated (hydrophobic) glass discs in multi-titer plates were carried out with the aim to compare the biofilm accumulation capacity if the mixed culture was used or if the five monocultures were used successively. After an incubation phase of 24 h, the total number of adhered bacteria in single-culture experiments was significantly different from the total number of adhered bacteria in the related mixed-culture experiments (Fig. 5.5). Furthermore, the results for both test surfaces have shown that the ratio between the total numbers of adhered bacteria on hydrophilic and hydrophobic glass surfaces observed in mixed cultures did not always correlate with the corresponding results for single cultures (Fig. 5.5-arrows). This indicates clearly both bacteria-specific attachment processes and interbacterial factors of influence during the initial adhesion process and the biofilm formation. Rijnaarts et al. have shown data dealing with the adhesion properties of seven bacterial strains on glass and Teflon. Comparative studies using single strains have shown differences in adhesion, without clear correlations (Rijnaarts et al., 1999). Triandafillu et al. showed that the adhesion of 18 different strains of *P. aeruginosa* after 2 h of incubation differs significantly between the microorganisms (Triandafillu et al., 2003), indicating that each bacterial model has to be validated according to the biofilm problem. Consequently, it seems to be a reasonable strategy when the bacterial model systems can be chosen on the basis of the respective real-life situation being addressed (Goeres et al., 2005).

Nonetheless, if the evaluation of biomaterials with regard to their capacity to form superficial biofilms is addressed, the requirement to employ application-oriented, reproducible, and stable microbiological models arises. To increase the practical or clinical relevance of biofilm test procedures, the application of mixed cultures was proposed especially for extended periods of time. However, the practical application of bacterial mixed cultures requires well-controlled culture tools to ensure the parallel cultivation of up to five single bacterial strains and the resulting mixed culture. For this purpose, bioreactor systems were introduced to allow the control of one or more environmental or operating variables under sterile conditions. This includes, e.g., temperature, pH, nutrient composition, medium composition and flow rate, metabolic concentration, and oxygen–carbon dioxide concentration.

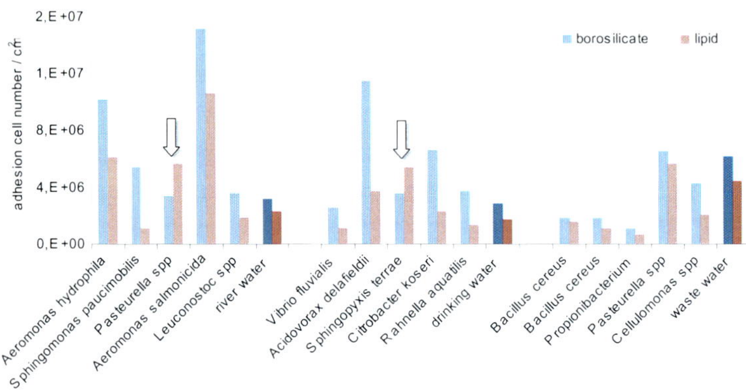

Figure 5.5 Results of bioadhesion analysis in monocultured and mixed-cultured biofilm models on hydrophilic uncoated (borosilicate glass) and lipid-coated (Tetraether lipid) surfaces.

The development of bioreactor technologies may be regarded as a breakthrough in the field of biofilm monitoring and testing. Two typical test scenarios based on bioreactor techniques are the establishment of a plaque model to simulate the microbial situation in the oral cavity and the establishment of an infection model to address the risk of implant-associated infections.

5.9 Examples for in vitro Biofilm Testing

5.9.1 Dental Plaque Formation

Dental plaque layers on teeth and dental biomaterials are one of the most important reasons for the degradation of tooth substance (caries, corrosion of dental biomaterials) and damages of the gingiva tissue (periodontitis, gingivitis). Therefore, the prevention of plaque formation represents an effective way to enhance the oral hygiene and to ensure the therapeutic effect of dental biomaterials. Regarding the materials applied in the mouth microenvironment, there are different strategies to enhance antimicrobial surface effects: selection of materials with surface-energetic parameters, which can inhibit or delay the initial adhesion of oral microorganisms; and minimization of surface roughness and antibacterial surface modifications by coupling antibacterial compounds such as defensins or enzymes. However, the fundamental prerequisite for the application of biomaterials and medical devices is their biocompatibility. According to the Medical Device Directive, the manufacturers have to guarantee that their products are not cytotoxic and compatible with the surrounded tissues. No severe disease should be caused by the material itself by possibly released degradation products. The required high quality standards are of special importance concerning new materials with antiplaque effects. The test methods recommended in international and national standards include, among others, different in vitro tests. However, in view of the current knowledge about biocompatibility testing, the presently employed in vitro tests recommended in the ISO standards can only insufficiently reflect the real interactions between biomaterial surfaces and the complex biological environment in the oral cavity. This is mainly due to a simplification of experimental designs recommended in standard regulations to ensure handling by a wide range of users and laboratories.

The authors have developed a flow-chamber-based in vitro plaque model for testing both initial bacteria adhesion on surfaces and long-term effects of material surfaces on the plaque accumulation and propagation. The system consists of a multivessel bioreactor for continuous cultivation of up to five bacterial single strains and an additional vessel for cultivation of mixed bacterial cultures. Temperature-controlled flow-through chambers with tailor-made geometry and size, sample arrays, and integrated measurement probes can be connected with the mixed bacterial culture and allow a continuous cross-flow under sterile and reproducible conditions over an arbitrary period of time. Especially for dental plaque simulations, the incubation period is restricted to 15 h. This is in good agreement with natural plaque formation processes observed in the oral cavity. The pH value (7.2), dissolved oxygen content (microaerophilic/anaerobic, aeration with 95% N_2, 5% CO_2), and temperature (37°C) can be adjusted automatically. For the simulation of natural dental plaque biofilm characteristics, the following bacterial strains are employed: *S. mutans*, *Streptococcus sanguinis*, *Actinomyces viscosus*, *Fusobacterium nucleatum*, and *Veillonella parvula* provided by commercial partners. All species will be cultivated separately as pure single cultures in species specific medium. Just before each adhesion test, a mixed bacterial suspension consisting of five dental bacteria will be prepared by mixing appropriate volume fractions of five suspended single cultures in a separate bioreactor vessel such that the total cell number is approximately 10^7 cells/ml. The mixed culture can be incubated continuously (D = 0.015 h^{-1},) in basal medium. Supplements such as albumin or sucrose to mimic natural saliva or diet cycles can be added on demand. The dental materials to be tested are fixed in the lower part of the flow chamber opposite to the window for optical observation integrated in the upper part. The bacterial suspension is pumped through the flow-through chamber, respectively, across the sample surface with low volume flow rates of about 0.3 ml/min. The calculated Reynolds number is significantly smaller by some orders of magnitude than the critical Reynolds number, which indicates a laminar flow within the flow chamber. Sterile sampling after incubation allows the analysis of the plaque formed on the top of the surfaces by suitable test methods. The samples are rinsed after incubation twice to remove nonadhered bacteria. The quantification of the adhered bacteria is achieved by counting after detachment by ultrasonic treatment, centrifugation, resuspension, and labeling by fluorescence probes (e.g., BacLight/Molecular Probes, consisting of Syto 9 for selective staining of living bacteria and propidium iodide for staining of dead bacteria). The total number of bacteria can be determined directly after labeling in a hemocytometer using a fluorescence microscope. Alternatively, the documentation of attached bacteria directly on the material surface is possible using CLSM or scanning electron microscopy (Fig. 5.6). It is needless to say that both techniques possess the capacity to provide data about the local biofilm thickness and the distribution of individual biofilm components on the surface. It is common practice to use specific measuring and rendering software tools to analyze the most important features of three-dimensional images taken from microscopic techniques and to validate surface effects on bacterial adhesion, bacterial activity, and biofilm formation.

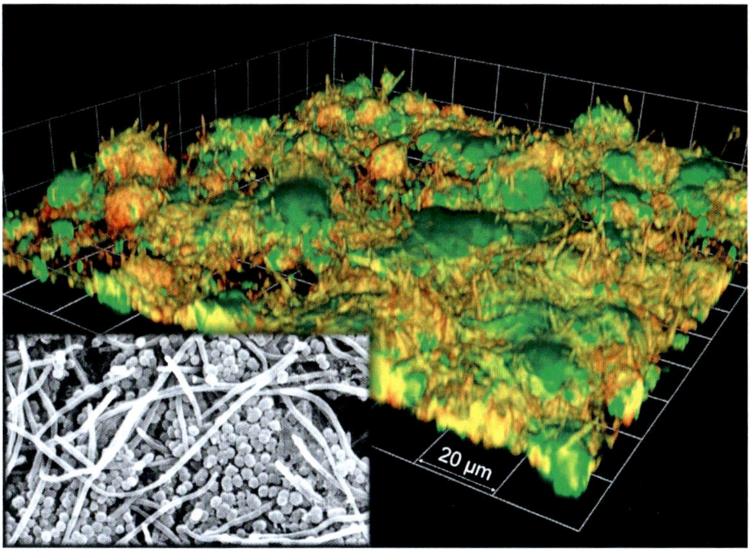

Figure 5.6 Dental plaque biofilm on biomaterial surface after 5 days of in vitro incubation under cross-flow conditions: confocal three-dimensional image after 5 days (green: living bacteria; red: dead bacteria) and SEM. The biofilm contains different bacteria (streptococci and fusobacteria), which are well organized in a typical early mushroom structure.

Due to its flexible design, this in vitro system was successfully applied for a couple of biofilm tests:

- Biomedical applications (plaque accumulation on dental biomaterials, biofilm formation on urinary catheters and cardiovascular stents, testing of antimicrobial agents such as photosensitizer and antiadhesive materials/surface modifications)
- Biotechnological applications (biofilm formation on bioreactor components, optical biosensors, and filtration materials)
- Water management (effect of surface modifications such as lipid coatings to increase the efficiency of filtration materials in bioremediation)

It can be concluded that the bioreactor-based flow chamber system represents an excellent experimental setup to evaluate dental materials referring to their potential of plaque accumulation in the frame of a preclinical test phase, without expensive and time-consuming clinical studies. Moreover, the established bioreactor system allows kinetic studies of the biofilm formation under reproducible conditions and optical in situ control. The in vitro system is clinically validated by means of comparative in vivo investigations of plaque accumulation on different materials used in dental practice (Schade, 2005; Wehle, 2004). In detail, the study was performed with dental alloys, ceramics, and various composites in the oral cavity of healthy human patients.

5.9.2 Biofilm-Related Infections

Biomaterial-associated infections represent an enormous potential health risk. Regardless of the medical device under consideration, it has been shown that the formation of a microbial biofilm and the presence of pathogenic bacteria are substantial prerequisites to cause severe complications. Biofilms in medical devices show characteristics distinctly different from biofilms in nature, such as a dense EPS matrix, tight association with a surface, altered growth rates, and a strongly decreased susceptibility to antimicrobial agents. In this process, the number of bacteria can fluctuate and often the concentration of surface-attached microorganisms may vastly exceed the number in the liquid phase. The exact mechanisms involved in implant-associated infections are still subject of intensive research.

Persistent infections caused by bacterial biofilm were reviewed by Costerton et al. (Costerton, 1999). It could be shown that biofilms develop preferentially on inert surfaces or on dead tissue surfaces, and occur commonly on medical devices and fragments of dead tissue. It can be estimated that 65% of hospital-acquired infections are related to surface-attached bacteria (Resch et al., 2005). An especially high infection potential is related to biofilms on specific devices: prosthetic heart valves, central venous catheters, urinary catheters, contact lenses, intrauterine devices, and dental implants (Donlan and Costerton, 2002). It is a fact that catheter-related infections show an extremely high risk compared with other nosocomial infections. Obviously, there is a direct correlation between the use of indwelling medical devices and the observed infection rate. About 35% of these patients die as a direct consequence of a nosocomial septicemia (Eggimann et al., 2004; Harbarth et al., 2003). Catheter-associated urinary tract infections (CAUTIs) are 80% of hospital-acquired urinary tract infection and contribute not only to increased morbidity and mortality but also to longer hospital stays and dramatically increased medical costs (Regev-Shoshani et al., 2010). To moderate the complexity of microbial infection analysis, research has to continue as a parts-based approach, which includes an intensive knowledge of various aspects of biofilm formation, such as the role of environmental conditions, the substrate characteristic, the influence on EPS formation or on intercellular communication (Karunakaran et al., 2011). With the aim to evaluate the infection potential of implant surfaces in close proximity to the clinical situation, a suitable technical platform is needed to perform the necessary biofilm experiments. With the same line of reasoning used already for the plaque experiments, bioreactor systems were introduced to allow the control of one or more environmental or operating variables under sterile conditions.

The basis for these dynamic investigations represents the simulation of natural test conditions by the application of a lab-scale bioreactor system coupled with flow-through chambers to allow for the online analysis of the microbial reactions directly on the material surface. Both the initial adhesion of selected pathogens and the subsequent biofilm formation in dependence of the incubation time and the test surface could be observed and evaluated by image-analysis and image-processing techniques. In the context of these investigations, suitable fermentation models (mixed cultures) have been established, which allow a clinically relevant simulation of the infective environment in the laboratory scale.

It is particularly notable that Peritonitis, an inflammation of the peritoneum, occurs often in connection with continuous ambulatory peritoneal dialysis. Therefore, Peritonitis represents a life-threatening infection associated with surfaces of indwelling medical devices, which might result in the loss of the catheter (Reimann et al., 2001; Yishak et al., 2001). In the hope of developing materials that are intrinsically colonization resistant, the original catheter surface (silicone) was coated by means of an ultrathin tetraether lipid coating to inhibit bacterial adhesion and biofilm formation. A mixed bacterial culture consisting of *S. aureus* (ATCC 12600, DSMZ, Germany) and *S. epidermidis* (PCM 2479, DSMZ, Germany) was applied in a simulated peritoneal dialysis medium (original dialysis medium, including nutrients, proteins, and supplements) and pumped through a specifically adapted flow-through chamber systems. A so-called "seed and feed" model for dynamic tests was established as follows: The experiment was subdivided into two phases—initial adhesion on surfaces during 2 h (seed phase) and monitoring of the subsequent biofilm growth during 18 h (feed phase), immediately after the seed phase. The study was performed by means of a special bioreactor system to guarantee a sterile test environment and a reproducible mode of operation. As a result, a significantly reduced bacterial adhesion for the lipid-coated silicone surfaces could be shown (Fig. 5.7). The results suggest that tetraether lipid coatings are effective in reducing initial bacterial adhesion on catheter surfaces for peritoneal dialysis (Frant et al., 2006).

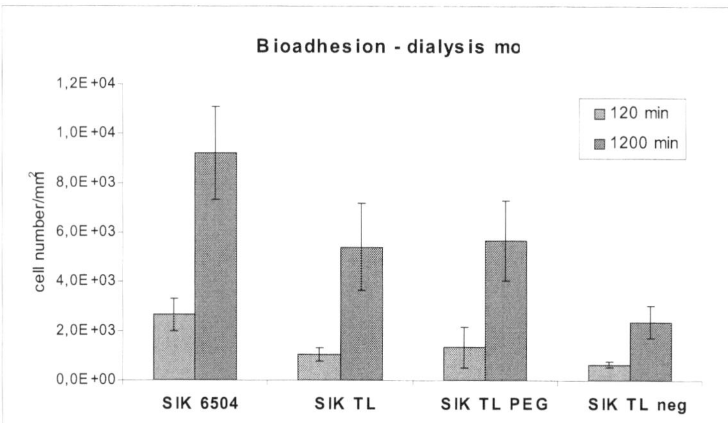

Figure 5.7 In vitro bioadhesion test in peritoneal dialysis model, flow chamber system on uncoated and lipid-coated silicone (Raumedic SIK 6504); TL: tetraether lipid; TL PEG: lipid modified with polyethylene glycol 3000; TL neg: lipid modified with taurine.

Staphylococcus species are often cited as usually infective microorganisms (Stobie et al., 2009). But not only Donlan et al. published a comprehensive list of different microorganisms commonly associated with biomaterials on medical devices (Donlan, 2001, 2002), more than 50 different organisms causing catheter-related infections were reported by Schünlin and Voss (Schünlin and Voss, 2005). While 80% of infections associated with short-term indwelling urinary catheters are caused by single organisms, infections in long-term catheters are predominantly polymicrobial.

It could be shown that 10% of these biofilms include more than five species, 77–95% are associated with two or more organisms (Warren, 2001). Stickler et al. confirmed the presence of mixed populations during urinary tract infections (UTIs). Several of these are capable of producing urease and lead to encrustation processes (Stickler, 2008).

It can be concluded that UTIs are one of the leading causes of nosocomial infections due to the fact that the causative microorganisms within indwelling catheters are effectively protected from the host defense and corresponding therapies. Medical devices such as catheters or ureteral stents are, therefore, particularly vulnerable to biofilm formation and encrustation. It is, therefore, a special challenge to develop a new catheter surface with anti-infective and antiencrustative properties and to establish a clinically relevant test environment that takes into account the real microbiological situation at site.

As part of a comprehensive study, a complex model was established and validated for UTI. This infection model comprised five bacterial strains: *S. aureus, S. epidermidis, E. coli, Enterococcus faecalis, and Ps. aeruginosa* cultivated in artificial urine based on a proposal by Griffith et al. (Griffith et al., 1976). To consider also the encrustation of urinary catheters, the laboratory model of urinary tract infection can be upgraded by encrustation components (Bithelis et al., 2004; Choong et al., 2001; Shaw et al., 2005). It is known that a urinary tract infection is induced above all by urease-producing bacteria. Among those bacteria related to UTI and encrustation, *Proteus mirabilis* plays obviously a dominant role in the encrustation process (Jones et al., 2007).

Consequently, the performance of the introduced in vitro model can be further improved if the pH value of the artificial urine can be triggered by the addition of urease. Following a test period of 14 days, the pH was enhanced in this way from 5.7 to 8.8, which allows the formation of crystalline deposits on the catheter surface (Fig. 5.8). It should be mentioned that the results of the in vitro experiments are comparable with the clinical findings gained during parallel in vivo experiments.

It is worth noting that any such investigations depend substantially on the availability of a bioreactor-based platform technology. With this in mind, many investigators started to design various configurations of bioreactor systems with different strategies to control the in vitro culture conditions. Two main conclusions can be drawn at this point:

1. Taking into consideration the whole process of biofilm formation from the initial bacterial adhesion up until later developmental stages, biofilms contain as a rule diverse microbial populations (multispecies biofilms). Consequently, the introduction of mixed bacterial cultures seems to be of higher clinical relevance than the application of monoculture biofilms. First in vitro models are available, but they are still in their infancy.
2. Complex biological test scenarios require an adequate technical setup to be able to establish clinically relevant in vitro models. Bioreactors represent a suitable and versatile platform technology to provide a closed culture environment and to implement all necessary control strategies to guarantee a reproducible operation during testing.

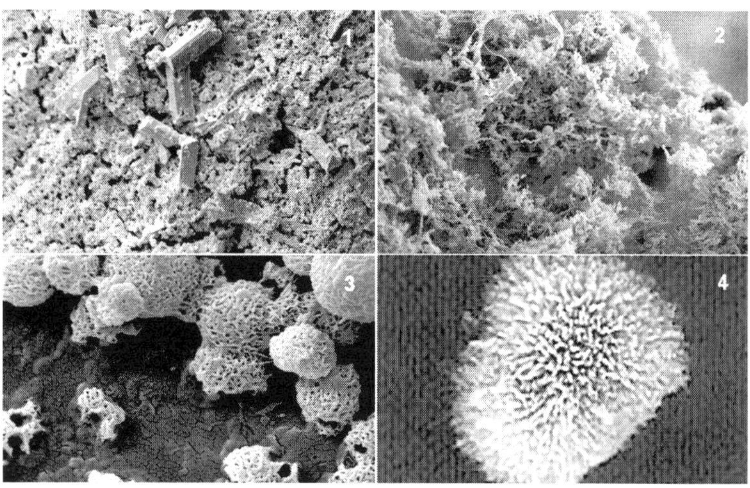

Figure 5.8 Urinary tract infection and encrustation model. SEM analysis: (1) encrustation after in vitro test on polyurethane (4 weeks); (2) encrustation after in vivo application on polyurethane (6 weeks); (3) ureate crystals after in vitro test (4 weeks); (4) ureate crystals after in vivo application (www.laboklin.com).

References

Abu-Lail, N., and Camesano, T. 2006. Specific and nonspecific interaction forces between *Escherichia coli* and silicon nitride, determined by Poisson statistical analysis. *Langmuir*, **22**(17): 7296–7301.

Adams, N., and Schubert, U.S. 2007. Poly(2-oxazolines) in biological and biomedical application contexts. *Adv Drug Deliv Rev*, **59**(15): 1504–1520.

Allion, A., Baron, J., and Boulange-Petermann, L. 2006. Impact of surface free energy and roughness in cell distribution and viability. *Biofouling*, **22**(5/6): 269–278.

Andersen, L.P., and Rasmussen, L. 2009. Helicobacter pylori-coccoid forms and biofilm formation. *FEMS Immunol Med Microbiol*, **56**(2): 112–115.

Banerjee, I., Pangule, R.C., and Kane, R.S. 2011. Antifouling coatings: recent developments in the design of surfaces that prevent fouling by proteins, bacteria, and marine organisms. *Adv Mater*, **23**(6): 690–718.

Baveja, J.K., et al. 2004. Biological performance of a novel synthetic furanone-based antimicrobial. *Biomaterials*, **25**(20): 5013–5021.

Benoit, M., et al. 2010. New device for high-throughput viability screening of flow biofilms. *Appl Environ Microbiol*, **76:** 4136–4142.

Berg, J.M., et al. 1994. Three-component Langmuir–Blodgett films with a controllable degree of polarity, *Langmuir*, **10:** 1225–1234"

Bithelis, G., et al. 2004. Assessment of encrustations on polyurethane ureteral stents. *J Endourol*, **18**(6): 550–556.

Boulange-Petermann, L., Baroux, B., and Bellon-Fontaine, M-N. 1993. The influence of metallic surface wettability on bacterial adhesion. *J Adhes Sci Technol*, **7**(3): 221–230.

Boulange-Petermann, L., et al. 2004. Influence of surface chemistry on the hygienic status of the industrial stainless steel. *Biofouling*, **20**(1): 25–33.

Branda, S., et al. 2006. A major protein component of the *Bacillus subtilis* biofilm matrix. *Mol Microbiol*, **59**: 1229–1238.

Brandes, N., et al. 2004. Adsorption physiologischer Proteine auf verschiedenen Keramikpartikeln. *Biomaterialien*, **5**(1): 22–27.

Bridier, A., et al. 2011. Resistance of bacterial to disinfectants a review. *Biofouling*, **27**(9): 1017–1032.

Buckingham-Meyer, K., et al. 2003. Alternative biofilm growth reactors, in *The Biofilm Laboratory :Step-by-step Protocols for Experimental Design, Analysis and Data Interpretation* (Hamilton, M., Heersink, J., Buckingham-Meyer, K., and Goeres, D., eds), Cytergy Publishing, Bozeman, pp. 31–51.

Burmolle, M., et al. 2010. Biofilms in chronic infections—a matter of opportunity—monospecies biofilms in multispecies infections. *FEMS Immunol Med Microbiol,* **59**(3): 324–336.

Busscher, H.J., and van der Mei, H.C. 2006. Microbial adhesion in flow displacement systems. *Clin Microbiol Rev,* **19**(1): 127–141.

Busscher, H.J., Cowan, M.M., and van der Mei, H.C. 1992. On the relative importance of specific and nonspecific approaches to oral microbial adhesion. *FEMS Microbiol Lett,* **88**: 199–209.

Cao, L., et al. 2007. Plasma deposited tetraglyme surfaces greatly reduce total blood protein adsorption, contact activation, platelet adhesion, platelet procoagulant activity, and in vitro thrombus deposition. *J Biomed Mater Res A,* **81A**: 827–837.

Chaudhury, M., et al. 2006. Settlement behavior of swimming algal spores on gradient surfaces. *Biointerphases,* **1**(1): 18–21.

Chen, S., et al. 2005. Strong resistance of phosphorylcholine self-assembled monolayer to protein adsorption: Insights into nonfouling properties of zwitterionic materials. *J Am Chem Soc,* **127**(41):14473–14478.

Choong, S., et al. 2001. Catheter-associated urinary tract infection and encrustation. *Int J Antimicrob Agents,* **17**: 305–310.

Coenye, T., and Nelis, H.J. 2010. In vitro and in vivo model systems to study microbial biofilm formation. *J Microbiol Methods,* **83**(2): 89–105.

Costerton, J.W., et al. 1995. Microbial biofilms. *Annu Rev Microbiol,* **49**(1): 711–745.

Costerton, J.W., Stewart, P.S., and Greenberg, E.P. 1999. Bacterial biofilms: A common cause ofpersistent infections. *Science,* **284**(5418): 1318.

Cucarella, C., et al. 2004. Role of biofilm-associated protein bap in the pathogenesis of bovine *Staphylococcus aureus. Infect Immun.* **72**: 2177–2185.

Dalsin, J., et al. 2003. Mussel adhesive protein mimetic polymers for the preparation of nonfouling surfaces. *J Am Ceram Soc,* **125**: 4253–4258.

Dawes, C., Jenkins, G., and Tonge, C. 1963. The nomenclature of the integuments of the enamel surface of teeth. *Br Dent J,* **16**: 65–68.

de Carvalho, C. 2007. Biofilms: Recent developments on an old battle. *Recent Pat Biotechnol,* **1**(1): 49–57.

Decho, A.W., Norman, R.S., and Visscher, P.T. 2010. Quorum sensing in natural environments: Emerging views from microbial mats. *Trends Microbiol,* **18**(2): 73–80.

Derjaguin, B., and Landau, L.1941. Theory of the stability of strongly charged lyophobic sols and of the adhesion of strongly charged particles in solutions of electrolytes. *Acta Physica Chimica,* **14**: 633.

Dickinson, R., Ruta, A., and Truesdail, S. 2000. Physicochemical basis of bacterial adhesion to biomaterial surfaces, in *Antimicrobial/Anti-infective Materials* (Sawan, S.P., and Manivannan, G., eds), Technomic Publishing Co. Inc., Pennsylvania, pp. 67–93.

Domenico, P., et al. 2001. Activities of bismuth thiols against staphylococci and staphyloccal biofilms. *Antimicorb Agents Chemother,* **45**(5): 1417–1421.

Donlan, R. 2001. Biofilms and device-associated infection. *Emerg Infect Dis,* **7**(2): 277–281.

Donlan, R. 2004. Model system for growing and quantifying *Streptococcus pneumoniae* biofilms in situ and in real time. *Appl Environ Microbiol,* **708**: 4980–4988.

Donlan, R.M. 2002. Biofilms: Microbial life on surfaces. *Emerg Infect Dis,* **8**(9): 881–890.

Donlan, R.M., and Costerton, J.W. 2002. Biofilms: Survival mechanisms of clinically relevant microorganisms. *Clin Microbiol Rev,* **15**(2): 167–193.

Eggimann, P., Sax, H., and Pittet, D. 2004. Catheter-related infections microbes. *Infect Immun,* **6**: 1033–1042.

Emoto, K., et al. 2000. Preparation of nonfouling surface through the coating with core polymerized block copolymer micelles having aldehyde-ended PEGshell. *Colloids Surf B Biointerfaces,* **18**: 337–346.

Feng, W., Brash, J., and Zhu, S. 2006. Nonbiofouling materials prepared by atom transfer radical polymerization grafting of 2-methacryloloxyethyl phosphorylcholine: Separate effects of graft density and chain length on protein repulsion. *Biomaterials,* **27**: 847–855.

Ferreiros, et al. 1989. Surface free energy and interactions of *Staphylococcus epidermidis* with biomaterials. *FEMS Microbiol Lett,* **60**: 89.

Filoche, S., Wong, L., and Sissons, C. H. 2010 .Oral biofilms: emerging concepts in microbial ecology. *J Dent Res,* **89**(1): 8–18.

Flemming, H., and Wingender, J. 2010. The biofilm matrix. *Nat Rev Microbiol,* **8**: 623–633.

Frant, M. 2008. Funktionalisierung von Biowerkstoffen durch biomimetische Strukturen auf der Basis von Tetraetherlipiden—ein Antifoulingkonzept. *Dissertation MLU Halle.*

Frant, M., et al. 2006. Anti-infective surfaces based on tetraether lipids for peritoneal dialysis catheter systems. *Mat.-wiss. u. Werkstofftech,* **37**(6): 538–545.

Friedrich, C.L., et al. 2001. Structure and mechanism of action of an indolicidin peptide derivative with improved activity against Gram-positive bacteria. *J Biol Chem,* **276**(26): 24015–24022.

Gallardo-Moreno, A.M., et al. 2009. In vitro biocompatibilty and bacterial adhesion of physicochemically modified Ti6AlV4 surface by means of UV radiation. *Acta Biomaterialia,* **3**: 181–192.

Giardi, C., et al. 2009. Nonionic polyoxazoline surfactants based on renewable source: Synthesis, surface and bulk properties. *React Funct Polym,* **69**(9): 643–649.

Gill, J., Deretic, V., and Chakrabarty, A. 1987. Alginate production by the mucoid *Pseudomonas aeruginosa* associated with cystic fibrosis. *Microbiol Sci,* **4**(10): 296–299.

Glantz, P-O. 1971. The adhesiveness of teeth. *J Colloid Interface Sci,* **37**(2): 281–290.

Goeres, D., et al. 2005. Statistic assessment of a laboratory method for growing biofilms. *Microbiology,* **151**: 757–762.

Gopal, J., et al. 2004. Photocatalytic inhibition of microbial adhesion by anodized titanium. *Biofouling,* **20**(3): 167–175.

Gottenbos, B., et al. 2003. Positively charged biomaterials exert antimicrobial effects on Gram-negative bacilli in rats. *Biomaterials,* **24**(16): 2707–2710.

Griffith, D., Musher, D., and Istin, C. 1976. The primary cause of infection induced urinary stones. *Invest Urol,* **13**(5): 346.

Gross, M., et al. 2001. Key role of teichoic acid net charge in *Staphylococcus aureus* colonization of artificial surfaces. *Infect Immun,* **69**(5): 3423–3426.

Gupta, A., et al. 2006. Glycocalyx-mimetic dextran-modified poly(vinyl amine) surfactant coating reduces platelet adhesion on medical-grade polycarbonate surface. *Biomaterials,* **27**: 3084–3095.

Haamann, D., et al. 2010. Antibacterial hydrogel coating for nonadhesive wound dressings, in *Proceedings of the Aachen-Dresden International Textile Conference,* Institute of Textile Machinery and High Performance Material Technology, Dresden.

Halperin, A., et al. 2007. Primary versus ternary adsorption of proteins onto PEG brushes. *Langmuir,* **23**: 10603–10671.

Hanson, S., et al. 1980. In vivo evaluation of artificial surfaces with a nonhuman primate model of arterial thrombosis. *J Lab Clin Med,* **95**(2): 289–304.

Hanzelka, B., and Greenberg, E. 1995. Evidence that the N-terminal region of the *Vibrio fischerii* LuxR protein constitutes an autoinducer-binding domain. *J Bacteriol,* **177**: 815–817.

Harbarth, S., Sax, H., and Gastmeier, P. 2003. The preventable proportion of nosocomial infections: An overview of published reports. *J Hosp Infect,* **54**: 258–266.

Hoffman, L., D'Argenio, D., and MacCoss, M. 2005. Aminoglycoside antibiotics induce bacterial biofilm formation. *Nature,* **436**(7054): 1171–1175.

Hojo, K., et al. 2009. Bacterial interactions in dental biofilm development. *J Dent Res,* **88**(11): 982–990.

Holland, N., et al. 1998. Biomimetic engineering of nonadhesive glycocalyx-like surfaces using oligosaccharide surfactant polymers. *Nature,* **392**(6678): 799–801.

Hubner, N.O., et al. 2010. Efficacy of chlorhexidine, polihexanide and tissue-tolerable plasma against *Pseudomonas aeruginosa* biofilms grown on polystyrene and silicone materials. *Skin Pharmacol Physiol,* **23 Suppl**: 28–34.

Hume, E., et al. 2004. The control of *Staphylococcus epidermidis* biofilm formation and in vivo infection rates by covalently bound furanones. *Biomaterials,* **25**: 5023–5030.

Ishihara, K., et al. 1994. Hemocompatibility of graft copolymers composed of poly(2-methacryloxyethyl phosphorylcholine) side chain and poly(n-butyl methacrylate) backbone. *J Biomed Mater Res,* **28**: 225–232.

Israelachvili, J. 1997. The different faces of poly*(ethylene glycol). Proc Natl Acad Sci USA,* **94**: 8378.

Ista, L.K., Mendez, S., and Lopez, G.P. 2010. Attachment and detachment of bacteria on surfaces with tunable and switchable wettability. *Biofouling,* **26**(1): 111–118.

Jang, C.H., et al. 2010. Effect of vancomycin-coated tympanostomy tubes on methicillin-resistant *Staphylococcus aureus* biofilm formation: In vitro study. *J Laryngol Otol,* **124**(6): 594–598.

Jeon, J.G., et al. 2011. Natural products in caries research: Current (limited) knowledge, challenges and future perspective. *Caries Res,* **45**(3): 243–263.

Jones, S.M., et al. 2007. Structure of *Proteus mirabilis* biofilms grown in artificial urine and standard laboratory media. *FEMS Microbiol Lett,* **268**(1): 16–21.

Juan, L., et al. 2010. Deposition of silver nanoparticles on titanium surface for antibacterial effect. *Int J Nanomedicine,* **5**: 261–267.

Kane, R., Deschateles, P., and Whitesides, G. 2003. Kosmotropes form the basis of protein-resistant surfaces. *Langmuir,* **19**: 2388–2391.

Kaplan, J.B. 2005. Antibiotic-induced biofilm formation. *Int J Artif Organs,* **34**(9): 737–751.

Karunakaran, E., et al. 2011. Biofilmology: A multidisciplinary review of the study of microbial biofilms. *Appl Microbiol Biotechnol,* **90**(6): 1869–1881.

Klee, D., et al. 2003. Surface modification of poly(vinylidenefluoride) to improve the osteoblast adhesion. *Biomaterials,* **24**(21): 3663–3670.

Kohnen, W., et al. 2003. Development of a long-lasting ventricular catheter impregnated with a combination of antibiotics. *Biomaterials,* **24**(26): 4865–4869.

Kolenbrander, P., et al. 2002. Communication among oral bacteria. *Microbiol Mol Biol Rev,* **66**(3): 486–505.

Krsko, P., and Libera, M. 2005. Biointeractive hydrogels. *Mater Today,* **8**(12): 36–44.

Lawrence, J., Swerhone, G., and Neu, T. 2000. A simple rotating annular reactor for replicated biofilm studies. *J Microbiol Methods,* **42**: 215–222.

Lee, J.H., Ju, Y.M., and Kim, D.M. 2000. Platelet adhesion onto segmented polyurethane film surfaces modified by adhesion and cross-linked of PEO-containing block copolymers. *Biomaterials,* **21**: 683–691.

Lewis, A.L., et al. 2003. Wettable phosphorylcholine-containing polymers useful in blood filtration. *J Mater Sci Mater Med,* **14**(1): 39–45.

Lopez, D., Vlamakis, H., and Kolter, R. 2010. Biofilms. *Cold Spring Harb Perspect Biol,* **2**(7): a000398.

Marechal, J.P., and Hellio, C. 2009. Challenges for the development of new nontoxic antifouling solutions. *Int J Mol Sci,* **10**(11): 4623–4637.

Marsh, P.D. 1994. Microbial ecology of dental plaque and its significance in health and disease. *Adv Dent Res,* **8**(2): 263–271.

Martinez, L.R., et al. 2010. Demonstration of antibiofilm and antifungal efficacy of chitosan against candidal biofilms, using an in vivo central venous catheter model. *J Infect Dis,* **201**(9): 1436–1440.

McCoy, W., et al. 1981. Observations of fouling biofilm formation. *Can J Microbiol,* **27**: 910–174.

Mehne, J., et al. 2008. Characterization of morphology of self-assembled PEG monolayers: A comparison of mixed and pure coatings optimized for biosensor applications. *Anal Bioanal Chem,* **391**(5): 1783–1791.

Miller, M.B., and Bassler, B.L. 2001. Quorum sensing in bacteria. *Annu Rev Microbiol,* **55**: 165–199.

Mohammadi, Z., and Abbott, P.V. 2009. The properties and applications of chlorhexidine in endodontics. *Int Endod J,* **42**(4): 288–302.

Montag, D., et al. 2012. Dependence of the initial adhesion of biofilm forming Pseudomonas putida mt2 on physicochemical material properties. *Biofouling,* **28**(3): 315–327.

Morra, M. 2000. On the molecular basis of fouling resistance. *J Biomater Sci Polym Ed,* **11**(6): 547–569.

Mozes, N., et al. 1987. Immobilization of microorganisms by adhesion: Interplay of electrostatic and nonelectrostatic interactions. *Biotechnol Bioeng,* **30**(3): 439–450.

Murata, H., et al. 2007. Permanent nonleaching antibacterial surfaces-2: How high density cationic surfaces kill bacteria. *Biomaterials,* **28**: 4870–4879.

Neu, T., and Lawrence, J. 2009. Extracellular polymeric substances in microbial biofilms, in *Microbial Glycobiology: Structures, Relevance and Applications* (Imoran, A., Brennan, P., Holst, O., and von Itzstein, M., eds), *Elsevier, San Diego,* pp. 735–758.

Neut, D., et al. 2003. Residual gentamicin-release from antibiotic-loaded polymethylmethacrylate beads after 5 years of implantation. *Biomaterials,* **24**(10): 1829–1831.

Ostuni, E., et al. 2001. Self-assembled monolayers that resist the adsorption of proteins and the adhesion of bacterial and mammalian cells. *Langmuir,* **17**(20): 6336–6343

Park, J.H., et al. 2003. Norfloxacin-releasing urethral catheter for long-term catheterization. *J Biomater Sci Polym Ed,* **14**(9): 951–962.

Park, K.D., et al. 1998. Bacterial adhesion on PEG modified polyurethane surfaces. *Biomaterials,* **19**(7–9): 851–859.

Pedri, L. 2004. Interaction of bacteria with hydrophobic and hydrophilic interfaces. *Dokument von Autor,* 1–24.

Peters, A., and Wimpenny, J. 1988. A constant-depth laboratory model film fermenter. *Biotechnol Bioeng,* **32**: 263–270.

Pidhatika, B., et al. 2008. Nonfouling surface coatings based on poly(2-methyl-2-oxacoline). *Chimia,* **62**(4): 264.

Quirenen, M., and Bollen, C.M.L. 1995. The influence of surface roughness and surface free energy on supra- and subgingival plaque formation in man. *J Clin Periodontol,* **22**: 1–14.

Ratner, B. 2007. The catastrophe revisited: Blood compatibility in the 21st century. *Biomaterials,* **28**: 5144–5147.

Regev-Shoshani, G., et al. 2010. Slow release of nitric oxide from charged catheters and its effect on biofilm formation by *Escherichia coli. Antimicrob Agents Chemother,* **54**: 273–279.

Reimann, D., et al. 2001. Peritonealdialyse-die Alternative in der Nierenersatztherapie. *Ärzteblatt Sachsen,* **11**: 509.

Resch, A., et al. 2005. Differential gene expression profiling of *Staphylococcus aureus* cultivated under biofilm and planktonic conditions. *Appl Environ Microb,* **71**: 2663.

Rijnaarts, H.H.M., et al. 1999. DLVO and steric contributions to bacterial deposition in media of different ionic strength. *Colloid Surface,* **14**: 179–195.

Romero, D., et al. 2010. Amyloid fibers provide structural integrity to *Bacillus subtilis* biofilms. *Proc Natl Acad Sci USA,* **107**: 2230–2234.

Roosjen, A., et al. 2006. Bacterial factors influencing adhesion of *Pseudomonas aeruginosa* strains to a poly(ethylene oxide) brush. *Microbiology,* **192**: 2673–2682.

Rose, S., et al. 2004. Biological responses to cationically charged phosphorylcholine-based materials in vitro. *Biomaterials,* **25**: 2125–2135.

Rosentritt, M., et al. 2008. Adhesion of *Streptococcus mutans* to various dental materials in a laminar flow chamber systems. *J Biomed Mater Res B Appl Biomater,* **86**(1): 36–44.

Ruegsegger, M., and Marchant, R. 2001. Reduced protein adsorption and platelet adhesion by controlled variation of oligomaltose surfaction polymer coating. *J Biomed Mater Res,* **56**: 156–167.

Saldarriaga-Fernandez, I.C., et al. 2007. The inhibition of the adhesion of clinically isolated bacterial strains on multicomponent cross-linked poly(ethylene glycol)-based polymer coatings. *Biomaterials,* **28**(28): 4105–4112.

Salta, M., et al. 2010. Designing biomimetic antifouling surfaces. *Philos Transact A Math Phys Eng Sci,* **368**(1929): 4729–4754.

Schade, R. 2005. Entwicklung eines in vitro Systems zur Prüfung der initialen Plaqueadhärenz an dentalen Biomaterialien, Thesis Jena.

Schmidt, D., et al. 2004. Contact angle hysteresis, adhesion and marine biofouling. *Langmuir,* **20**: 2830–2836.

Schünlin, T., and Voss, A. 2005. Miscellaneous organisms, in *Catheter-Related Infection,* 2nd ed (Seifert, H., Jansen, B., and Farr, N.M., eds), Marcel Dekker, New York, pp. 222–255.

Sharma, S., Johnson, R., and Desai, T. 2004. XPS and AFM analysis of antifouling PEG interfaces for microfabricated silicon biosensors. *Biosens Bioelectron,* **20**: 227–239.

Shaw, G., Choong, S., and Fry, C. 2005. Encrustation of biomaterials in the urinary tract. *Urol Res,* **33**: 17–22.

Sheludko, A., et al. 2008. The effect of mutations in the synthesis of lipopolysaccharides and calcofluor-binding polysaccharides on biofilm formation by *Azospirillum brasilense. Mikrobiologiia,* **77**: 358–363.

Sissons, C.H. 1997. Artificial dental plaque biofilm model systems. *Adv Dent Res,* **11**(1): 110–126.

Som, A., et al. 2008. Synthetic mimics of antimicrobial peptides. *Biopolymers,* **90**(2): 83–93.

Steinberg, D., et al. 1995. Adsorption of human salivary proteins to titanium powder. I. Adsorption of human salivary albumin. *Biomaterials,* **16**(17): 1339–1343.

Stickler, D. 2008. Bacterial biofilms in patients with indwelling urinary catheters. *Nat Clin Pract Urol,* **5**(11): 598–608.

Stobie, N., et al. 2009. Silver-doped perfluoropolyether-urethane coatings: Antibacterial activity and surface analysis. *Colloids Surf B Biointerfaces,* **72**(1): 62–67.

Subramanyan, S., et al. 2000. A chemically intelligent infection-resistant coating, in *Antimicrobial/Anti-Infective Materials* (Sawan, S.P., and Manivannan, G., eds), Technomic Publishing Co. Inc., Pennsylvania, pp. 220–238.

Taylor, M., et al. 2004. Evidence for acryl homoserine lactone signal production in bacteria associated with marine sponges. *Appl Env Microb,* **70**(7): 4387–4389.

Teodioso, J., et al. 2011. Flow cell hydrodynamics and their effects on *E. coli* biofilm formation under different nutrient conditions and turbulent flow. *Biofouling,* **27**(1): 1–11.

Tielker, D., et al. 2005. *Pseudomonas aeruginosa* lectin LecB is located in the outer membrane and is involved in biofilm formation. *Microbiology,* **151**: 1313–1323.

Tiller, J.C., et al. 2001. Designing surfaces that kill bacteria on contact. *Proc Natl Acad Sci USA,* **98**(11): 5981–5985.

Todar, K. Online textbook of bacteriology. *Mechanisms of Bacterial Pathogenicity.* http://textbookofbacteriology.net/pathogenesis_3.html: p. 3.

Tosatti, S., et al. 2003. Peptide functionalized poly(L-lysine)-g-poly(ethylene glycol) on titanium: Resistance to protein adsorption in full heparinized human blood plasma. *Biomaterials,* **24**(27): 4949–4958.

Triandafillu, K., et al. 2003. Adhesion of *Pseudomonas aeruginosa* strains to untreated and oxygen-plasma treated PVC from endotracheal intubation devices. *Biomaterials,* **24**: 1507–1518.

Tziampazis, E., Kohn, J., and Moghe, P. 2000. PEG-variant biomaterials as selectivity adhesive protein templates: Model surfaces for controlled cell adhesion and migration. *Biomaterials,* **21**: 511–520.

Upadhyayula, V.K., and Gadhamshetty, V. 2010. Appreciating the role of carbon nanotube composites in preventing biofouling and promoting biofilms on material surfaces in environmental engineering: A review. *Biotechnol Adv,* **28**(6): 802–816.

Vacheethasanee, K., and Marchant, R. 2000. Surfactant polymers designed to suppress bacterial (*Staphylococcus epidermidis*) adhesion on biomaterials. *J Biomed Mater Res,* **50**: 302–312.

van Dijk, L. J., Gadsweer, R., and Busscher, H. J. 1988. Interfacial free energy as a driving force for pellicle formation in the oral cavity: An in vivo study in beagle dogs. *Biofouling,* **1**: 19–25.

van Merode, A.E., et al. 2006. Influence of culture heterogeneity in cell surface charge on adhesion and biofilm formation by *Enterococcus faecalis. J Bacteriol,* **188**(7): 2421–2426.

van Oss, C. J. 1994. *Interfacial Forces in Aqueous Media,* Marcel Dekker, New York, 440 pp.

Vasilev, K., Cook, J., and Griesser, H.J. 2009. Antibacterial surfaces for biomedical devices. *Expert Rev Med Devices,* **6**(5): 553–567.

Verway, E.J.W., and Overbeek, J.Th.G. 1948. *Theory of the Stability of Lyophobic Colloids,* Elsevier, New York.

Vogler, E.A. 1993. Interfacial chemistry in biomaterials science, in *Wettability* (Berg J.C., ed), Marcel Dekker, New York, Basel, Hong Kong, pp. 183–250.

Vogler, E.A. 1998. Structure and reactivity of water at biomaterial surfaces. *Adv Colloid Interfac Sci*, **74**: 69–117.

Vogler, E.A. 1999. Water and the acute biological response to surfaces. *J Biomater Sci Polym Ed*, **10**(10): 1015–1045.

Wagner, V.E., Koberstein, J.T., and Bryers, J.D. 2004. Protein and bacterial fouling characteristics of peptide and antibody decorated surfaces of PEG-poly(acrylic acid) copolymers. *Biomaterials*, **25**(12): 2247–2263.

Wang, Y., et al. 2011. Investigation of the role of hydrophilic chain length in amphiphilic perfluoropolyether/poly(ethyleneglycol) networks: Toward high performance antifouling coatings. *Biofouling*, **27**(10): 1139–1150.

Warren, J. 2001. Catheter-associated urinary tract infections. *Int J Antimicrob Agents*, **17**: 299–303.

Waschinski, C., et al. 2005. Influence of satellite groups on telechelic antimicrobial functions of polyoxazolines. *Macromol Biosci*, **5**: 149–156.

Waters, C., and Bassler, B. 2005. Quorum sensing: Cell-to-cell communication in bacteria. *Annu Rev Cell Dev Biol*, **21**: 319–346.

Wehle, J. 2004. Klinische Studie zur initialen In-vivo-Plaqueakkumulation aufverschiedenen dentalen Werkstoffen, Thesis, Göttingen.

Werner, C., Maitz, M., and Sperling, C. 2007. Current strategies towards hemocompatible coatings. *J Mater Chem*, **17**: 3376–3384.

Xu, L.C., and Siedlecki, C.A. 2007. Effects of surface wettability and contact time on protein adhesion to biomaterial surfaces. *Biomaterials*, **28**(22): 3273–3283.

Yang, W.J., et al. 2011. *Biomimetic anchors for antifouling and antibacterial polymer brushes on stainless steel. Langmuir*, **27**(11): 7065–7076.

Yang, Y.F., Wan, L.S., and Xu, Z.K. 2010. Surface hydrophilisation and antibacterial functionalization for microporous polypropylene membranes. *Water Sci Technol*, **61**(8): 2053–2060.

Yim, G., Wang, H., and Davies, J.C. 2007. Antibiotics as signaling molecules. *Philos Trans R Soc Lond B Biol Sci*, **362**: 1195–1200.

Yishak, A., et al. 2001. The outcome of peritonitis in patients on automated peritoneal dialysis. *Adv Perit Dial*, **17**: 205–208.

Zasloff, M. 2002. Antimicrobial peptides of multicellular organisms. *Nature*, **415**(24): 389–395.

Zhang, L., Rozek, A., and Hancock, R.E.W. 2001. Interaction of cationic antimicrobial peptides with model membranes. *J Biol Chem*, **276**(38): 35714–35722.

Zhao, L., et al. 2009. Antibacterial coatings on titanium implants. *J Biomed Mater Res B Appl Biomater*, **91**(1): 470–480.

Chapter 6

Antimicrobial Implant Coating

Klaus-Dieter Kühn
Department of Orthopaedic Surgery, Medical University of Graz, Auenbruggerplatz 5, 8036 Graz, Austria
Klaus.kuehn@medunigraz.at

Novel antimicrobial coating concepts of implant surfaces are described in this review. Some orthopedic implants with special antimicrobial coatings have achieved a CE-notification as a medical device class III product (e.g., marrow nails, sutures). Several R&D groups work in this field to find a solution aimed at preventing bacterial colonization of medical implants. This achievement may constitute an additional advantage for the coated device in a highly competitive market. Plastics or slightly rough metallic surfaces, such as implants made of titanium, have shown an inherent property to be colonized by germs if a bacterial contamination has occurred, e.g., during the surgery. In a process called biofilm formation, many pathogens such as *Staphylococcus aureus* and *Staphylococcus epidermidis* may easily start to colonize the implant by adhering to serum proteins coating the implant surface. Because of the subsequent production of a dense glycocalyx layer and the reduction of their metabolic activity,

Biofunctional Surface Engineering
Edited by Martin Scholz

ISBN 978-981-4411-60-8 (Hardcover), 978-981-4411-61-5 (eBook)
www.panstanford.com

such biofilm-associated bacterial growth forms are well protected from the host's immune defense system and the antimicrobial action of antibiotics. As a consequence, even high local concentrations of antibiotics do not succeed in completely eradicating bacteria in biofilms. It is, therefore, of great importance to prevent by all means the bacterial adhesion on biomaterial surfaces. This can be achieved with antimicrobial surface coating.

6.1 Introduction and Economical Aspects of Implant-Related Infection

A variety of different devices and biomaterials (see Table 6.1) used in modern medicine ensure longer survival and better quality of life for patients with a multitude of medical conditions. However, the more and more extensive use of devices has one major drawback: the growing number of infections associated with medical devices. Particularly older and multimorbid patients, who benefit the most from new treatment options, face the highest risk of infection. As a consequence, the majority of cases of infections in critically ill patients are related to medical devices (Darouiche, 2001; von Eiff et al., 2005).

Table 6.1 Medical implants

	Medical implants
Angiology	Peripheral catheter Central catheter (tunneled, non-tunneled) Pulmonary catheter Implanted catheter Drainage
Cardiology	Valve prostheses Implantable defibrillators Pacemaker Vascular prostheses Artificial hearts/ventricular assist devices (VADs) Coronary stents Implantable monitors Mechanical heart valve

Medical implants	
Urology	Penile prostheses Urethral implants
Gynecology	Breast implants
Neurosurgery	Ventricular shunts Ommaya reservoir Intracranial pressure gauge Neurostimulators Spinal implants
Orthopedic/trauma surgery	Joint prostheses, hip, knee, shoulder, elbow, cups Reconstructive implants Spinal implants Screws, nails, plates, pins Bone substitutes Surgical sutures Hernia meshes Fixateur Collagen fleeces, felts Kirschner wires
Otolaryngology	Cochlear implants Middle ear implants
Ophthalmology	Intraocular lenses Glaucoma tube
Dentistry	Implants

Depending on the device, infection may cause a high mortality rate and require prolonged antibiotic therapy and/or repeated surgical interventions (Darouiche, 2004). Patients with cardiac devices and ventricular shunts face the highest rate of mortality related to infection. Moreover, bacterial contamination of a ventricular shunt poses a high risk of intellectual, cognitive, and neurological deficits to the survivors. While infections of orthopedic devices are rarely life threatening, they may cause serious disabilities and a significant reduction of the patient's mobility and quality of life. The same applies to penile and mammary implants, which necessitate complete removal and can cause major disfigurement and psychological trauma in the event of infection (Darouiche, 2004; Choux et al., 1992; Barrack et al., 2000). The additional morbidity of infected central vascular catheters, urinary catheters, and sutures is relatively low compared to other devices; however, it still necessitates prolonged medical treatment (Patton et al., 1991; O'Grady et al., 2011; Kathju et al., 2009).

In addition to the often severe clinical consequences, infection does also increase the treatment expenses. The main cost generators of device-related infections (Bozic and Ries, 2005; Ferguson et al., 1996; Kirkland et al., 1999; Warren et al., 2006) are

- Additional surgical procedures
- Increased length of hospitalization
- Prolonged treatment with antibiotics
- And the implantation of new, often expensive devices

The treatment costs per patient can easily exceed $50,000 (Table 6.2). In consideration of these facts, it seems only logical that authorities aim for the minimization of their expenses in terms of potentially avoidable infections. For example, Medicare stopped reimbursing hospital-acquired infections—so-called "never events"—from 1 October 2008 (Department of Health and Human Services, 2008). These changes have two major consequences. First, additional reimbursement is not provided for any infection acquired during the current hospitalization and those for which substantial documentation to determine if the condition was present at admission is unavailable. Second, hospitals will receive reduced payments if they do not report such an event. In the context of growing financial pressure on health-care systems all around the world, it seems likely that more countries will follow this example in the near future.

One of the most efficient and practical approaches aimed at reducing the frequency of medical-device-related infections is the addition of antimicrobial agents to the device. The oldest example for such a successful symbiosis of biomaterials and antimicrobials is the antibiotic-loaded PMMA bone cement, an acrylic material for the fixation of metallic implants in the body. The addition of antibiotics to PMMA cement began in 1969 (Buchholz and Engelbrecht, 1970; Wahlig and Buchholz, 1972; Kühn, 2000; Frommelt and Kühn, 2005; Kühn, 2007). At a later point, we will describe the principle of bone cements containing antibiotics as an excellent basis for the medical implants coating concept. As a proof of concept for the anti-infective properties of antibiotic-loaded cement, a recent meta-analysis has

Table 6.2 Economic data of medical device infection in the US health care system

Device	Materials*	Implanted devices (per year)	Rate of infection (%)†	Number of infections (per year)	Costs per infection ($)‡	Annual costs ($)	Mortality◊	Literature
Cardiac devices								
Mechanical heart valve	Reprocessed tissue, stainless steel, carbon	85	4	3.4	50	170,000	High	Darouiche, 2001; Darouiche, 2004; Cooke, 2004; Ferguson et al., 1996
Vascular graft	Dacron, Teflon, polyutherane	450	4	16	40	720,000	Moderate	Darouiche, 2001; Darouiche, 2004; Cooke, 2004; Ferguson et al., 1996
Pacemaker –defibrillator	Titanium, titanium alloy	300	4	12	35	420,000	High	Darouiche, 2001; Darouiche, 2004; Cooke, 2004; Ferguson et al., 1996

(*Continued*)

Table 6.2 *(Continued)*

Device	Materials*	Implanted devices (per year)	Rate of infection (%)†	Number of infections (per year)	Costs per infection ($)‡	Annual costs ($)	Mortality ◊	Literature
Catheters								
Central vascular catheters ℓ	Silicone rubber, Teflon, polyutherane	250	5	12	10	125,000	Moderate	Darouiche, 2004; Cooke, 2004; Veenstra et al., 1999
Urinary catheters	Silicone rubber, Teflon, polyutherane	5,000	20	1,000	0.5	500,000	Low	Darouiche, 2004; Cooke, 2004; Patton et al., 1991
Dental implants								
Dental implants	Titanium, Ti–Al–V alloy, stainless steel, polyethylene, calcium phosphate	1,000	5	50	N/A	N/A	Low	Darouiche, 2001; Cooke, 2004

Device	Materials[*]	Implanted devices (per year)	Rate of infection (%)[†]	Number of infections (per year)	Costs per infection ($)[‡]	Annual costs ($)	Mortality[◊]	Literature
Hernia								
Meshes (incisional hernia)	Polypropylene, polyester, polytetrafluoro ethylene	100	4	4	3⊤	6,000	Low	O'Grady et al., 2011; Kirkland et al., 1999; Finan et al., 2009; Demir et al., 2005
Neurosurgical								
Ventricular shunt	Silicone rubber, Teflon, polyutherane	40	6	2	50	120,000	High	Darouiche, 2004; Cooke, 2004; Choux et al., 1992
Orthopedics								
Internal and external osteosynthetic devices[⌂]	Stainless steel, cobalt-chromium alloy	2,000	5	100	15	1,500,000	Low	Darouiche, 2001; Darouiche, 2004; Cooke, 2004

(*Continued*)

Table 6.2 *(Continued)*

Device	Materials*	Implanted devices (per year)	Rate of infection (%)†	Number of infections (per year)	Costs per infection ($)‡	Annual costs ($)	Mortality◊	Literature
Hip joint	Titanium, Ti-Al-V alloy stainless steel polyethylene	250	1	2	95	237,500	Low	Cooke, 2004; Bozic and Ries, 2005; Kim, 2008; Kurtz et al., 2008
Knee joint		500	2	10	30	300,000	Low	Cooke, 2004; Barrack et al., 2000 Kim, 2008; Kurtz et al., 2008
Plastic								
Mammary implant (pair)	Silicone	130	2	2	20	52,000	Low	Darouiche, 2004; Dunn et al., 1992
Suture material								
Sutures ¶	Collagen, gut, nylon, silk	45,000	1	1,350	3⊤	4,050,000	N/A	Kirkland et al., 1999; Greenwald et al., 1994

Device	Materials*	Implanted devices (per year)	Rate of infection (%)†	Number of infections (per year)	Costs per infection ($)‡	Annual costs ($)	Mortality◊	Literature
Urologic								
Inflatable penile implant	Bioflex, ultrex	15	3	0.45	35	15,750	Low	Darouiche, 2004; Hellstrom et al., 2010

Note: Based in parts on the work of references 1 and 3.

* Commonly used materials for the type of medical device.

† Rate of infection in initially inserted implants. The risk of infection is significantly greater in revision procedures.

‡ Combined costs of medical and surgical treatment.

◊ Semi-quantitative scale for attributable mortality: low, <5%; moderate, 5%–25%; high, >25%.

ℓ Infection rates based on catheters without antimicrobial coating.

⊤Based on costs for the treatment of SSI.

⌂Fracture-fixation devices include intra-medullary nails, external-fixation pins, plates, and screws.

¶All inpatient surgeries. The development of the infection is not necessarily due to suture material. Infection rate based on devices without antimicrobial coating.

concluded that its use led to a reduction in the infection rate in primary hip arthroplasty by 50% compared to plain cement (Parvizi et al., 2008). While medical devices with antimicrobial agents are initially more expensive, long-term cost reductions have become evident in various cases. On the basis of the calculated reductions in the prevalence of prosthetic joint infections, it has been shown that despite the additional costs involved for using antibiotic-loaded bone cement on a routine basis in primary hip replacements, the overall cost savings may get to $200 per patient (Cummins et al., 2009). Similar savings can be achieved with antimicrobial coatings on central venous catheters, which resulted in reduced expenses of $196 per catheter used (Veenstra et al., 1999a). Even in the case of urinary catheters, where infections cause little to insignificant morbidity, more costly silver-impregnated devices may result in modest savings (Rupp et al., 2004). Similar successes in reducing infection rates were observed in silver-coated urinary catheters and antiseptic-impregnated suture material (Rupp et al., 2004; Justinger et al., 2011; Rasić et al., 2011).

In the recent past, other devices were successfully combined with anti-infective agents. One example is the impregnation of central venous catheters with chlorhexidine and silver sulfadiazine, which helps to reduce the risk of catheter-related blood stream infections by 40% (Veenstra et al., 1999b). Significant reductions in the infection rates can be achieved by combining devices with antimicrobial agents particularly in clean-contaminated surgery, such as the implantation of a penile prosthesis (Wilson et al., 2007).

Considering the precarious financial situation of health-care systems all over the world and the potentials for savings, research activities aimed at avoiding infections at biomaterial surfaces with anti-infective coatings will certainly receive greater attention in the future. For a high antimicrobial efficacy, implant coatings are required to have the properties summarized in Table 6.3.

6.2 Formation of Biofilm on Implant Surfaces

Implants may harbor bacteria, which may persevere on the surface in organized biofilms over many years. However, all foreign bodies such as medical implants are not capable of actively combating the bacteria and thus the formation of the biofilm. The following project, therefore, explains why the coating of implants represents a sensible and necessary strategy in the antimicrobial equipment of implants. In addition, it lists the agents generally deployed to combat microorganisms and thus suitable for the coating of implants.

Table 6.3 Basic coating requirements

- ➢ It should adhere well to rough and smooth surfaces.
- ➢ It should provide at least a temporary barrier for germs.
- ➢ It should not have receptors to facilitate the adherence of germs.
- ➢ It should dispense active ingredients from the coating and/or implant surface.
- ➢ It should initially ensure high local concentration of active ingredients.
- ➢ It should counteract the formation of biofilm (at least 48 h to 10 days).
- ➢ It should exhibit a temporary local effect (5–10 days).
- ➢ It should contain active ingredients of tissue, bone and, at best, capable of entering cells.
- ➢ If possible, it should not require any unknown and toxic substances.
- ➢ The active ingredients should develop a specific effect against bacterials only.
- ➢ The active ingredient should ensure fast metabolism and/or expulsion.
- ➢ The active ingredients should be applicable in a broad spectrum for prophylaxis.
- ➢ The active ingredients should be applicable in a narrow spectrum for therapy.

6.3 Germ Invasion

The human organism consists of approximately 10 billion cells and exists in peaceful cohabitation with a significantly greater amount of microorganisms (approximately by the power of 10). Many of these microorganisms take on vital tasks for the host. Evolution has successfully molded this cohabitation of microorganisms and humans over millions of years and ensured the formation of a symbiotic connection of the highest precision and quality, ensuring mutual survival.

However, if microorganisms enter the body and take possession of somatic cells, which are not adapted to the evolutionary trained connection, the human defense mechanism cannot cope in the long term and the aggressiveness of the invader exceeds the tolerance level of the host.

This imbalance can lead to disease, whereby the host organism is also excellently equipped against such microbial attacks. For this purpose, the immune systems has developed intelligent recognition and destruction strategies and is always capable of initiating respective counter measures to successfully ward off the invader. The body's own defense system furthermore ensures that a recognition cascade is initiated in the event of a repeat confrontation with the foreign organism, which quickly leads to the disbursement of all necessary molecules serving for the protection of the host.

However, the immediate counter strategy of the body following a germ invasion is always critical if the microorganisms have the potential to escape the defense system of the host organism. For example, this is the case if the germs discover refuges within the body, which cannot be penetrated by the immune cells, resulting in the fact that the invaders are no longer recognizable for the system. Next to "natural refuges," such as hematoma, carious teeth, dead skin particles or bone splinters after fractures, and particularly the dreaded sequesters, meaning devitalized bone tissue surrounded by involucre (the cambium layer of the periosteum) formed new bones, germs prefer using foreign objects and/or implants for rapid colonization. Thus the human immune system increasingly loses control over the invading germs and considers itself safe, since there is no feedback to the system telling it whether to become active or not.

6.4 Colonization of an Implant Surface

To circumvent the defense system of a host, microorganisms have developed excellent strategies, permitting them to establish within the host unrecognized. Immediately after entering, the germs are capable of adhering to the surface of foreign objects. Such reversible adhesion is facilitated by specific receptors and proteins (adhesive factors), which are highly complex and extremely specialized. If the surface is considered suitable, the bonding force suddenly increases, ensuring the irreversible bonding to the "substrate." The activity of the bacteria adhering to the surface is increased extremely, and it inevitably leads to proliferation and maturing of the organisms with the development of an ideally arranged network. The consolidation and interaction of this network with increasingly stronger cell layers create a well-organized matrix of polysaccharides (Fig. 6.1). A continuous stream of bacteria invade this gelatinous structure, including not only those that have created this biofilm, but also other, less aggressive or biofilm-forming organisms.

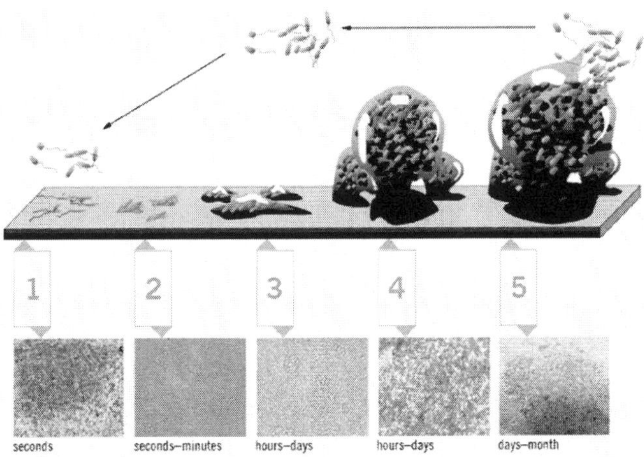

Biofilm formation	
Phases 1 and 2: Adhesion	The adhesion of microorganisms on solid surface is a common natural phenomenon (Costerton et al. 1999; Costerton et al. 1987), for example in the colonization of epithelial cells. Adhesion to an implant takes approximately 1–2 h. It is determined by numerous factors, for example by the type of cell surface and the receptors of the microorganism, the physiochemical properties of the surface, or the environment (Dunn et al., 1992). In this respect, the bacteria compete with the host cells in the colonization of the surface (Gristina and Costerton 1985).
Phase 3: Proliferation	After approximately 2–3 h, the bacteria begin to proliferate. The increasing proliferation and maturing of the bacteria and the formation of a network comprising several cell layers result in greater adhesion to the foreign material (von Eiff 1999).
Phase 4: Maturing	After a further day, the stable biofilm itself takes form, with the formation of a gel matrix comprising several layers in which the bacteria embed themselves (Donlan and Costerton, 2002). Nutrients are reserved and bacteria protected against immune response or antibiotics (Patel et al. 2007).
Phase 5: Separation	Individual bacteria may separate from the biofilm, colonize remote regions, and establish additional sources of infection (Kong et al. 2006).

Figure 6.1 Biofilm formation.

6.5 Biofilm

The microorganisms are perfectly protected within a biofilm, are no longer recognizable, and reduce their metabolism to an essential minimum. The outer layers serve as a protective wall against the body's own defense mechanisms such as proteins or enzymes as well as a barrier for bacteria-destroying macrophages. The penetration of substances to this interior of the biofilm is made extremely difficult, so that anti-infective agents are barely able to penetrate the matrix or are completely prevented from doing so. This requires such high concentrations of antibacterial substances—up to a 1000-fold concentration—to even affect bacteria in the biofilm. However, these extreme doses of active ingredients are generally highly toxic for the human organism and are thus not indicated. What remains are excellently organized bacteria structures at the surface of an implant, which at times remain inconspicuous for many years. Germs that detach themselves from the biofilm and pass from the sessile form of the matrix to the planctonic and freely movable form to reach the bloodstream are dreaded. From there they are capable of colonizing in far removed regions of the body and form sources of infection. The excess detachment of germs from the biofilm can lead to sepsis if the host's immune system is weakened.

There is a large body of evidence suggesting that the vast majority (more than 85%) of all implant-associated infections are initiated during or immediately after the surgical intervention (Nasser, 1999). It has also become clear that implant-associated infections require only an extremely low number of germs inoculated during the operation to colonize the surface of the foreign body (Elek and Conen, 1957; Kaiser et al., 1992).

Among these biofilm-related pathogens are in particular germs of the natural skin flora, which now meet a new terrain within the organism and develop surprisingly quickly effective survival strategies there. Even before the body's defense system is able to recognize a germ invasion, the organism initially reacts to the foreign body itself. This reaction is always related to an excessive complement activation. At the same time, the body's own immune response is significantly reduced and the elimination of the invaders is sharply reduced by phagocytosis. As a consequence, everything is biased toward the survival of the germs in the organism and the inevitable colonization of the foreign implant surface, which occurs faster than its colonization with somatic cells. This competition for the implant surface was also described as the "race for the surface." It is of further notice that because of the formation of biofilms, the detection of the pathogens is a particular challenge (Fig. 6.2).

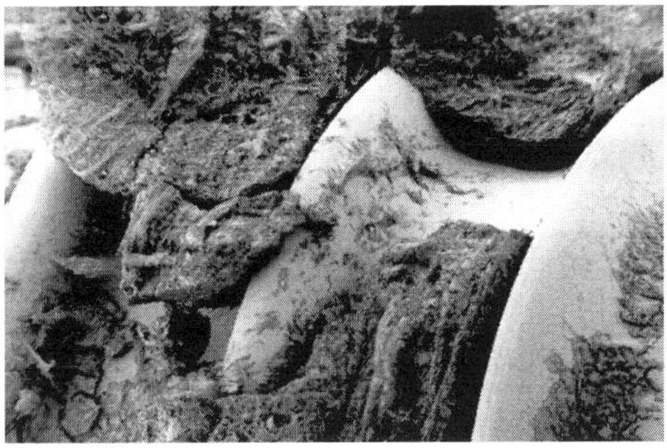

Figure 6.2 Biofilm on metal implant.

6.6 Germ Detection

A correct diagnosis aimed at detecting possible germs on metallic implants and/or related polymeric material is the precondition for initiating the appropriate clinical treatment strategies. Until now, the microbiological detection from joint aspirate or from a joint biopsy is considered the gold standard in diagnosis. Recently, a novel method involving sonication of the implant has been suggested to increase the sensitivity of the germ detection (Bjerkan et al., 2009; Kobayashi et al., 2009; Trampuz et al., 2007, see Table 6.4).

Table 6.4 Sonication

= Microbiological culture of biopsies – gold standard
Additional use of ultrasound treatment and/or vortexing
A short ultrasound treatment of the removed implants and/or vortexing removed cement fragments increases the release of bacteria adhering to the biofilm.
The sensitivity of the microbiological analysis increases significantly with the implementation of these methods compared with the "classic" scraping off of samples.

6.7 Medical Biofilms

The classic and most prominent biofilm is dental plaque, which causes caries, gingivitis, and periodontitis. A connection between the germs in the biofilm in case of periodontitis and various systemic illnesses such as cardiovascular and respiratory diseases as well as diabetes is being discussed. Bacterial biofilms on the eardrum in children could be the cause for constantly recurring chronic ear infections (Otis media). The tissue of many patients with sinusitis also contains organized biofilms. Fibronectin is considered to create the prerequisite for biofilms, whereby these substances are released in heart-valve patients with defects of the vascular endothelium. Biofilms were also detected in biopsy material from males with prostatitis such as mucoviscidosis patients (Christoph et al., 2005).

Depending on the body region where which germs are the issue for an implant-associated infection, different antimicrobial agents can and must be equipped with coatings.

6.8 Antimicrobial Agents

The procedures applied to reduce the number of germs on a surface are well-known. To avoid infections during surgical procedures, surgeons and microbiologists can avail themselves of various antimicrobial substances, which are summarized in the following sections (Mims et al., 2006).

6.9 Antiseptic Agents

Antiseptics sum up chemical substances that are essentially applied as disinfection agents (reduction by at least 5 log units of microorganisms; sterilization is equal to the reduction of at least 6 log units, see Table 6.5). In medicine, antiseptics are used in case of wound infections, e.g., to prevent sepsis. Antiseptics can be subdivided into heavy metal ions, agents containing halogens, organic ammonium salts, phenols and phenol derivatives, and alcohols.

Table 6.5 Germ-reduction procedure

Procedure	Reduce of germs	Survivor
Cleaning	Reduction by 0–2 power of 10	Viruses, bacteria, fungus/ fungus spores
Disinfection	Reduction by 3–5 power of 10	Viruses, bacteria, fungus/ fungus spores
Sterilization	Reduction by more than 6 power of 10	Particularly bacterial spores
Decontamination	Elimination of living and dead microorganisms, including endotoxins	

6.10 Heavy Metal Ions

Although heavy metals, such as silver ions, copper ions, mercury ions, or zinc, possess an excellent broad antimicrobial impact, they prefer to randomly attack S–H groups and are not capable of differentiating whether it is a bacterial protein with an S–H group or a vital protein of the host cell with an S–H group.

This random mode of action has to be considered a disadvantage. Furthermore, the statement that there are no resistance mechanisms against heavy metal ions is not sustainable (Hasman et al., 2006). Alternately, antibiotics attack specifically only the microorganism that tries to rapidly spread within the body without poisoning the host organism in the process.

All these antiseptic agents based on chemical toxins have the disadvantage that they randomly attack a central molecular structure within the body and destroy it. In contrast to chemical toxins, antibiotics are antibacterial substances that attack a specific target in the cell. For example, they specifically block an important metabolic process of the bacterial organism. As a consequence, the bacteria are no longer viable.

6.11 Antiseptics Containing Halogen

These antiseptic substances are characterized by iodine containing compounds and hypochlorites (salts of hypochloric acid, HClO). For example, the "mild" iodine-containing antiseptics typically used for the disinfection of skin were developed on the basis of the knowledge that they were capable of quickly killing germs by completely encapsulating the bacteria. On the other hand, hypochlorites were used for surface disinfection and are a component of the "respiratory burst" in the context of the cellular defense of microorganisms. There they are formed by the neutrophilic myeloperoxidase and released into the phagolysosom (Löffler et al., 2007).

In addition, chlorine-, bromine-, or iodine-containing solutions can be utilized for antiseptic surface treatment and are used topically for smaller wounds and wound dressings. However, these antiseptics work unspecifically, can attack, e.g., sulfur compounds, and thus lead to the deactivation of microorganisms.

6.12 Organic Ammonium Salts

Quaternary ammonium compounds, such as benzalkonium chloride, appear in disinfection agents (Sagrotan®) and in algicides as active ingredient. In medicine, they also serve as a means for the preventive treatment of mucous infections due to dermatophytes and are applied in antiseptic mouthwashes and particularly as a preservative. As a cationic surfactant, cetyltrimethylammonium bromide represents a further ammonium salt. Octenidine is characterized by its broad-spectrum effectiveness against Gram-positive and Gram-negative germs, yeasts, fungal infection, and encapsulated viruses. It is sufficiently active against MRSA without disturbing wound healing. Its application in the medical field includes gynecology and urology. It does not attack mucous membranes and is active in very low dosages as well as not being neurotoxic. Dequalinium chloride is used in medicine in vaginal tablets, lozenges, as a solution for gargling, and in nose drops (e.g., Fluomizin®, Anginova®). Chlorhexidine (CHX) contains two benzene rings and appears as chloride, acetate, or gluconate. It is characterized by its extremely broad active spectrum. Hardly any substance is described as thoroughly as chlorhexidine. It adheres perfectly to teeth and can easily penetrate mucous membranes. Chlorhexidine is almost completely discharged without being metabolized. Its effect is the destruction of the bacterial cell membrane. As a pharmaceutical product, chlorhexidine is applied in the so-called PerioChip® (36% chlorhexidine). In dentistry, chlorhexidine is found in a multitude of mouthwashes and in the topical application in wound ointments and powders. Polyhexanide is used medically for the rinsing of infected wounds and in wound dressings. Due to its good tissue tolerance and wound-healing promotion, polyhexanide is often applied in case of badly healing wounds. It particularly serves as preservative for cosmetics. Polyhexanide possesses a broad active spectrum, including being effective against methicillin-resistant *Staphylococcus aureus* (MRSA).

6.13 Phenols and Phenol Derivatives

Phenol is the simplest of benzene-derived phenol with only one hydroxy group and the molecular formula C_6H_5OH. Interesting out of this group is triclosan as a derivative of phenol, since it is already on the market in a licensed medical device (suture material). It possesses an active spectrum that is effective against Gram-positive germs. It does not have a broad spectrum and is capable of chemically transforming to produce chlorinated benzo-furan and chlorinated benzo-dioxine. It negatively affects the central nervous system and is linked to increased allergies and asthma. It is also likely to promote bacterial resistance and induce cross-resistance. It may degrade into dioxin, which is toxic and has to be highly pre-purified to prevent formation of chlorinated benzo-dioxine. Further antiseptics are found among the chinolin derivatives (e.g., oxichinolin) and among the benzochinon derivatives (e.g., ambazon).

6.14 Alcohols

Isopropanol, ethanol, and propanole can be utilized as antiseptics. A certain content of water is required in case of ethanol 70–80% to be an optimal disinfectant. It is regarded as an ideal means for the disinfection of hands. Proteins are encapsulated by alcohol and unfurl, which causes their protective cover to disintegrate, denaturing the proteins in the process.

6.15 Chemotherapeutics/Anti-Infective Agents

Chemotherapeutics are low-molecular, naturally appearing, or synthetically manufactured chemical compounds used for the most selective possible damage of somatic cells and/or pathogens. Cytostatika are utilized as drugs in the treatment of cancer; pharmaceutical products and/or drugs combating infectious diseases are characterized as anti-infective agents. Depending on the type of the causative agent, differentiation is made between antibiotics (against bacteria), virostatic agents (against viruses), antimycotic agents (against fungi), and anthelmintic agents (against worms).

The classical subdivisions of chemotherapeutics particularly distinguish between the chemical structures of the substances as well as their mechanism of action (target). Among the chemotherapeutics, particularly antibiotics are interesting for the coating of implants; for this reason, we examine this substance group in detail below. Antibiotics work selectively against bacteria and hereby attack various positions of the microorganism.

6.15.1 Inhibition of Cell Wall Biosynthesis

(ß-Lactam-antibiotics, Glykopeptide, Fosfomycin)
For example, these antibiotics inhibit murein-biosynthesis: fosfomycin, cycloserin, terizidon, bacitracin, vancomycin, ß-lactame antibiotics such as methicillin, peniciline, cephalosporine, monobactame, carbapeneme (imipenem, meropenem), many penicillins and cephalosporine (e.g., Ceftibuten).

6.15.2 Blocking of Protein Synthesis

(Aminoglykoside, Tetracycline, Chloramphenicol, Macrolide, Lincosamide)
Inhibitors of protein-biosynthesis form aminoglycosides such as streptomycin, neomycin, kanamycin, gentamicin, amikacin, tobramycin; tetracycline such as tetracyclin, minocyclin, doxycyclin, oxytetracyclin; macrolide such as erythromycin, clarithromycin, roxithromycin, azitromycin, spiramycin; chloramphenicol; das lincosamid-antibiotice clindamycin; fusidin acid and linezolid (oxazolidon-antibiotic).

6.15.3 Suppression of Nucleic Acid Synthesis

(Rifampicin (Ansamycin-antibiotic), Sulfonamide, Gyrase inhibitors)

Gyrase inhibitors such as fluorochinolone: norfloxacin, pefloxacin, ciprofloxacin, ofloxacin, sparfloxacin, moxifloxacin; folic acid antagonists such as sulphonamides: sulfadiazin, sulfamethoxazol, sulfalen, and diamino-benzylpyrimidine: trimethoprim, pyrimethamin; nitroimidazol derivations such as metronidazol, nimorazol, tinidazol; flucytosin, antiviral polymerase inhibitors.

6.15.4 Interference with Permeability of Cytoplasma Membrane

(Polyen antibiotics, Polypeptid antibiotics)
Polypetides such as colistine and lipopetides such as daptomycin (depolarization of membrane potentials) destroy bacterial structures by the changing permeability.

6.16 Bacteriostasis/Bacteriocidal

Antibiotics can inhibit the growth and/or reproduction of bacteria (bacteriostasis) or ensure the destruction of the microorganisms (bacteriocidal). These include those which always (sulfonamides) and those which predominately (tetracyline) work bacteriostatic. However, aminoglycosides are always bactericide, and penicillin kills bacteria only during the reproduction phase.

6.17 Mechanism of Action of Antibiotics

Antibiotics selectively attack molecular structures of pathogenic bacteria. For example, sulfanilamid attacks only a single bacterial enzyme in the nucleotide synthesis of the bacterium and is thus harmless for the human body. Many microorganisms in the ground emit antibiotics specifically to secure a competitive advantage for themselves. They are resistant themselves and kill their direct competitors.

Penicillin produced by mould fungi selectively blocks the enzyme that synthesizes the peptidoglycan layer of the bacterial cell wall. In the process, the bacterial cell loses its outer protective layer and can be easily attacked by the host organism and metabolized. The human body does not possess such peptidoglycan structures; therefore, only the bacterial cell is being attacked. It is, therefore, the objective of antibiotic research to find such processes that occur only in pathogenic organisms and to equip the antibiotic active ingredients in such a manner to ensure that they destroy exactly these processes. Chloramphenicol and streptomycin selectively attack the bacterial ribosomes that are made of completely different structures—30s and 60s subunits—than those of the human ribosomal organelle, which consists of 40s and 80s subunits.

6.18 Rifampicin

With excellent bone and cell penetration, rifampicin attacks the mRNA polymerase of pathogens and is systematically applied in case of infected revisions such as in combination with chinolon antibiotics (combination therapy). It possesses verifiably excellent activity against sessile bacteria in the biofilm and is characterized by the greatest effect against *Staphylococcal* of all currently available antibiotics. Rifampicin possesses the same bioavailability in oral as well as intra venous administration; there are currently hardly any primary resistance known against *Staphylococcal*. However, in a monotherapy, rifampicin produces extremely quick resistance and so a combination with a chinolon, such as levofloxacin, is recommended. Rifampicin has significant side effects and is a reserve antibiotic.

6.19 Resistance

Resistance describes the property of microorganisms to reduce or completely neutralize the effect of antibiotics. The fact that every bacterium is resistant against some antibiotics (such as cephalosporins against *Enterococci*) is known as natural (intrinsic) resistance. For example, Gram-negative bacteria possess an outer membrane, which represents a barrier against the penetration of antibiotics (Donlan, 2001). The bacterium could furthermore lack a transport system for the antibiotic or the metabolic pathway against which the antibiotic is supposed to work.

Opposed to natural resistance is the phenomenon of acquired resistance in which originally sensitive bacteria become resistant against certain antibiotics due to changes in their genetic makeup. This type of acquired resistance is known in *Staphylococci*, which became resistant against penicillin upon extensive exposure to the antibiotic (Jefferson, 2004).

Bacteria are capable of acquiring resistances against all anti-infective chemical and biological substances. The microorganisms developed excellent strategies also for this purpose. Thus a particular organelle of the bacterial cell can initiate an increased pump mechanism (flux), which ejects the "poison" that entered the bacterial cytoplasm. Such active transports are described for heavy metals such as silver, copper, and others just as for the classic antibiotics (Hasman et al., 2006). Other bacteria can actively close their pores and thus prevent the intrusion of antibiotic toxins. In addition, nature always produces mutations, which are encoded in the genetic structure of the bacteria cell and naturally also passed on through the generations. Tuberculosis bacteria are especially devious; although they are easily recognized and phagocytized by the macrophages once they have entered the body of the host, they cannot be killed by the host cells. They are able to survive in the cytoplasm within the macrophage to develop resistances and to be delivered into the blood stream from the macrophages in case of a weak immune system. Resistant bacteria are furthermore capable to synthesize a defense enzyme that can even eliminate antibiotics. For example, bacteria can produce a penicillin-splitting enzyme that ferrets out, splits, and deactivates the antibiotic. The synthesis of this particular enzyme represents a modified form of a normal digestive enzyme and is encoded on small DNA plasmid rings of the bacterial cell. Unfortunately, these mobile genetic elements facilitate an information exchange from one bacteria to the next, ensuring quick spreading of the resistance gene within a bacteria population (Table 6.6). This transfer mechanism is particularly problematic in organized biofilms as they harbor a large number of bacteria of various species; the various types of bacteria are capable of receiving the resistance information from several sources leading often to cross-resistances. An additional viral attack of the bacteria cells is particularly dramatic in this context. The viruses infect the bacterium, and the altered genomes hereby adopt possible resistance genes of the bacterium and transfer these to the entire bacterial colony. Therefore, many research efforts that stand in constant battle with the resistance development of bacteria focus on the plasmids and their information cascade. The objective is to interrupt them intelligently, thus preventing the transmission of information (Goodsell, 2010).

Table 6.6 Resistance mechanisms

The mechanisms of bacterial resistance in biofilm are based on a number of factors:
Intrinsic resistance:
➢ Reduced penetration of anti-microbial substances through the biofilm
➢ Chemically-altered micro-environment, e.g. lack of oxygen, changes in the pH value
Acquired resistance:
➢ Reduced growth rate of the bacteria in the biofilm
➢ Modified, multi resistant phenotypes with resistance gene expression
➢ "Persister cells" and "small-colony variants"
For example:
1. Enzyme: they split and deactivate antibiotics - e.g. Escherichia coli
2. Pumps: molecular structures of the cell wall which actively, quickly eject antibiotics before they can affect the cell - e.g.pseudonomas aerugionosa,
3. Replacing the bacterial target structure of the antibiotic: lack of recognition - e.g. staphylococcusaerues. VRSA

Others, in turn, explore the living conditions of the bacteria and try to specifically intervene in the close-knit supply system of the bacteria. Particularly siderophores, linked to beta-lactam antibiotics, are capable of significantly improving their antibacterial activity. Siderophore antibiotic conjugates were used as a "Trojan Horse" strategy to overcome penetration-mediated bacterial antibiotic resistance (Miller and Malouin, 1994). Such structures are bacterial iron chelators, mostly containing catecholate or hydroxamate groups as chelating ligands. They are expressed under iron starvation conditions and sequester extracellular ferric ions (Winkelmann et al., 1987). Specific bacterial outer membrane receptors recognize the iron-complexed siderophores and initiate the active transport into the bacterial cell. Wittmann et al. (2002) investigated this phenomenon and found that most of the conjugates with beta-lactams showed high in vitro activity against Gram-negative bacteria, especially *Pseudomonas aeruginosa, Escherichia coli, Klebsiella pneumoniae, Serratia marcescens,* and *Stenotrophomonas maltophilia.* The compounds with enhanced antibacterial activity use active iron uptake routes to penetrate the bacterial outer membrane barrier, demonstrated by assays with mutants deficient in components of the iron transport system.

6.20 Methicillin-Resistant *Staphylococcus Aureus*

Methicillin, a close derivative of penicillin, was successfully used in 1959 as an antibiotic against bacteria, which became impervious to penicillin, thus also *Staphylococcus aureus and Streptococcus pneumoniae.* As early as 1961, the first methicillin-resistant *S. aureus* (MRSA) became known. In the 1980s, MRSA was widespread in hospitals and care facilities and later also beyond such establishments. Until today, treatment is difficult because an uninhibited systemic spread is often found in the entire body. Alas, MRSA is furthermore resistant against almost all beta-lactam antibiotics such as cephalosporine and derivatives of penicillin, meaning an antibiotic group that is particularly important in therapy and is often applied. Of all things, MRSA produces an enzyme that splits and deactivates beta-lactam. The often chosen answer is the reserve antibiotic vancomycin. However, strains of MRSA are already resistant against this glycopeptide antibiotic. VRSA is characterized by several resistance genes, which were acquired in a so-called gene cassette. These genes encode special enzymes that exchange the original target structure for vancomycin in the cell wall. Vancomycin is no longer able to dock on and fails.

6.21 Resistance in Biofilms

Bacteria organized in the biofilm are usually "mute" due to the extreme cell density and are characterized by a severely reduced metabolism. The multilayered mucous coat of polysaccharide works like a barrier for the body's own immune system and, in addition, lastingly inhibits the activities of the immune cells (Costerton et al., 1987; von von Eiff et al., 1999). In case of primary (intrinsic) resistance, reduced cell growth and reduced nutrient intake due to decelerated diffusion pathways inside the biofilm result in the fact that also anti-infective substances can penetrate such protected layers of the biofilm only limitedly and in very low concentration. This decelerated disposition provides bacteria with the optimal opportunity to develop resistances (Tresse et al., 1995). The bacteria in the biofilm tolerate extremely high antibiotic concentration (up to 1000 fold) compared to plantonic life forms, obviously due to the reduced growth of the germs (Jefferson, 2004; Costerton et al., 1999). The acquired resistance is created by an intelligent cell-to-cell communication system (quorum sensing) and is based on phenotypical differences of the bacteria in the biofilm, which may particularly affect the growth rate and gene expression (Donlan, 2001). The exchange of genetic materials is significantly facilitated and enables the transfer of antibiotic-resistant phenotypes.

6.22 Small-Colony Variants and Persister Cells

Specialized germ subpopulations can form in the biofilm with increasing development, which serve as a nutrient and oxygen barrier. These are obviously capable of entering dormant metabolic phases. These so-called "small-colony variants" are characterized by reduced sensitivity toward anti-infective agents (Neut et al., 2007). In addition, further specialized representatives may form, which neither distinguish themselves nor die in the presence of anti-infective agents (persister cells)(Lewis, 2008; Stewart, 2002; Cogan, 2006). Small-colony variants as well as persister cells are attributed with the ability to develop into viable bacteria after an antibiotic therapy and to significantly contribute to the development of resistances (Lewis et al., 1991; Roberts and Stewart, 2005).

6.23 Coating Strategies of Implants

Infections during surgical procedures are steadily increasing and endanger health and life of the patients involved. Furthermore, subsequent treatment, as previously illustrated, causes extremely high costs, which strain the health-care system long term. Operations related to implant-associated infections are always major and time-consuming medical challenges for the treating physicians. Causes for implant-associated infections are the constantly increasing number of operations with implants. This does not only concern the increasing number of younger patients, but that of older, weakened, and multi-morbid people in an ever-changing society, where patients are subject to therapeutic measures due to previous illnesses, which significantly weaken the body's defense system. Another peculiarity is a significant increase in revision surgery and difficult and complicated operations with a high risk of infection. The increase of the appearance of problem germs and multi-resistant bacteria in hospitals is also noteworthy. Lacking understanding for hygiene and further education of specialists, but also economic measures in the operating theatre due to increasing cost pressure, add to the unsatisfactory situation. Against this background, it becomes an issue that options are available at all to sensibly equip implants with antimicrobial substances. The following contemplations particularly concentrate on combining metallic implants, which generally remain within the body for quite a long period of time, with antimicrobial substance on the surface of the implant.

6.24 Antimicrobial Protection of Biomaterials

Implants are biomaterials and consist of various materials. Biomaterials are synthetic or natural materials that support and/or replace various bodily functions of a special type in medicine and are in direct interaction with the human biological systems. The affinity of various biomaterials and/or their materials toward microorganisms is quite different and depends on the material and its surface on one hand and the location of the implant within the body on the other (Thull, 2004). Bacteria such as *Staphylococcus epidermidis* can obviously colonize polymers and, e.g., hydroxylapatite a little easier than metals, for which in turn *Staphylococcus aureus* seems to be more interesting (Fig. 6.3). The rougher a polymer or metallic surface, the greater the likelihood of it being colonized by microorganisms.

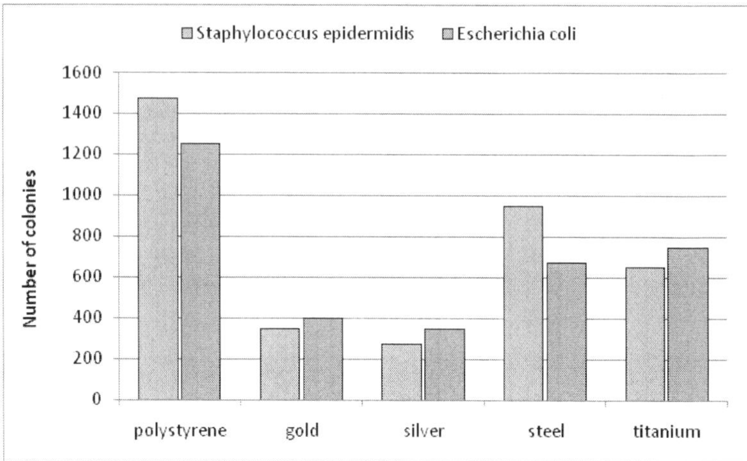

Figure 6.3 Affinity of germs to biomaterial surfaces (Thull 2004).

6.25 Systemic Antibiotic Administration

Despite the implementation of strict hygienic measures in the operating theatre, systemic antibiotics are administered in any surgical intervention to prevent surgical site infection to occur. The preferred antibiotic agents are cephalosporins, such as cephazoline, cefuroxime, or cefoxitine. A single shot is usually administered shortly before the operation (30–60 min prior to incision, see Table 6.7). It is absolutely mandatory that a sufficiently high antibiotic concentration is achieved in the serum and in the surgical site before the incision takes place. Since patients with implants are at a generally higher risk for infections, an optimal systemic antibiotic prophylaxis is particularly important in this group, given the fact that an infection may stem not only from nearby contamination sites but also from remote areas from which bacteria travel via the blood stream (hematogenous infections).

6.26 Local Antibiotic Administration

Since the sole systemic antibiotic administration is not always sufficient to reduce the risk of an implant-associated infection, on the long term it should be combined with the administration of a locally delivered antibiotic agent. The operational use of osteosynthesis material or bone-anchored implants in "difficult-to-access" regions of the body represents a worst-case scenario. Bone tissue pharmacologically represents a functional lower "compartment" and the systemically administered antibiotics are often not capable of penetrating into deeper tissues because of the following reasons (Table 6.8).

Table 6.7 Antibiotic administration in primary surgeries without infection

- ➢ Systemic antibiotic administration (preventive)
- ➢ Is preferred in the prohylaxis = e.g. broad spectrum cephelosporins
- ➢ Single shot
- ➢ Immediately following initiation of anaesthesia - and again after approx. 30 minutes
- ➢ Cephalosporins have a broad and fast mode of action
- ➢ Also oxacilline
- ➢ Local administration = e.g. gentamicin-containing (broad spectrum) Palacos® cement

Table 6.8 Systemic antibiotic administration: barriers

Molecules, membranes, cells, tissues, and organs are penetrated or bypassed
Active ingredients: toxic for certain organs
Active ingredients: low affinity to the destination
Premature inactivation
Expulsion
Diffusion and penetration barriers at the infection location

In addition, the various antibiotics in hospital use vary greatly in their ability to penetrate bone. Pharmacocinetic tests revealed, e.g., that the lincosamid antibiotic clindamicin, which is particularly used in dentistry, has excellent bone-penetration properties (Table 6.9).

Table 6.9 Systemic antibiotic treatment: pharmacokinetic bone (Mader and Adams, 1988)

Antibiotic	Concentration		
	Serum (μg/ml)	Infected bone (μg/g)	Serum (%)
Clindamycin (70 mg/kg)	12.1 ± 0.6	11.9 ± 1.9	98.3
Vancomycin (30 mg/kg)	36.4 ± 4.6	5.3 ± 0.8	14.5
Nafcillin (40 mg/kg)	21.8 ± 4.6	2.1 ± 0.3	9.6
Moxalacram (40 mg/kg)	65.2 ± 5.2	6.2 ± 0.7	9.5
Tobramycin (5 mg/kg)	14.3 ± 1.3	1.3 ± 0.1	9.1
Cefazolin (15 mg/kg)	67.2 ± 2.6	2.6 ± 0.2	6.1
Cefazolin (5 mg/kg)	45.6 ± 3.2	2.6 ± 0.2	5.7
Cephalothin (40 mg/kg)	34.8 ± 2.8	1.3 ± 0.2	3.7

For best clinical efficacy, the combined systemic and local antibiotic administration has become standard of care in cemented arthroplasty. The best clinically studied and commercially available drug delivery device for controlled local release of antibiotics was gentamicin-sulfate-containing Palacos® R (Buchholz and Engelbrecht, 1970). Based on the experiences with gentamicin-containing Palacos® R, the PMMA beads were developed in the 1980s. Due to their high active ingredient content and the ideal spherical surface, these PMMA chains were successfully used as local agent carrier in the treatment of bone infections in the two-stage arthroplasty exchange and in soft tissue infections, such as after corrected fracture repair. The PMMA bone cement polymer serves as carrier matrix for the incorporated active ingredients. The PMMA beads were strung onto surgical wire and temporarily inserted at the infection site. However, for some applications, the undegradable PMMA polymer, which has to be extracted in a second operation, is not always the ideal carrier of active ingredients. As a consequence, new absorbable biomaterials have been developed to circumvent this problem of a second intervention. To this class belong a wide variety of materials such as the bone graft substitutes on a calcium basis (e.g., hydroxylapatite or calcium sulfate and/or tri-calcium phosphate), gelatines, and/or collagen fleeces, all loaded with various anti-infective ingredients.

6.27 PMMA Bone Cements as Local Carriers of Active Ingredients

As mentioned before, a US meta study retrospectively showed that local antibiotics in PMMA bone cements can reduce the risk of infection in primary cemented arthroplasty by more than 50%. The PMMA matrix contains finely dispersed antibiotic particles, which are locally released after the implantation and act peri- and postoperatively as a bacterial colonization barrier and even anti-infective treatment support (Parvizi et al., 2008).

For cemented prostheses, the addition of antibiotics, especially gentamicin sulfate, to PMMA bone cements is a clinically proven and successful method for approximately 30 years. Thermostability as well as high water solubility properties of the antibiotics in the PMMA matrix are fundamental requirements for high efficient ingredient elution. It is of greatest importance to stick to the recommendation to add the antibiotics only to the cement powder, never to the liquid component of PMMA cements. After the implantation, the cured PMMA bone cement fulfill a double function: anchoring of the metallic implant and local release of antibiotics.

The principle of the local antibiotic treatment (GB) in bone cement was described in detail by Wahlig in 1987 (Fig. 6.4). The elution behavior of the gentamicin-containing Palacos® R was investigated. Comparably high gentamicin concentrations were measured locally. Up to 47 μg/ml was detectable in spongious bone, 11 μg/ml of gentamicin was found in cancellous bone, and still 1 μg/ml was found in cortical bone; 17 μg/ml was detected in connective tissue in the interface. The measured gentamicin concentrations were hardly detectable systemically and amounted to 0.7 μg/ml in the serum and 17 μg/ml in urine. In comparison, only a minimal local concentration of 0.4 μg/ml could be detected following a single intramascular shot of 1 × 80 mg gentamicin sulfate solution, while comparably higher gentamicin concentrations of approximately 5 μg/ml were detected in the serum and approximately 200 μg/ml in the urine. As an alternative or partner of gentamicin, several other antibiotics are used in bone cement (Table 6.10) (Wahlig, 1987).

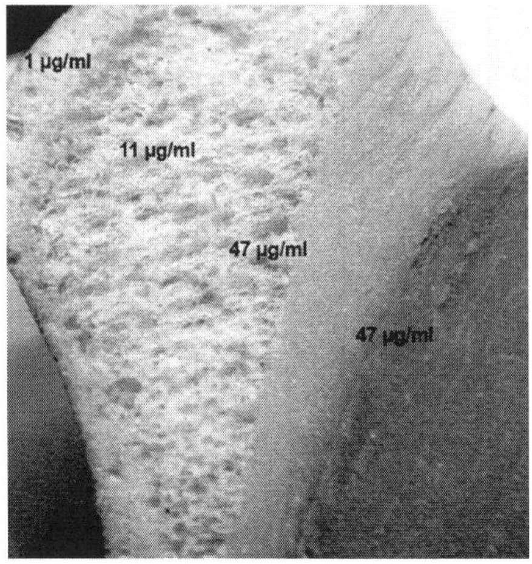

Figure 6.4 PMMA: Principle of antibiotic release

The antibiotic release from the PMMA bone cements is initiated when the polymer comes into contact with secretion and blood. The incorporated water penetrates into the cement surface and diffuses further into the cement matrix. During this process, the antibiotic dissolves into the areas close to the surface and diffuses to the cement surface. This means the release of the antibiotic from the cement matrix depends on the surface and follows the rules of diffusion. This process is also closely related to the hydrophilic properties of the bone cement. As a consequence, the active agent release proceeds proportionally to the water absorption on the one hand and the available cement surface on the other. The composition of the polymers in the bone cement and thus the water absorption of the cement significantly influences the release of the active agent.

6.28 Metallic Implants

The local antimicrobial protection of the surface of cementless prostheses, osteosynthetic screws, plates, nails, or fixations, dental implants, or spine implants has more or less been disregarded until today. As well as several steel alloys, particularly titanium and/or titanium alloys, are used, which represent a particularly interesting and suitable implant material for such prostheses due to their relatively low E-modulus and the passivation layer on the surface.

Table 6.10 Antibiotics in commercially available PMMA cements

Antibiotic	Class	Bactericidal [+], bacteriostatic [–]	Target	Effective against	Gram-positive [+], Gram-negative [–]	Example
Gentamicin	Aminoglycoside	+	Inhibits bacterial protein synthesis; formation of nonsense proteins; disturbs the reading of mRNA on 30s ribosomes	Staphylococcus spec., *E. coli*, Enterobacter, Pseudonomads, Klebsiella, Proteus	+/–	Palacos® R+G
Tobramycin	Aminoglycoside	+	Inhibits bacterial protein synthesis; disturbs the reading of mRNA on 30s ribosomes	Staphylococcus spec., *E. coli*, Enterobacter, Pseudonomads, Klebsiella, Proteus	+/–	Simplex® with Tobramycin

(*Continued*)

Table 6.10 (*Continued*)

Antibiotic	Class	Bactericidal [+], bacteriostatic [–]	Target	Effective against	Gram-positive [+], Gram-negative [–]	Example
Clindamycin	Lincoamide	– to +	Inhibits bacterial protein synthesis; binding on 50s ribosomes and inhibits protein synthesis	Streptococcus, Staphylococcus, Anaerobia, Propioni	+/–	Copal® G+C
Vancomycin	Glycopeptid	+	Inhibits the bacterial cell wall cross-link	Staphylococcus spec., MRSA, MRSE	+	Copal® G+V
Erythromycin	Makrolide	–	Inhibits the protein synthesis on ribosomes	Streptococcus, Staphylococcus, Anaerobe, Corynebacteria	+	Simplex®AKZ
Colistine	Polypetide	+	Changes permeability of the cytoplasm membrane	Pseudonomads, not Proteus	–	Simplex®AKZ

Some methods for the local antimicrobial protection of such metallic implant surfaces are known:

1. Polymer-layer-forming carrier system with incorporated antibiotics/antiseptics/peptides
2. Antibiotics/antiseptics/peptides included in porous hydroxylapatite or calcium phosphate coatings
3. Coating with heavy metal/heavy metal salts with or without an additional layer
4. Coating with self-adhesive, low soluble antibiotic/antiseptic salts

In the following section, the major coating strategies are described in detail using metallic implants as example. Subsequently, further metallic and nonmetallic biomaterials are introduced, which essentially feature similar coating strategies (Kühn and Vogt, 2007, see Table 6.11).

6.29 Polymer-Layer-Forming Carrier System with Incorporated Antibiotics/Antiseptics

One option of a local implant protection is the integration of antimicrobial substances into a polymer-layer-forming carrier system (Kanellakopoulou and Giamarellos-Bourboulis, 2000; Anderson, 2003; Lucke et al., 2003; Gollwitzer et al., 2003) with incorporated antibiotics. These coatings are made of biodegradable polyesters such as polylactide, including gentamicin sulfate as an antibiotic. These coatings provide the benefit that different soluble antibiotics/antiseptics can be included without the necessity of chemical modifications of the active substance and that registered polymers such as polylactide can be applied as layer-forming material. The device registration process is, therefore, less extensive compared to new carrier systems or active agents. Nonetheless, these coatings also have their disadvantages. Active substance suspensions are usually utilized for the coating process. The purpose of the active substance suspensions is the provision of homogeneity during the coating process to achieve reproducible loading concentrations. Basically, the active substance release does not proceed concurrently with the forming of the polymer layer. The formation of acid-degradation

Table 6.11 Coating strategies: advantages and disadvantages

Approach	Advantages	Disadvantages
Polymer layer-forming carrier with incorporated antibiotics	➢ Antibiotics may be highly soluble in water ➢ Different antibiotics may be used without modification ➢ Use of approved layer-forming material	➢ Coating technology with suspensions complex ➢ Release of antibiotics not synchronic with layer degradation ➢ Polymer layer-forming materials (PLLA) degrade slowly, releasing degradation products (acid release) ➢ Layer as additional barrier to bone growth
Antibiotics in porous hydroxyl apatite coatings	➢ Use of easily soluble antibiotics ➢ No modification required ➢ No polymer layer-forming material ➢ No degradation products ➢ Use of typical HA-coated implants	➢ Limited protraction of antibiotic release ➢ Easily soluble antibiotics are quickly dissolved from the surface ➢ Limited to HA-coated implants
Coating with heavy metals or heavy metal salts	➢ Silver or copper (ions) with broad antimicrobial effect ➢ Relatively cost-saving	➢ Silver and copper ions are potentially cytotoxic ➢ Unspecific effect ➢ Silver ions react with human proteins ➢ Silver ions from hardly soluble salts ➢ Silver ions are easy to reduce
Coating with self-adhesive low-soluble antibiotic salts	➢ No polymeric layer ➢ No acidic degradation products ➢ Antibiotic release synchronic with layer degradation ➢ Simple coating technology	➢ Sparingly soluble salts of antibiotics accessible by ion exchange ➢ Problem of registration/approval

products has to be considered in the application of polymer layer formation based on hydroxycarboxylic acid.

Currently, an entire series of further biodegradable substances applied to an implant in the form of a spray or immersion process are tested in trials . Dissolved active ingredients are subsequently released. For example, biopolymers on cellulose basis (polysaccharide, chitosan, starch, glycogen, collagen), polyhydroxyalkanoate (PHB), proteins, and peptides as well as metallic Mg-compounds and, e.g., spider silk are pulverized and processed into scaffolds. Anti-infective substances are incorporated into the scaffolds as early as during manufacture, or it is done via subsequent coating of the scaffolds. Generally, a multitude of microbial agents can be combined with such materials (Sripriya et al., 2004; Prabu et al., 2006). As well as the degradation products and the possible occurrence of endotoxins, also the interaction between carrier and active ingredients, have to be considered in such products. To achieve a sensible retard effect of the eluted active ingredient from such carriers, additional substances have to be utilized at times or the matrix has to be subjected to special treatment.

Marrow nails are currently available in the market, which are equipped with a polylactide layer suspended in gentamicin sulfate as antimicrobial ingredient. The polymer layer adheres well to the smooth metallic surface of the implant (Fig. 6.5). However, the layer quite easily shears off during the implantation and the original surface protection does no longer exist.

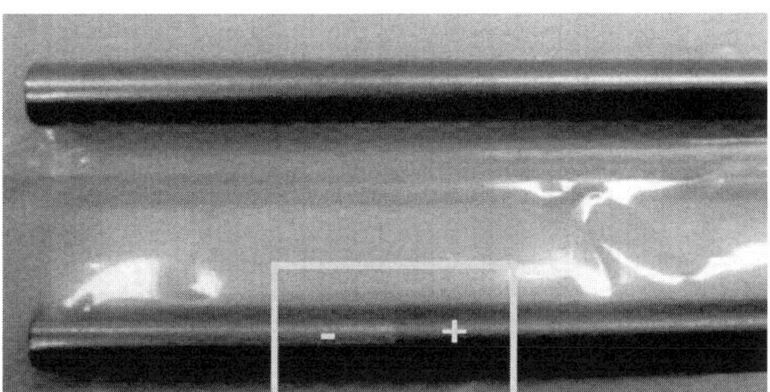

– means without coating; + means PLLA/G-coating

Figure 6.5 Marrow nail coated with PLLA/gentamicin (Gollwitzer et al. 2003).

Newly developed polymer pockets are offered in the USA in cardiology, consisting of dual components (resorbable and nonresorbable), being sterile prostheses designed with an open-pore weave, knotted filaments of lightweight polypropylene mesh and coated with a resorbable polymer (AIGISRx). The nonresorbable mesh substrate is a large-pore mesh knitted from monofilament polypropylene filaments, similar in composition and diameter to 5–0 suture (Fig. 6.6). The knitted mesh represents over 90% of the entire AIGISRx® device by weight. The bioresorbable and biocompatible polymer based on the amino acid tyrosine breaks down linearly, primarily via hydrolysis and is resorbed within approximately 140 days. This bio-resorbable polymer breaks down into naturally occurring components. Its primary purpose is to act as a carrier for the antimicrobial agents. The tyrosine polymer and drug combination, which is spray coated onto the polypropylene mesh, represents the remaining 10% of the AIGISRx® device by weight.

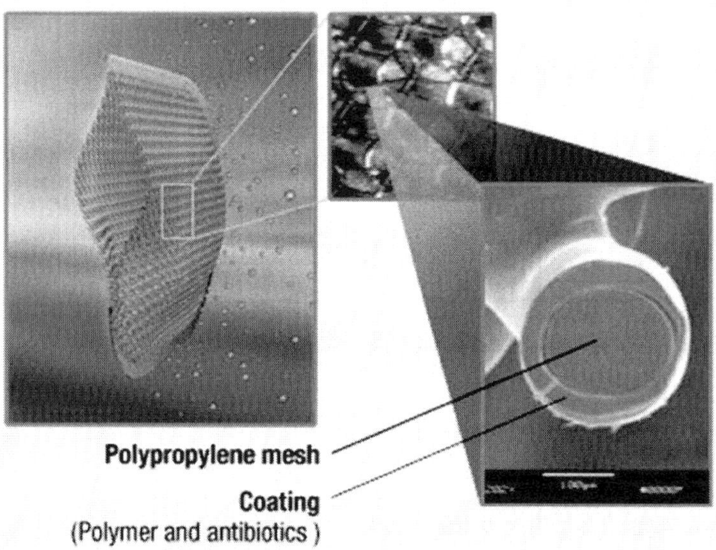

Figure 6.6 AIGISRx® device: principle.

The resorbable polymer carries two distinct antibiotics, namely, minocycline and rifampin (Fig. 6.6). Once the pacemaker or defibrillator is placed into the surgically created pocket, the resorbable polymer begins to break down and releases both antibiotics. The agents are released for 7 to 10 days to reduce the likelihood of an infection. The body absorbs the resorbable polymer over the next approximately 140 days, leaving only the nonresorbable lightweight polypropylene mesh to hold and stabilize the device (Klug et al., 1997; Sohail et al., 2007; Lekkerkerker et al., 2009).

The material is approved by the FDA and is claimed to "help reduce the possibility of infection"! The combination of these active ingredients is not unproblematic in this context, since particularly rifampicin, but also minocycline, is considered reserve antibiotics. Furthermore, the remaining nonresorbable polymer pocket within the body constitutes a further disadvantage, as this pocket represents another ideal retreat for germs. However, the basic principle seems sensible and logical.

6.30 Antibiotics/Antiseptics Included in Porous Hydroxylapatite Coatings

Highly porous implant coatings are not only easily penetrated by germs, but also provide ample surface for antimicrobial active ingredients. Alt et al. (2006) published their experiences with implants that were equipped with a porous hydroxylapatite coating, including gentamicin sulfate and gentamicin crobefat in their cavities. The antibiotics used in these tests are gentamicin salts, which are also used in a commercial collagen fleece. Due to its fast solubility, gentamicin sulfate provides high initial elution peak, while the slowly soluble gentamicin crobefat is responsible for the protracted release of the aminoglycoside gentamicin. Both gentamicin derivatives merely display minor adhesion to surfaces! However, similar to other inorganic coatings, an HA surface coated with such a salt mixture (50:50) exhibits an agent elution under in vitro conditions, which is detectable for only a short time: 60% of the Gentamicin is released within the first two hours, while the residual gentamicin was eluted in the subsequent hours. In total, a release lasting only 24 h could be observed. Vancomycin coatings on calcium phosphate layers (50–80 μm) produced similar results. The calcium phosphate layer was applied to titanium by means of electrophoresis and subsequently sintered at 900°C. Vancomycin was applied by immersion (at 37°C for up to 24 h). It was also released within a few hours. A tobramycin calcium phosphate layer (approximately 40 μm through biometric coating) displayed similar results, while a number of other antibiotics such as cephalothine, carbenicilline, or cefamondole produced good results in this test series (Stigler et al., 2002). Campbell et al. (2000) described an HA+CHX (chlorhexidin) coating, which is supposed to serve for the prevention of infection.

Porous HA layers on implants are characterized by extremely large, but hardly reproducible surfaces. This option provides the advantage that the formation of polymer layers is not required, thus avoiding the imponderability of degradation products. It also permits the utilization of commercially available hydroxylapatite-coated prostheses and implant devices. However, this method has the disadvantage that the retarded release of active substances is only possible with the application of low-soluble active substances. The adhesion of commercially registered antibiotics in the hydroxylapatite layer is relatively low. The loading capacity is mainly determined by the pore volume of the hydroxylapatite coating.

As well as in the coating of the surface of a prosthesis equipped with an additional layer of inorganic salts for the improvement of osteointegration, porous moulds and granulates made of HA, TCP, calcium sulfate, or other calcium compounds are used as coating surface or bone replacement material. The coating concept is comparable; also here the extreme internal surface can be used as depot for active ingredients.

Synthacer® (pure HA) bone substitute, which consists of a high micro as well as macro-porous structure resembling cancellous bone (Schnürer et al., 2003), was coated with gentamicin fatty acid (G-sodium dodecylsulfate, SDS). The pores can be several hundreds of micrometers in diameter and permit incorporation and integration of bone. The initially high release of antibiotic (approximately 60% of the total amount of antibiotic) is followed by a prolonged elution for up to four weeks at a lower rate, which is still microbiologically effective. The more hydrophobic the fatty acid used, the slower is the burst release, yet the longer the protracted release (Teller et al., 2006, see Fig. 6.7). Another degradable composite, namely, pellets of calcium sulfate and nanoparticulate HA (PerOssal®), showed release properties of antibiotics for approximately 10 days (Englert et al., 2007).

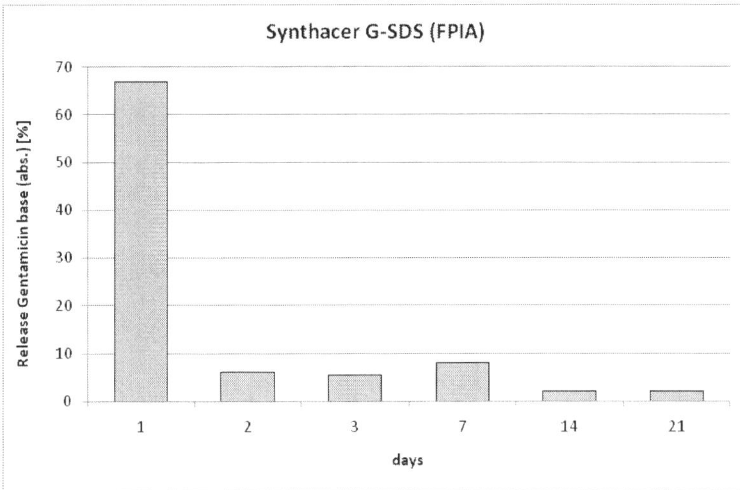

Figure 6.7 Release of gentamicin from Synthacer® loaded by gentamicin fatty acid salt (SDS) (Teller et al. 2006).

6.31 Coating with Heavy Metal/Heavy Metal Salts

A further method is to coat medical implants with heavy metal/heavy metal salts (Illingworth et al., 2000; Ambrosius et al., 1998; Darouiche, 1999; Trerotola et al., 1998; Grzybowski and Trafny, 1999; Ziegler et al., 2003). The application of heavy metals and heavy metal salts as microbiocides has received considerable attention. Among them is, in particular, silver in the form of nanoparticles as well as low soluble silver, because silver as well as copper, zinc, etc., have proven to provide excellent broad antimicrobial properties at relatively low costs.

For example, silver, silver salts (Ag sulfadiazin) or Ag-nanoparticles are used in diverse medical devices:

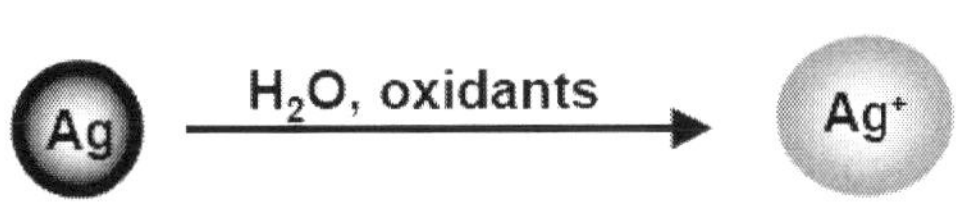

In the process, Ag^+ ions interact with functional groups of proteins (–SH, –S–S, NH_2, –COOH, –OH groups), which may cause damage to the cell membrane and important enzymes. Interactions with cellular DNA and the substitution of other metal ions (Ca, Zn) by Ag in vital enzymes have also been established.

Furthermore, heavy metals and heavy metal salts can be applied to a variety of surfaces or integrated into implants, providing an effectual metal concentration at the surface of the implant (Table 6.12) However, the low selectivity of heavy metals constitutes a clear drawback of this technology. Heavy metal ions, such as silver ions, do not specifically react with microbial structures but will most likely react with human or animal cells and cell components as described above. Therefore, the antimicrobial depth effect of silver ions, particularly in the bone or hard tissues, is limited because heavy metal ions may react with components of bone tissue leading to the formation of low soluble salts in the process. Furthermore, silver ions, similar to other heavy metal ions, are chemically easily reduced. It is, therefore, expected that heavy metal ions released from the surface will most likely react with blood components such as sulfates and phosphates to silver sulfates and/or silver phosphates. These almost insoluble salts are evacuated and stored in body tissue with the following consequences:

1. Heavy metal ions are quickly neutralized and can thus become ineffective against bacteria.
2. Heavy metal ions are not or not easily eliminated from the body and thus remain in the body tissue.

Copper ions may also be considered suitable anti-infective coating material as they occur naturally in our organism. However, copper appears exclusively bound in complex structures and free copper ions may also be highly toxic for the human body. Diverse copper coatings have been described so far in literature. For example, TiO_2 layers are produced with Cu^{2+} ion endowment. A sol-gel system based on tetrabutoxytitanat/s-butanol was chosen as the carrier layer. Cu(II)-acetate was introduced into the sol, and drying and calcification occurred at 500°C. The layer was applied to Ti_6Al_4V test specimens by way of dip coating (construction of multilayers (1x to 4x). A good bactericide effect against MRSA strains (up to 6 log units) as well as minimal cytocompatibility was observed in vitro. Furthermore, excellent mechanical stability of the coating could be verified (Haenle et al., 2011).

Table 6.12 Coating procedure with heavy metal ions (Schnabelrauch, 2011)

PVD procedure (magnetron-sputtering)
Plasma-immersion-ions implantation
CVD procedure (including CCVD, atmospheric pressure CVD)
Electro-chemical procedure
Sol-Gel procedure
Biomimetic separation procedure
Nano(micro) particle based procedure

Heidenau et al. (2005) examined coatings of implants with Ag and Cu ions. LD 50 cell numbers of fibroblasts subject to the concentration of the metal ions as well as the inhibition of growth of *S. epidermidis* in vitro were tested. In the process, heavy metal concentrations were described, which only showed minor toxicity compared with fibroblast cells in vitro and simultaneously exhibited effectiveness against *S. epidermidis* (Table 6.13).

Table 6.13 Metal-ion-containing coatings (Heidenau et al., 2005)

Metal ions	LD_{50} (L929-fibroblasts) (mmol/l)	LD_{50} (Reduction of bacterial growth)
Ag^+	3.5×10^{-3}	0.93
Zn^{2+}	3.6×10^{-3}	1.11
Hg^{2+}	4.2×10^{-3}	7.58
Cu^{2+}	2.3×10^{-1}	2.5×10^4
Co^{2+}	3.4×10^{-2}	1.42
Al^{3+}	1.8	0.46

However, these in vitro tests also leave many questions unanswered: On one hand, it is interesting how many SM ions will still have to be released to ultimately kill all bacteria, on the other, it will then have to be demonstrated how many fibroblasts will still survive. Such tests can mimic the real situation in the human body only to a limited extent.

In summary, the considerable potential of cytotoxicity should be always kept in mind if heavy metals/heavy metal salts are considered to be used as a component in antimicrobial coatings.

Currently, some medical devices incorporating silver ions, such as venous catheters, bladder catheters, endotracheal tubes, tumor endoprosthetics, wound covers for burn injuries, cardiovascular implants (heart valves), surgical masks, medical instruments, tissue prostheses, and hernia netting are commercially available.

6.32 Coating with Self-Adhesive, Low-Soluble Antibiotic Salts

Combinations of antibiotics and fatty acids were the first antimicrobial coating of metallic implants described (Kühn et al., 2003, Vogt et al., 2005). Particularly those antibiotics that are based on aminoglycosides feature a broad range of efficacy. The bactericidal antibiotics gentamicin and tobramycin are aminoglycoside antibiotics and used successfully in PMMA bone cements for many years. Gentamicin as well as tobramycin are utilized in the form of sulfates.

The most frequently used antimicrobial agent in PMMA bone cement is gentamicin sulfate; it consists of a mixture of gentamicin C2, C1a, and C2a+b and is highly soluble. It does not exhibit substantial adhesion to metal surfaces. As it is a cationic antibiotic, it possesses five proton amino groups. Gentamicin attaches itself to the bacterial ribosome, thus disrupting and inhibiting the bacterial protein synthesis. The result is the creation of nonsense proteins, which damage bacterial membranes.

The technique of transferring water-soluble gentamicin sulfate into low-soluble gentamicin fatty acid salts is a prerequisite for using it as coating material. Ion exchange easily facilitates the conversion of gentamicin sulfate into gentamicin fatty acid salts. This process replaces sulfate ions with fatty acid anions (Fig. 6.8). Suitable fatty acid anions include laurate, myristate, and palmitate. During the ion exchange process, the protonic gentamicin base remains unaltered. The process does not chemically alter the antimicrobial active gentamicin base (Kühn et al., 2003; Vogt et al., 2005). Furthermore, the ratio of gentamicin C1 to C1a and C2a+b is not modified. Gentamicin fatty acid salts are waxy solids exhibiting extensive adhesion properties on a multitude of surfaces in thin layers. Fatty acid anions are nontoxic and are metabolized in the human organism by ß-oxidation, thereby generating carbon dioxide and aqua (Kühn and Vogt, 2007).

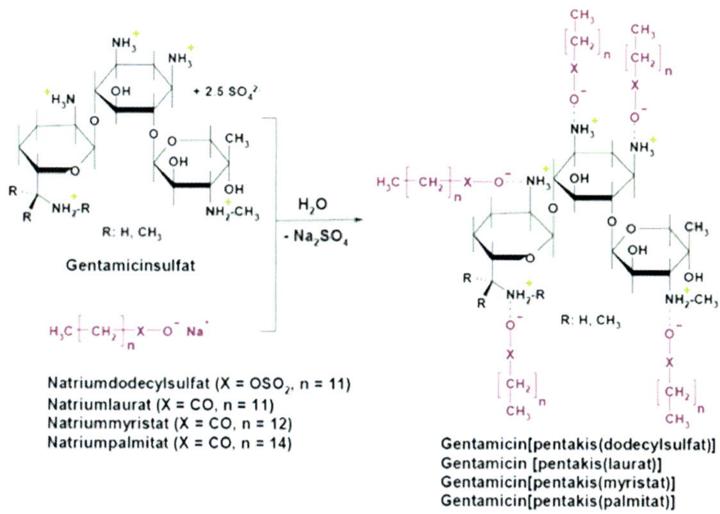

Figure 6.8 Gentamicin fatty acids (Vogt et al. 2005).

Gentamicin palmitate is particularly interesting. It is chemically a gentamicin derivate substance; the salt is a colorless to yellowish waxy solid, which is soluble in organic solvents. It may be applied to the surface of cementless prostheses via spray coating or dip coating. The loading capacity is quite variable (up to 300 µg gentamicin base/cm^2). Depending on the roughness of the surface, the technique of coating as well as the manufacturing of the coating solution and test conditions, the gentamicin (base) release takes place within a period of 5 to 10 days under in vitro conditions (Kühn, 2010).

The coated prostheses can be sterilized by gamma radiation or EtO. The sterilization process has no influence on the coated implant or the coating itself. First trials conducted in an animal test model investigating the osteointegration capacity of gentamicin-palmitate-coated sand-blasted titanium bars did not produce any undesired side effects. The osteointegration of the coated titanium bars was comparable to that of noncoated titanium bars (Table 6.14)

Table 6.14 Gentamicin-palmitate-coated titanium discs

Animal study: rabbit model
Experimental conditions
Specimens: Titanium pin, length 14 mm, diameter 2 mm
Coating: Gentamicin palmitate = 0.6–1.3 mg/cm^2
Fixation: 2 mm drilling in the femur
Test duration: 4 weeks
Six animals with coated and 6 animals with uncoated titanium pin
Result
No osteolysis
No inflammable reaction
Osteointegration = no difference:
- Coated = **54.5%**
- Reference uncoated = **55.5%**

The gentamicin content and its release profile are adjustable and ideally depend on the elution profile of PMMA bone cements such as the gold-standard Palacos® R+G. A comparison between the gentamicin base release of gentamicin-palmitate-coated titanium plates with that of gentamicin sulfate in Palacos® R+G showed a continuous gentamicin release from the gentamicin palmitate coat, which proved to be similar to that from Palacos® R+G (Fig. 6.9). Therefore, it can be assumed that the local protection capability of the gentamicin palmitate coat on the implant surface is similar to the antimicrobial protection provided by the cement surface of Palacos® R+G. Both the gentamicin sulfate in PMMA bone cements and the gentamicin palmitate coating show comparable anti-infective behavior within the proliferation assay according to ISO DIN EN 17025. Furthermore, the gentamicin palmitate coating is biocompatible according to ISO DIN EN 10993 (Kühn and Brünke, 2010).

The inhibitor test clearly shows the antimicrobial efficacy of gentamicin palmitate as coat on titanium compared with GS in the bone cement. For this purpose, small round moulds are produced. The titanium discs (diameter 15.6 mm) are also generally used in the production of commercially available uncemented prostheses (roughness: stems Ra 7 μm, cups Ra 70+/- 10 μm). They are hereby

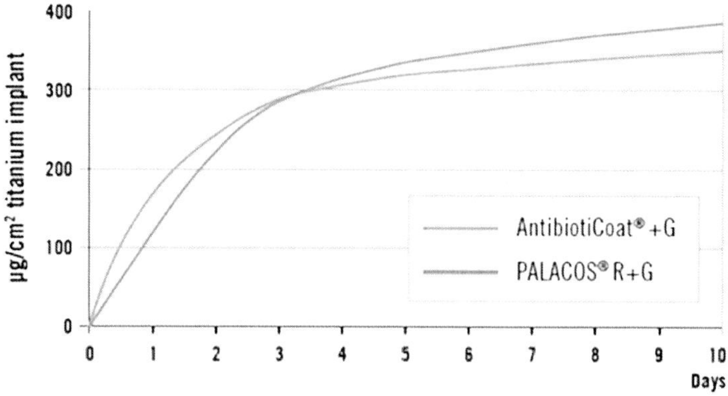

Figure 6.9 Antibiotic release of gentamicin-containing Palacos R+G vs gentamicin–palmitate-coated titanium discs (Stemberger and Kühn 2010).

coated with 220 μg/cm^2 G and in the test compared with moulds from bone cement containing antibiotics. An uncoated titanium disc is used as reference. For the purpose of the test, 0.5 McFarland was diluted 1:100 and swabbed over Müller Hinton Agar plates. The discs were moistened with 10 μl of PBS on the agar contact side and were allowed to sit for one hour at room temperature to facilitate adherence. After 24 h of incubation at 37°C, diameters were measured on the bottom side of the Petri dishes. Inhibiting areolas were comparable in all discs; merely the PMMA moulds showed slightly reduced diameters with 88% of the diameter of titanium discs coated with gentamicin palmitate. The reference discs (uncoated) did not display any inhibiting areolas (Kühn, 2010; Kittinger et al., 2011, see Fig. 6.10).

Almost all metallic implants can be coated with gentamicin palmitate. As well as dental implants made of titanium (Stemberger et al., 2007), also spinal implants can be successfully equipped with anti-infective agents (Fig. 6.11). Gentamicin palmitate displays excellent adhesion even in plastic implants made of PEEK and ensures the protection against local colonization by pathogenic germs. The surfaces of titanium prostheses are usually rough, allowing the coating material to easily penetrate the inner surface of the titanium layer. The flat surfaces of external fixation screws as well as pins and wires coated with gentamicin palmitate can also be utilized to inhibit bacterial colonization. External fixation by means of screws and pins allows good access for bacteria. So-called "pin-track infections" occur in 57% to 75% of all cases (Emami et al., 1995; McDonald et al., 1994). It is possible to obtain homogeneous coatings of 2.5 mg/cm^2 by using gentamicin palmitate (4% solution) with airbrush technique on screws consisting of steel and titanium. The gentamicin base release was comparable to bone cement containing gentamicin during the first days.

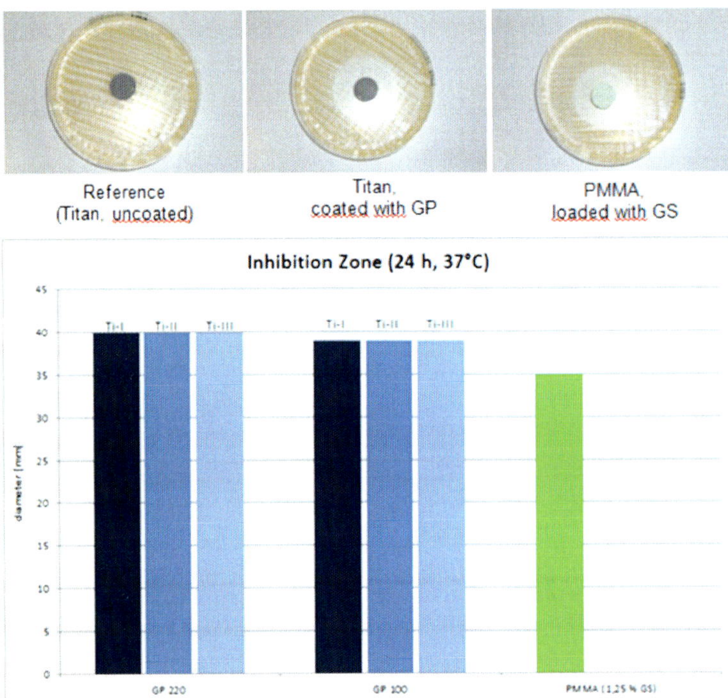

Figure 6.10 Inhibition areolas of gentamicin-palmitate-coated titanium discs vs PMMA with gentamicin sulfate (Kittinger et al. 2011).

6.33 Other Implants

6.33.1 Vascular Grafts

In the event of impending loss of arterial circulation, natural blood vessels can be replaced by so-called stents. The most common

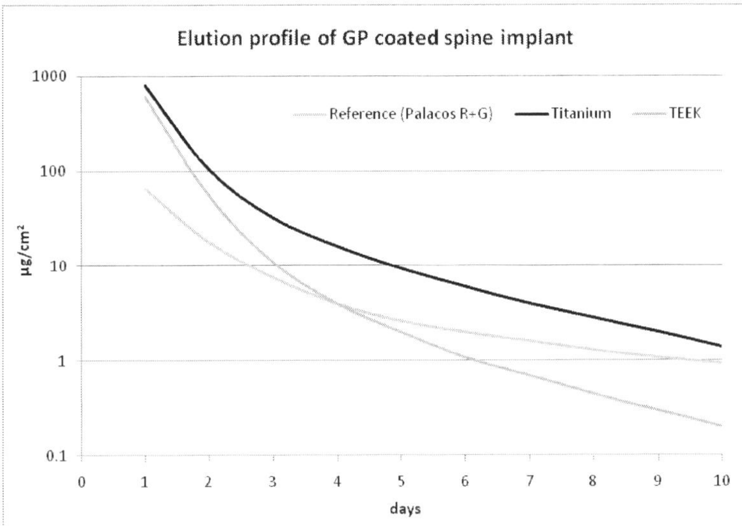

Figure 6.11 Release of gentamicin-palmitate-coated titan and PEEK spine implants.

causes for the medical failure of blood vessels are aneurysmatic changes, arteriosclerotic diabetes mellitus, and nicotine abuse or traumatic events. Synthetic prostheses can fail post-operatively due to bleeding, seroma formation, blocking of the vascular lumen due to thrombotic deposits, or the excessive formation of a neo-intima (Seeger et al., 1990) as well as infections and have to be revised quickly. Infections originating during the vascular reconstruction as a consequence of an intraoperative contamination of the wound or the post-operative colonization by, e.g., hematogenically scattering germs, represent a life-threatening situation for the patient. Analyses of septic complications in 410 autogenic and alloplastic vascular bridging crafts show a complication ratio of up to 11%, which co-affects the implant in infrainguinal surgical procedures at 80% and as deep infections at 67%. Twenty-five percent of patients affected by deep infections lost an extremity as a direct consequence, and 11% of them died due to the infections (Pounds et al., 2005). In view of these dramatic observations, various coating technologies are examined to equip vascular prostheses with antimicrobial agents. Dacron vascular prostheses are, e.g., protected from infections by using various gelatine coatings (= barrier effect). However, it has been shown that these coatings displayed only weak resistance against an *S. epidermidis* colonization (Farooq et al., 1999). As alternative, Dacron vascular prostheses can also be dipped in a rifampicin bath (Goeau-Brissonniere et al., 1994; Lachapelle et al., 1994; Sardelic et al., 1996). In animal trials, the combination of rifampicin with gelatine or albumin proved to be more effective than the combination of a coating with gelatine or albumin with other antibiotics such as vancomycin and teicoplanin (Galdbart et al., 1996; Malassiney et al., 1996). A gelatine coating containing gentamicin produced very effective protection (Ginalska, 2005; Edmiston et al., 2006). Vascular prostheses are also combined with silver. A comparison in animal tests between a silver acetate coating applied to a PTFE vascular prosthesis and a gelatine–rifampicin coating was not able to verify an advantage of the silver over the untreated prostheses. In comparison, the rifampicin coating produced an effective antimicrobial protection (Vicaretti et al., 1998; Goeau-Brissonniere et al., 2002). The verified germ reduction in vitro in a coating combination of silver and ciprofloxacine is solely attributed to the antibiotic (Benvenisty et al., 1988). Other coatings to affix hydrophile-active ingredients onto the lipophilic surfaces of the grafts, e.g., consist of benzalconium chloride (Greco et al., 1995; Harvey and Greco, 1981), tridodecylmethylammonium chloride (Harvey et al., 1982), gentamicin sulfate or teicoplanin (Matl et al., 2008). Coatings of absorbable carrier material on polylacid basis were also used. However, PTFE prostheses can also be easily coated by dipping them in various gentamicin salts of lauric acid and palmitic acid, as described before. The release can be easily influenced, particularly through the choice of fatty acids (Fig. 6.12); the gentamicin palmitate also displays hemocompatible characteristics (Matl et al., 2008).

6.33.2 Hernia Meshes

Tests of explanted hernia meshes showed that colonies of bacteria can quickly colonize the surface of the mesh during the surgery. These germs use the hernia as a retreat and guide rail, which easily causes a relapse. *Staphylococcus epidermidis* is, in particular, responsible for delayed infections. These delayed infections occur months, in rare occasions also years, after the operation (Avtan et al., 1997). Hernia meshes consist of varied materials, in most cases nonabsorbable plastics (PP, PE, PVDF, and/or combinations of material) where at times also individual components can be resorbed (PLA), to sustainably reduce the weight of the implanted hernia after the operation. The surface is furthermore roughened and thus extremely enlarged (Fig. 6.13). Meshes such as these are also quite easily and effectively coated by dipping them in an active ingredient—fatty acid solution.

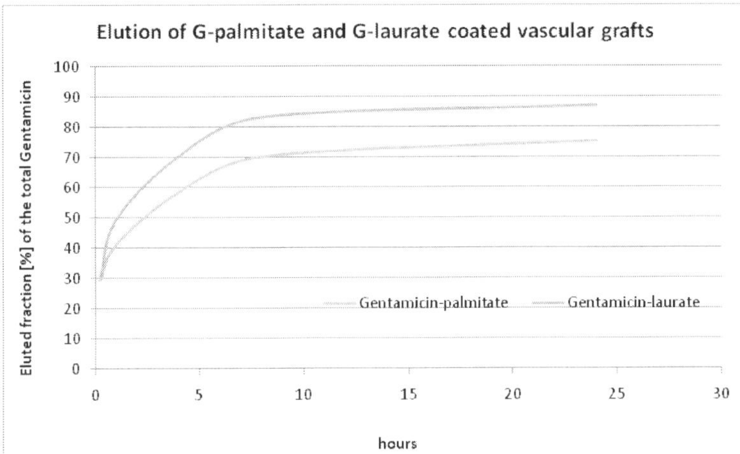

Figure 6.12 Elution of gentamicin-palmitate- and gentamicin-laurate-coated vascular grafts (Matl et al. 2008).

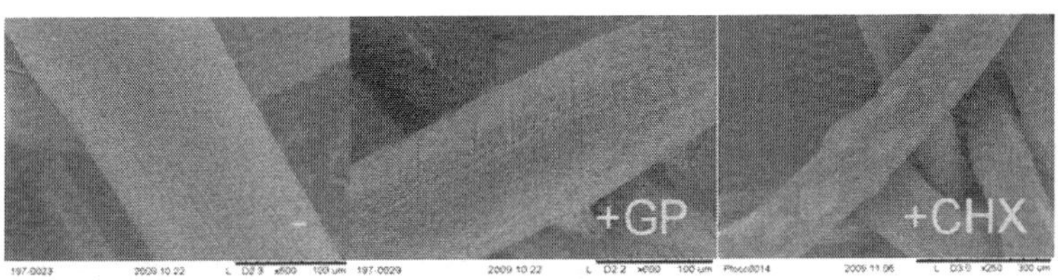

PP = polypropylene; – without coating

Figure 6.13 Gentamicin-palmitate- (GP) and CHX-coated hernia (PP) mesh (SEM).

CHX as well as gentamicin as palmitate adheres well to hernia surfaces in the example of hernias made of polypropylene fibers. The samples were examined under an electron microscope. The samples treated with gentamicin palmitate displayed a relatively even coating of the polypropylene fibers with gentamicin palmitate. The gentamicin palmitate layer had a slightly grainy structure, which is strongest on the sample with the highest loading. In contrast, the CHX fatty acid coatings form completely differently and adhere selectively to the hernia surface (Fig. 6.13).

The release kinetic of antibiotics and/or antiseptics from hernia plastic mesh illustrates a two-phase process much like other coated biomaterials. Thus, approximately 60% of the introduced gentamicin is initially released within the first 48 h. This is followed by lesser elution, which releases the incorporated antibiotic to over 90% after approximately 5 days. The release behavior of CHX is similar, however with a stronger retard effect. Here it is remarkable that the CHX release of the CHX palmitate coating lasts relatively long, while the CHX from the pharmaceutical product PeriChip (as CHX-gluconate, 36%) was released almost completely within the first 24 h.

6.33.3 Sutures

Surgical sutures are the main reason for wound infections. The surface of the suture functions as a guide for bacteria (Mangram et al., 1999; Gilbert et al., 2002). Wound infection is a dreaded complication in post-operative treatment. One of the most common surgery suture materials, VicylPlus®, is coated with the antiseptic triclosan. The coating helps "**to reduce the incidence of surgical site infections.**"

As an antiseptic agent, triclosan has some disadvantages in comparison with other antiseptics such as octenidine or chlorhexidine. Matl et al. (2009) examined PGA sutures, which were equipped with CHX-di-palmitate (CHX-P) and CHX-di-laurate (CHX-L) as well as octenidine hydrochloride with palmatic (OH) by dip coating. All coatings tested showed continuous drug release with the first 96 h (up to about 10 days). Due to lesser solubility of palmitic acid, CHX-P was dissolved significantly slower from the suture surface, while the more hydrophilic combination of CHX with lauric acid was dissolved faster. It could also be demonstrated that the composition of the active ingredient—fatty acid combination—also had a great influence on the release behavior. The greater the proportion of active ingredient, the higher the eluted amount of active ingredient (Fig. 6.14). Sutures coated with octenidine showed similar results, whereby OH-2 is released in minor amounts and shows excellent effectiveness against *S. aureus*. Bacterial growth in high concentration of 2×10^6 cfu/ml could be reduced with all coated sutures tested in this investigation. CHX-P (90 μg/cm suture)- and OH (28 μg/cm suture)-coated sutures showed a germ reduction of more than 99% after 24 h, whereas VicrylPlus® coated with triclosan showed a reduction of bacterial growth of approximately 34% after 24 h (Fig. 6.15a–c).

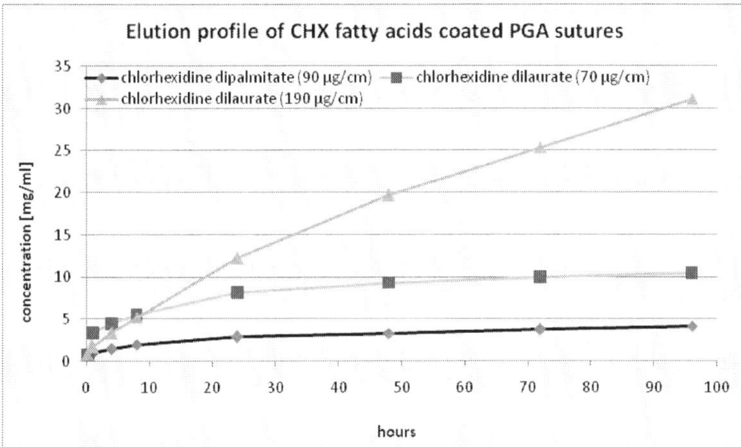

Figure 6.14 Elution profile of CHX-fatty-acids-coated PGA sutures.

6.33.4 Fleeces and Felts

Besides suture materials, other biomaterials are manufactured on PLA basis. Particularly fleeces and felts applied for hemostasis are equipped with anti-infective ingredients, if required, to ensure a high local level (Price et al., 1996) Fleeces on a collagen basis with antibiotics are already available in the market as medical devices Class III. Fleeces on PLA basis can similarly be equipped with, e.g., gentamicin palmitate. However, it must be observed that the fleeces are not completely coated with a hydrophobic fatty acid active ingredient, as it may negatively influence the hemato-typical characteristics of the fleece (Fig. 6.16). Some tests showed that a selective coating of PGA fleeces with gentamicin palmitate is possible by means of simple dipping and that the release is easily adjustable with respect to duration of coating, effective ingredient content, and combination with suitable fatty acids.

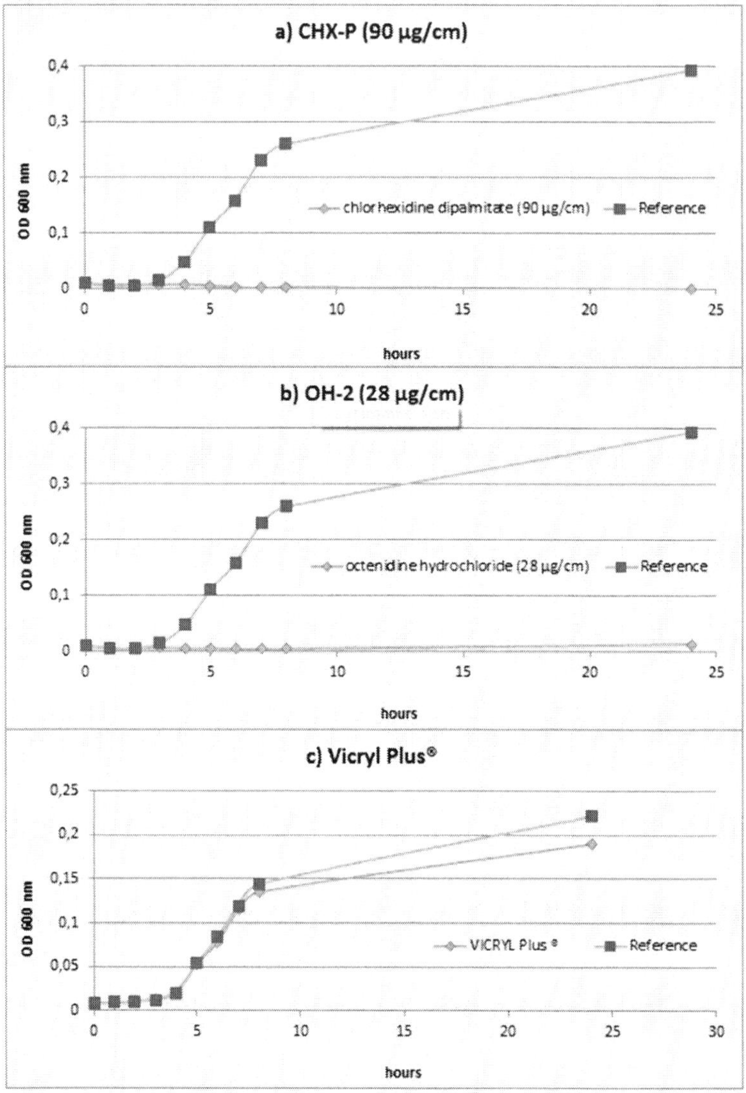

Figure 6.15 (a–c) Antimicrobial characteristics of coated sutures.

6.33.5 Pacemaker/Defibrillator

Pacemakers are electrodes directed to the heart and positioned endocardium, which emit stimulation impulses. Defibrillators create electrical defibrillation fields. The artificial impulses create heartbeats as soon as the heart works too slow (bradycardiac arrhythmia), while the electrical defibrillation fields interrupt pathological forms of a too-fast heartbeat (tachycardiac arrhythmia). Therefore, pacemakers only deliver impulses, while defibrillators create impulses as well as electrical defibrillation fields, so-called defibrillation shocks. The design of pacemakers and defibrillators is quite similar. Electronic controls and a battery are located in a titanium casing. The main components are connected with the electrodes via the head of pacemaker or defibrillator. Such implants are possible under sterile conditions in a cardiac catheter laboratory. Prior to the surgical procedure, the patient is administered a light sedative and, preventatively, antibiotics for the protection against infections. Although such infections occur rarely, they are extremely dangerous complications.

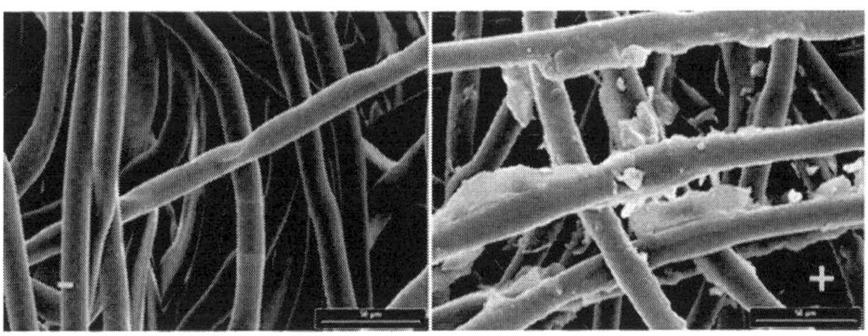

– = uncoated; + = coated with GP

Figure 6.16 Resorbable fleeces/felts fibers coated with gentamicin palmitate (GP).

Besides using a pocket made of various polymers, in which the casings are placed prior to an implantation, pacemakers or defibrillators, as described above, can also be equipped with an antibiotic/antiseptic fatty acid layer directly on the surface of the casings. The coating can be applied to both, the metallic casing material, particularly titanium, and also to the electrodes. The electrodes are encased by various plastics, which are easily coated despite their smooth surface and furthermore release active ingredients over several days after the operation (Fig. 6.17).

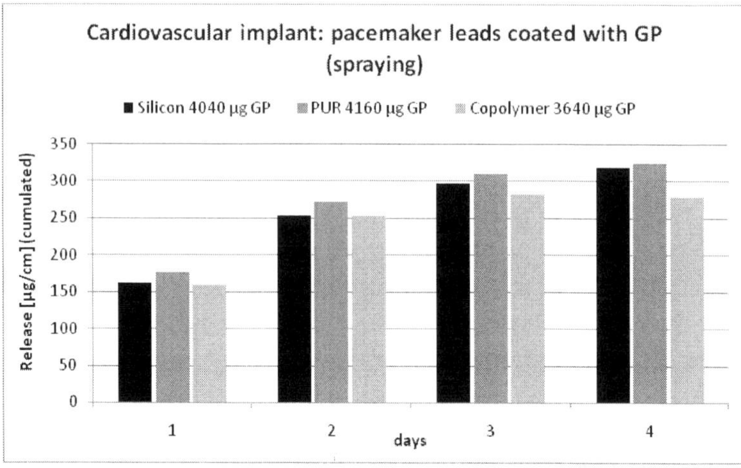

Figure 6.17 Elution profile of gentamicin-palmitate-coated pacemaker leads.

6.34 Further Biomaterial Coatings

Further coating strategies for biomaterials are covalent or ionic fixation of an active ingredient via anchor and/or spacer groups, adsorption of an active ingredient on the surface of the implant, or the embedding of the active ingredient in an organic or inorganic polymer layer or mesh. Jeon et al. (1991) describes an interesting model of an antiadhesive polymer coating. For example, polyethylenglycol chains (PEG-chains) are applied via their end groups on the surface of an implant by prior activation (Fig. 6.18). These chains align themselves and become a dense matrix refractive for cells due to water storage through hydrogen bridges. This works as an adhesive layer, and cells such as proteins can no longer adhere to the surface of the implant (Banerjee et al., 2011). While such PEG chains create a rather hydrophilic matrix, it is quite possible to imagine other adjusted chain structures, which construct a hydrophobic adhesive surface.

Long-chained biocide polymer structures (Fig. 6.19) with a positive charge, e.g., ammonium ions, can be applied to the surface of the implant via a functional group. These quaternary polymers form a cationic barrier, which interacts after cell penetration. Hereby, the positively charged polymer ends react with the negatively charged cell membrane structures, causing a massive malfunction at the cell membrane up to lysis (Fig. 6.20). The cell is positively killed following contact with the surface of the implant (Tiller et al., 2001; Tiller et al., 2002; Milovic et al., 2005).

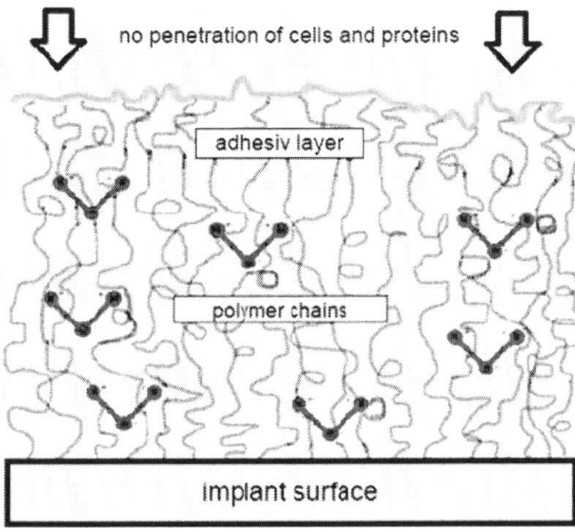

Figure 6.18 Antiadhesive protection of implant surfaces (Jeon et al. 1991; Banerjee et al. 2011).

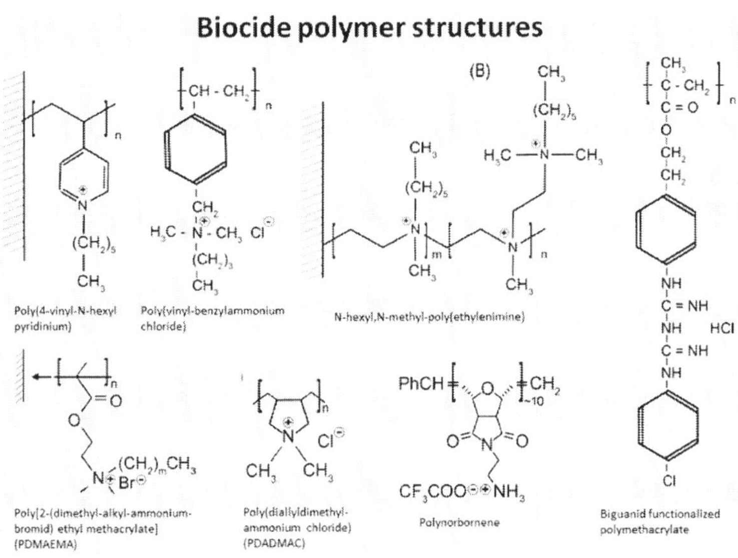

Figure 6.19 Biocide polymer structures (Schnabelrauch 2011).

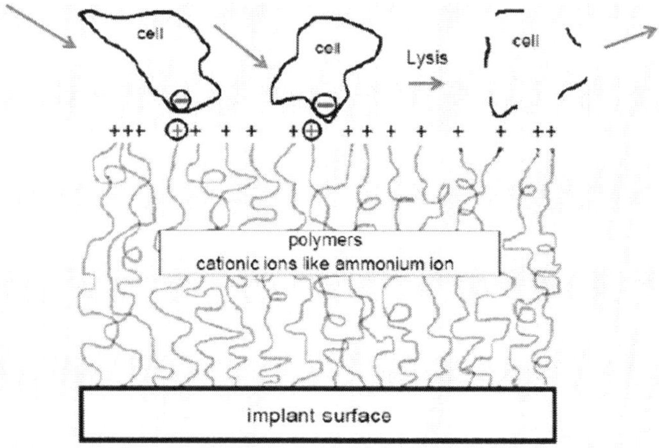

Germ		Germ reduction rate [%]				
		HDPE	LDPE	PP	NYLON	PET
S. aureus	Gram +	96 ± 3	97 ± 1	90 ± 3	92 ± 2	95 ± 1
E. coli	Gram −	97 ± 1	96 ± 2	98 ± 1	98 ± 2	95 ± 1

Figure 6.20 Biocide protection of implant surfaces (Tiller et al. 2002; Lewis and Klibanov 2005).

For example, polyethylene glycol chains are arranged on the surface of the implant in case of antiadhesive polymer layers, to which further layers can subsequently adhere, such as self-oriented layers (SAMs), zwitterionic structures, peptide layers, self-cleaning (nanostructured) layers, or ultra-hydrophobic layers.

Acknowledgements

A special thank you from the author goes to Mrs. B. Eckl for the translation, Mr. S. Böhm for her help in the establishment of the illustrations, Mr. A. Kontekakis and Mr. S. Gaiser for the preparation of economic issues, Dr. Chr. Berberich and Dr. S. Vogt and Dr. M. Schnabelrauch for the scientific review.

References

Alt V, et al. 2006. The effects of combined gentamicin-hydroxyapatite coating for cementless joint prostheses on the reduction of infection rates in a rabbit infection prophylaxis model. *Biomaterials*, **26**: 4627–4634.

Ambrosius WT, Harris VJ, and Snidow JJ. 1998. Tunneled hemodialysis catheters: Use of a silver-coated catheter for prevention of infection—a randomized study. *Radiology*, **2:** 491–496.

Anderson AB. 2003. Combining local drug delivery and implantable medical devices. *Med Device Technol,***14**(7): 16–19.

Avtan L, Avci C, Bulut T, and Fourtanier G. 1997. Mesh infections after laparoscopic inguinal hernia repair. *Surg Laparosc Endosc*, **7**(30): 192–195.

Banerjee G, Car S, Scott-Craig JS, Hodge DB, and Walton JD. 2011. Alkaline peroxide pretreatment of corn stover: Effects of biomass, peroxide, and enzyme loading and composition on yields of glucose and xylose. *Biotechnol Biofuels*, **4**: 16.

Barrack RL, Engh G, Rorabeck C, Sawhney J, and Woolfrey M. 2000. Patient satisfaction and outcome after septic versus aseptic revision total knee arthroplasty. *J Arthroplasty*, **15**(8): 990–993.

Benvenisty AI, Tannenbaum G, Ahlborn TN, Fox CL, Modak S, Sampath L, Reemtsma K, and Nowygrod R. 1988. Control of prosthetic bacterial infection: Evaluation of an easily incorporated, tightly bound, silver antibiotic PTFE graft. *J Surg Res*, **44**: 1–7.

Bjerkan G, Witso E, and Bergh K. 2009. Sonication is superior to scraping for retrieval of bacteria in biofilm on titanium and steel surfaces in vitro. *Acta Orthop*, **80**(2): 245–250.

Bozic KJ and Ries MD. 2005. The impact of infection after total hip arthroplasty on hospital and surgeon resource utilization. *J Bone Joint Surg Am*, **87**(8): 1746–1751.

Buchholz HW and Engelbrecht H. 1970. Über die Depotwirkung einiger Antibiotika bei Vermischung mit dem Kunstharz Palacos. *Chirurg*, **40**: 511–515.

Campbell AA, Song L, Li XS, Nelson BJ, Bottoni C, Brooks DE, and DeJong ES. 2000. Development, characterization and anti-microbial efficacy of hydroxyapatite-chlorhexidine coatings produced by surface-induced mineralization. *J Biomed Mater Res*, **53**(4): 400–407.

Choux M, Genitori L, Lang D, and Lena G. 1992. Shunt implantation: Reducing the incidence of shunt infection. *J Neurosurg*, **77**(6): 875–880.

Christoph A, Fux J, and William Costerton UA. 2005. Survival strategies of infectious biofilms. *Trends Microbiol*, **13**(1): 34–40.

Cogan NG. 2006. Effects of persister formation on bacterial response to dosing. *J Theor Biol*, **238**: 694–703.

Cooke FW. 2004. Bulk properties of materials, in *Biomaterial Science: An Introduction to Materials in Medicine* (Ratner BD, Hoffman AS, Schoen FJ, Lemons JE, eds), 2nd ed, Elsevier Academic Press, California, pp 23–32.

Costerton JW, et al. 1987. Bacterial biofilms in nature and disease. *Annu Rev Microbiol,* **41**: 435–464.

Costerton JW, Stewart PS, and Greenberg EP. 1999. Bacterial biofilms: A common cause of persistent infections. *Science,* **284**: 1318–1322.

Cummins JS, Tomek IM, Kantor SR, Furnes O, Engesaeter LB, and Finlayson SRG. 2009. Cost-effectiveness of antibiotic-impregnated bone cement used in primary total hip arthroplasty. *J Bone Joint Surg Am,* **91**(3): 634–641.

Darouiche RO. 1999. Anti-infective efficacy of silver-coated medical protheses. *Clin Infect Dis,* **29**(6): 1371–1377.

Darouiche RO. 2001. Device-associated infections: A macroproblem that starts with microadherence. *Clin Infect Dis,* **33**: 1567–1572.

Darouiche RO. 2004. Treatment of infections associated with surgical implants. *N Engl J Med,* **350**: 1422–1429.

Demir U, Mihmanli M, Coskun H, Dilege E, Kalyoncu A, Altinli E, Gunduz B, and Yilmaz B. 2005. Comparison of prosthetic materials in incisional hernia repair. *Surg Today,* **35**(3): 223–227.

Department of Health and Human Services. 2008. Medicare program; changes to the hospital in patient prospective payment systems and fiscal year 2009 rates. Fed Regist 2008; 73:48433. Available at: http://edocket.access.gpo.gov/ http://edocket.access.gpo.gov/**2008/pdf/E8–17914**.pdf. Accessed 29 November, 2011

Donlan RM and Costerton JW. 2002. Biofilms: Survival mechanisms of clinically relevant microorganisms. *Clin Microbiol Rev,* **15**: 167–193.

Donlan RM. 2001. Biofilm formation: A clinically relevant microbiological process. *Clin Infect Dis,* **33**: 1387–1392.

Dunn KW, Hall PN, and Khoo CTK. 1992. Breast implant materials: Sense and safety. *Br J Plast Surg,* **45**: 315–321.

Edmiston CE Jr, Goheen MP, Seabrook GR, Johnson CP, Lewis BD, Brown KR, and Towne JB. 2006. Impact of selective antimicrobial agents on staphylococcal adherence to biomedical devices. *Am J Surg,* **192**: 344–354.

Elek SD and Conen PE. 1957. The virulence of Staphylococcus pyogenes for man: A study of the problems of wound infection. *Br J Exp Pathol,* **38**: 573–586.

Emami A, Mjoeberg B, Karlstroem G, and Larsson S. 1995. Treatment of closed tibial shaft fractures with unilateral external fixation. *Injury,* **26**(5): 299–303.

Englert C, Angele P, Fierlbeck J, Dendorfer S, Schubert T, Mueller R, Lienhard S, Zellner J, Nerlich M, and Neumann C. 2007. Conductive bone substitute material with variable antibiotic delivery. *Unfallchirurg,* **110**(5): 408–413.

Farooq M, Freischlag J, Kelly H, Seabrook G, Cambria R, and Towne J. 1999. Gelatin-sealed polyester resists *Staphylococcus epidermidis* biofilm infection. *J Surg Res,* **87**: 57–61.

Ferguson TB Jr, Ferguson CL, Crites K, and Crimmins-Reda P. 1996. The additional hospital costs generated in the management of complications of pacemaker and defibrillator implantations. *J Thorac Cardiovasc Surg,* **111**(4): 742–752.

Finan KR, Kilgore ML, and Hawn MT. 2009. Open suture versus mesh repair of primary incisional hernias: A cost-utility analysis. *Hernia,* **13**(2): 173–182.

Frommelt L and Kuehn KD. 2005. Properties of bone cement: Antibiotic-loaded cement, in *The Well Cemented Hip Arthroplasty* (Breusch S and Malchau H, eds), Springer, Heidelberg, pp 86–92.

Galdbart JO, Branger C, Andreassian B, Lambert-Zechovsky N, and Kitzis M. 1996. Elution of six antibiotics bonded to polyethylene vascular grafts sealed with three proteins. *J Surg Res,* **66**: 174–178.

Gilbert P, McBain AJ, Storch ML, Rothenburger SJ, and Barbolt TA. 2002. Literature-based evaluation of the potential risk associated with impregnation of medical devices and implants with triclosan. *Surg Infect,* **3**(suppl 1): S55–S63.

Ginalska G, Osinska M, Uryniak A, Urbanik-Sypniewska T, Belcarz A, Rzeski W, and Wolski A. 2005. Antibacterial activity of gentamicin-bonded gelatin-sealed polyethylene terephthalate vascular prostheses. *Eur J Vasc Endovasc Surg,* **29**: 419–424.

Goeau-Brissonniere O, Mercier F, Nicolas MH, Bacourt F, Coggia M, Lebrault C, and Pechere JC. 1994. Treatment of vascular graft infection by in situ replacement with a rifampin-bonded gelatin-sealed Dacron graft. *J Vasc Surg,* **19**: 739–741.

Goeau-Brissonniere O, Fabre D, Leflon-Guibout V, Di Centa I, Nicolas-Chanoine M, and Coggia M. 2002. Comparison of the resistance to infection of rifampin-bonded gelatin-sealed and silver/collagen-coated polyester prostheses. *J Vasc Surg,* **35**: 1260–1263.

Gollwitzer H, Ibrahim K, Meyer H, Mittelmeier W, Busch R, and Stemberger A. 2003. Antibacterial poly (D,L-lactic acid) coating of medical implants using a biodegradable drug delivery technology. *Antimicrob Chemother,* **51**(3): 585–591.

Goodsell DS. 2010. Wie Zellen Funktionieren: Wirtschaft und Produktion in der molekularen Welt. 2. Auflage, *Spektrum Verlag.*

Grzybowski J and Trafny EA. 1999. Antimicrobial properties of copper-coated electroconductive polyester fibers. *Polim Med,* **29(**1–2): 27–33.

Greco RS, Kim HC, Donetz AP, and Harvey RA. 1995. Patency of a small vessel prosthesis bonded to tissue plasminogen activator and iloprost. *Ann Vasc Surg,* **9**(2): 140–145.

Greenwald D, Shumway S, Albear P, and Gottlieb L. 1994. Mechanical comparison of 10 suture materials before and after in vivo incubation. *J Surg Res,* **56**(4): 372–377.

Gristina AG and Costerton JW. 1985. Bacterial adherence to biomaterials and tissue. The significance of its role in clinical sepsis. *J Bone Joint Surg Am,* **67**: 264–273.

Haenle M, Fritsche A, Zietz C, Bader R, Heidenau F, Mittelmeier W, and Gollwitzer H. 2011. An extended spectrum bactericidal titanium dioxide (TiO_2) coating for metallic implants: In vitro effectiveness against MRSA and mechanical properties. *J Mater Sci Mater Med,* **22**(2): 381–387.

Harvey RA, Alcid DV, and RS Greco. 1982. Antibiotic bonding to polytetrafluoroethylene with tridodecylmethylammonium chloride. *Surgery,* **92**: 504–512.

Harvey RA and Greco RS. 1981. The noncovalent bonding of antibiotics to a polytetrafluoroethylene-benzalkonium graft. *Ann Surg,* **194**: 642–647.

Hasman H, Kempf I, Chidaine B, Cariolet R, Ersbøll AK, Houe H, Bruun Hansen HC, and Aarestrup FM. 2006. Copper resistance in *Enterococcus faecium,* mediated by the tcrB gene, is selected by supplementation of pig feed with copper sulfate. *Appl Environ Microbiol,* **72**(9): 5784–5789.

Heidenau F, Mittelmeier W, Detsch R, Haenle M, Stenzel F, Ziegler G, and Gollwitzer H. 2005. A novel antibacterial titania coating: Metal ion toxicity and in vitro surface colonization. *J Mater Sci Mater Med,* **16**(10): 883–888.

Hellstrom WJ, Montague DK, Moncado I, Carson C, Minhas S, Faira G, and Krishnamurti S. 2010. Implants, mechanical devices and vascular surgery for erectile dysfunction. *JSM,* **7**(1), 501–523.

Ilingworth B, Bianco RW, and Weisberg S. 2000. In vivo efficacy of silver-coated fabric against staphylococcus epidermidis. *J Heart Valve Dis,* **9**(1): 135–141.

Jefferson KK. 2004. What drives bacteria to produce a biofilm? *FEMS Microbiol Lett,* **236**: 163–173.

Jeon SI, Lee JH, Andrade JD, and Degennes PG. 1991. Protein surface interactions in the presence of polyethylene oxide. 1. Simplified theory. *J Coll Interf Sci,* **142**: 149–158.

Justinger C, Schuld J, Sperling J, Kollmar O, Richter S, and Schilling MK. 2011. Triclosan-coated sutures reduce wound infections after hepatobiliary surgery: A prospective non-randomized clinical pathway driven study. *Langenbecks Arch Surg,* **396**(6): 845–850.

Kaiser AB, Kernodle DS, and Parker RA. 1992. Low-inoculum model of surgical wound infection. *Infect Dis,* **166**(2): 393–399.

Kanellakopoulou EJ and Giamarellos-Bourboulis EJ. 2000. Carrier systems for the local delivery of antibiotics in bone infections. *Drugs,* **59**(6): 1223–1232.

Kathju S, Nistico L, Hall-Stoodley L, Post JC, Ehrlich GD, and Stoodley P. 2009. Chronic surgical site infection due to suture-associated polymicrobial biofilm. *Surg Infect (Larchmt),* **10**(5): 457–461.

Kim S. 2008. Changes in surgical loads and economic burden of hip and knee replacements in the US: 1997–2004. *Arthritis Rheum,* **59**(4): 481–488.

Kirkland KB, Briggs JP, Trivette SL, Wilkinson WE, and Sexton DJ. 1999. The impact of surgical-site infections in the 1990s: Attributable mortality, excess length of hospitalization, and extra costs. *Infect Control Hosp Epidemiol,* **20**(11): 725–730.

Kittinger C, Marth E, and Windhager R et al. 2011. Antimicrobial activity of gentamicin palmitate against high concentrations of *Staphylococcus aureus. J Mater Sci Mater Med,* **22**(6): 1447–1453.

Klug D, Lacroix D, Savoye C, Goullard L, Grandmougin D, Hennequin JL, Kacet S, and Lekieffre J. 1997. Systemic infection related to endocarditis on pacemaker leads: Clinical presentation and management. *Circulation,* **95**(8): 2098–2107.

Kobayashi H, Oethinger M, Tuohy MJ, Procop GW, and Bauer TW. 2009. Improved detection of biofilm-formative bacteria by vortexing and sonication: A pilot study. *Clin Orthop Relat Res,* **467**: 1360–1364.

Kong KF, Vuong C, and Otto M. 2006. Staphylococcus quorum sensing in biofilm formation and infection. *Int J Med Microbiol,* **296**: 133–139.

Kühn KD. 2000. *Bone cements. Up-to-date comparison of physical and chemical properties of commercial materials*, Springer-Verlag, Heidelberg.

Kühn KD, Vogt S, and Schnabelrauch M. 2003. Porous implants with antibiotic coating, their preparation and use. EP 1374923 B1.

Kühn KD. 2010. In-vitro release of gentamicinpalmitate coating in uncemented titanium implants. *Int J Nano Biomater*, **3**: 94–106.

Kühn KD and Brünke J. 2010. Effectiveness of a novel gentamicin palmitate coating on biofilm formation of *Staphylococcus aureus* and *Staphylococcus epidermidis*. *Int J Nano Biomater*, **3**: 107–117.

Kühn KD, Weber C, Kreis S, and Holzgrabe U. 2008. Evaluation of the stability of gentamicin in different antibiotic carriers using a validated MEKC method. *J Pharm Biomed Anal*, **48**(3): 612–618.

Kühn KD. 2007. Antibiotic-loaded bone cements: Antibiotic release and influence on mechancical properties, in *Local Antibiotics in Arthroplasty: State of the Art from an Interdisciplinary Point of View* (Walenkamp GHIM, ed), Thieme-Verlag, pp 47–57.

Kühn KD and Vogt S. 2007. Antimicrobial implant coating in arthroplasty, in *Local Antibiotics in Arthroplasty: State of the Art from an Interdisciplinary Point of View* (Walenkamp GHIM, ed), *Thieme-Verlag*, pp 23–30.

Kurtz SM, Lau E, Schmier J, Ong KL, Zhao K, and Parvizi J. 2008. Infection burden for hip and knee arthroplasty in the United States. *J Arthroplasty*, **23**(7): 984–991.

Lachapelle K, Graham AM, and Symes JF. 1994. Antibacterial activity, antibiotic retention, and infection resistance of a rifampin-impregnated gelatin-sealed Dacron graft. *J Vasc Surg*, **19**: 675–682.

Lekkerkerker JC, van Nieuwkoop C, Trines SA, van der Bom JG, Bernards A, van de Velde ET, Bootsma M, Zeppenfeld K, Jukema JW, Borleffs J-W, Schalij MJ, and van Erven L. 2009. Risk factors and time delay associated with cardiac device infections: Leiden device registry. *Heart*, **95**: 715–720.

Lewis K and Klibanov AM. 2005. Surpassing nature: Rational design of sterile-surface materials. *Trends Biotechnol*, **23**(7): 343–348.

Lewis K. 2008. Multidrug tolerance of biofilms and persister cells. *Curr Top Microbiol Immunol*, **322**: 107–131.

Lewis LA, et al. 1991. Genetic and molecular analysis of spontaneous respiratory deficient (res) mutants of *Escherichia coli* K12. *Microbiol Immunol*, **35**: 289–301.

Löffler G, Petrides PE, and Heinrich PC (eds). 2007. *Biochemie und Pathobiochemie*, Springer Medizin Verlag, Heidelberg, p 974.

Lucke M, et al. 2003. Gentamicin coating of metallic implants reduces implant-related osteomyelitis in rats. *Bone,* **32**(5): 521.

Mader JT and Adams KR. 1988. Experimental osteomyelitis, in *Orthopedic Infection* (Schlossberg D, ed), Springer, New York, pp 39–48.

Mangram AJ, Horan TC, Pearson ML, Silver LC, and Jarvis WR. 1999. Guideline for prevention of surgical site infection. *Infect Control Hosp Epidemiol,* **20**: 247–278.

Malassiney P, Goeau-Brissonniere O, Coggia M, and Pechere JC.1996. Rifampicin loading of vascular grafts. *J Antimicrob Chemother,* **37**: 1121–1129.

Matl FD, et al. 2008. New anti-infective coatings of medical implants. *Antimicrob Agents Chemother* 52(6): 1957–1963.

Matl FD, et al. 2009. New anti-infective coatings of surgical sutures based on a combination of antiseptics and fatty acids. *J Biomater Sci Polym Ed,* **20**(10): 1439–1449.

McDonald DE, Palmer RH, Hulse DA, Neigut JS, Hyman WA, and Slater MR. 1994. Holding power of threaded external fixation pins in the near and far cortices of cadaveric canine tibiae. *Vet Surg,* **23**(6): 488–493.

Miller M and Malouin F. 1994. Siderophore-mediated drug delivery: The design, synthesis, and study of siderophore-antibiotic and antifungal conjugates, in *The Development of Iron Chelators for Clinical Use* (Bergeron BJ and Brittenham GM, eds), CRC Press, Boca Raton.

Milovic NM, Wang J, Lewis K, and Klibanov AM. 2005. Immobilized N-alkylated polyethylenimine avidly kills bacteria by rupturing cell membranes with no resistance developed. *Biotechnol Bioeng,* **90**(6): 715–722.

Mims C, Dockrell HM, Goering RV, Roitt I, Wakelin D, and Zuckerman M. 2006. *Medizinische Mikrobiologie - Infektiologie mit StudentConsult-Zugang: mit Virologie, Immunologie,* Urban and Fischer Verlag, Elsevier GmbH, München.

Nasser S. 1999. The incidence of sepsis after total hip replacement arthroplasty. *Semin Arthroplasty,* **5**(4): 153–159.

Neut D, van der Mei HC, Bulstra SK, and Busscher HJ. 2007. The role of small colony variants in failure to diagnose and treat biofilm infections in orthopedics. *Acta Orthop,* **78**: 299–308.

O'Grady NP, Alexander M, Burns LA, Dellinger EP, Garland J, Heard SO, Lipsett PA, Masur H, Mermel LA, Pearson ML, Raad II, Randolph A, Rupp ME,

Saint S, and Healthcare Infection Control Practices Advisory Committee (HICPAC). 2011. *Guidelines for the Prevention of Intravascular Catheter-Related Infections*, Centers for Disease Control and Prevention, Atlanta, p 83.

Patel JD, Ebert M, Ward R, and Anderson JMS. 2007. Epidermidis biofilm formation: Effects of biomaterial surface chemistry and serum proteins. *J Biomed Mater Res A,* **80**: 742–751.

Parvizi J, Saleh KJ, Ragland PS, Pour AE, and Mont MA. 2008. Efficacy of antibiotic-impregnated cement in total hip replacement. *Acta Orthop,* **79**(3): 335–341.

Patton JP, Nash DB, and Abrutyn E. 1991. Urinary tract infection: Economic considerations. *Med Clin North Am,* **75**(2): 495–513.

Pounds LL, Montes-Walters M, Mayhall CG, Falk PS, Sanderson E, Hunter GC, and Killewich LA. 2005. A changing pattern of infection after major vascular reconstructions. *Vasc Endovascular Surg,* **39**: 511–517.

Prabu P, Dharmaraj N, Aryal S, Lee BM, Ramesh V, and Kim HY. 2006. Preparation and drug release activity of scaffolds containing collagen and poly(caprolactone). *J Biomed Mater Res A,* **79**(1): 153–158.

Price JS, Tencer FA, Arm DM, and Bohach GA. 1996. Controlled release of antibiotics from coated orthopaedic implants. *Biomed Mater Res,* **30**: 281.

Rasić Z, Schwarz D, Adam VN, Sever M, Lojo N, Rasić D, and Matejić T. 2011. Efficacy of antimicrobial triclosan-coated polyglactin 910 (Vicryl* Plus) suture for closure of the abdominal wall after colorectal surgery. *Coll Antropol,* **35**(2): 439–443.

Roberts ME and Stewart PS. 2005. Modelling protection from antimicrobial agents in biofilms through the formation of persister cells. *Microbiology,* **151**: 75–80.

Rupp ME, Fitzgerald T, Marion N, Helget V, Puumala S, Anderson JR, and Fey PD. 2004. Effect of silver-coated urinary catheters: Efficacy, cost-effectiveness, and antimicrobial resistance. *Am J Infect Control,* **32**(8): 445–450.

Sardelic F, Ao PY, Taylor DA, and Fletcher JP. 1996. Prophylaxis against Staphylococcus epidermidis vascular graft infection with rifampicin-soaked, gelatin-sealed Dacron. *Cardiovasc Surg,* **4**: 389–392.

Schnabelrauch M. 2011. Antimikrobielle Beschichtungen für Medizinprodukte. 7. Thüringer Grenz- und Oberflächentage und 8. *Thüringer Biomaterial-Kolloquium, Zeulenroda-Triebes, Plenarvortrag.*

Schnürer SM, Gopp U, Kühn KD, and Breusch S. Knochenersatzwerkstoffe. 2003. *Orthopäde* **32**(1): 2–10.

Seeger J, Borgeson M, and Lawson G. 1990. Pseudointimal thrombogenicity changes in small arterial grafts. *Surgery*, **107**: 620–626.

Sohail MR, Uslan DZ, Khan AH, Friedman PA, Hayes DL, Wilson WR, Steckelberg JM, Stoner SM, and Baddour LM. 2007. Risk factor analysis of permanent pacemaker infection. *Clin Infect Dis*, **45**(2): 166–173.

Sripriya R, Kumar MS, and Sehgal PK. 2004. Improved collagen bilayer dressing for the controlled release of drugs. *J Biomed Mater Res B Appl Biomater*, **70**(2): 389–396.

Stemberger AW, et al. 2007. New antibiotic carriers and coatings in surgery, in *Local Antibiotics in Arthroplasty: State of the Art from an Interdisciplinary Point of View* (Walenkamp GHIM, ed), *Thieme-Verlag*, pp 13–22.

Stemberger A and Kühn KD. 2010. Anti-infective protection of implants. *Biomaterialien*, **11**: 47.

Stewart PS. 2002. Mechanisms of antibiotic resistance in bacterial biofilms. *Int J Med Microboil*, **292**: 107–113.

Stigter M, de Groot K, and Layrolle P. 2002. Incorporation of tobramycin into biomimetic hydroxyapatite coating on titanium. *Biomaterials*, **23**: 4143–4153.

Teller M, Gopp U, Neumann H-G, and Kühn KD. 2006. Release of gentamicin from bone regenerative materials: An in vitro study. *J Biomed Mat Res, part B Appl Biomater*, **81B:** 23–29.

Thull R. 2004. Implantatoberfläche und biofilm, in Septische Knochen-und Gelenkchirurgie (Hendricht C, Frommelt L, and Eulert J, eds), Springer Verlag, Heidelberg, pp 203–210.

Tiller JC, Liao C-J, Lewis K, and Klibanov AM. 2001. Designing surfaces that kill bacteria on contact. *Proc Natl Acad Sci USA*, **98**: 5981–5985.

Tiller JC, Lee SB, Lewis K, and Klibanov AM. 2002. Polymer surfaces derivatized with poly(vinyl-*N*-hexylpyridinium) kill airborne and waterborne bacteria. *Biotechnol Bioeng*, **79**: 465–471.

Trampuz A, Piper KE, Jacobson MJ, Hanssen AD, Unni KK, Osmon DR, Mandrekar JN, Cockerill FR, Steckelberg JM, Greenleaf JF, and Patel R. 2007. Sonication of removed hip and knee prostheses for diagnosis of infection. *N Engl J Med*, **357**: 654–663.

Trerotola SO, Johnson MS, Shah H, Kraus MA, McKusky M, Ambrosius WT, Harris VJ, and Snidow JJ. 1998. Tunneled hemodialysis catheters: Use of a silver-coated catheter for preventation of infection—A randomized study. *Radiology,* **207**: 491–496.

Tresse O, Jouenne T, and Junter GA. 1995. The role of oxygen limitation in the resistance of agarentrapped, sessilelike *Escherichia coli* to aminoglycoside and betalactam antibiotics. *J Antimicrob Chemother,* **36**: 521–526.

Veenstra DL, Saint S, Saha S, Lumley T, and Sullivan SD. 1999a. Efficacy of antiseptic-impregnated central venous catheters in preventing catheter-related bloodstream infection: A meta-analysis. *JAMA,* **281**(3): 261–267.

Veenstra DL, Saint S, and Sullivan SD. 1999b. Cost-effectiveness of antiseptic-impregnated central venous catheters for the prevention of catheter-related bloodstream infection. *JAMA,* **282**(6): 554–560.

Vicaretti M, Hawthorne WJ, Ao PY, and Fletcher JP. 1998. An increased concentration of rifampicin bonded to gelatin-sealed Dacron reduces the incidence of subsequent graft infections following a staphylococcal challenge. *Cardiovasc Surg,* **6**: 268–273.

Vogt S, Kühn KD, Gopp U, and Schnabelrauch M. 2005. Resorbable antibiotic coatings for bone substitutes and implantable devices. *Materialwissenschaft und Werkstofftechnik,* **36**: 814–819.

von Eiff C, Heilmann C, and Peters G. 1999. New aspects in the molecular basis of polymerassociated infections due to staphylococci. *Eur J Clin Microbiol Infect Dis,* **18**: 843–846.

von Eiff C, Jansen B, Kohnen W, and Becker K. 2005. Infections associated with medical devices: Pathogenesis, management and prophylaxis. *Drugs,* **65**(2): 179–214.

Wahlig H and Buchholz HW. 1972. Experimental and clinical studies on the release of gentamicin from bone cement. *Chirurg,* **43**: 441–445.

Wahlig H. 1987. Über die Freisetzungskinetik von Antibiotika aus Knochenzementen Ergebnisse vergleichender Untersuchungen in vitro und in vivo. *Chirurgie und Orthopädie,* **31**: 221–226.

Warren DK, Quadir WW, Hollenbeak CS, Elward AM, Cox MJ, and Fraser VJ. 2006. Attributable cost of catheter-associated bloodstream infections among intensive care patients in a nonteaching hospital. *Crit Care Med,* **34**(8): 2084–2089.

Wilson SK, Zumbe J, Henry GD, Salem EA, Delk JR, and Cleves MA. 2007. Infection reduction using antibiotic-coated inflatable penile prosthesis. *Urology* **70**(2): 337–340.

Winkelmann G, van Helm D, and Neilands JB (eds). 1987. *Iron Transport in Microbes, Plants and Animals*, Chemie-Verlagsgesellschaft, Weinheim

Wittmann S, Schnabelrauch M, Scherlitz-Hofmann I, Möllmann U, Ankel-Fuchs D, and Heinisch L. 2002. New synthetic siderophores and their beta-lactam conjugates based on diamino acids and dipeptides. *Bioorg Med Chem*, **10**(6): 1659–1670.

Ziegler G, Gollwitzer H, Heidenau F, Mittelmeier W, and Stenzel F. 2003. Anti-infectious, biocompatible titanium oxide coatings for implants, and method for the production thereof. WO2004/026346 A2.

Chapter 7

Small-Angle X-Ray Spectroscopy as a Method to Monitor the Three-Dimensional Structure of Immobilized Biomolecules on Medical Device Scaffolds during Production

Rupert Tscheliessnig and Alois Jungbauer
University of Natural Resources and Applied Life Sciences,
Austrian Centre of Industrial Biotechnology,
Faculty of Physics, University of Vienna, Vienna, Austria
alois.jungbauer@boku.ac.at

The demand to develop convergent technology platforms, such as biofunctional medical devices, is rapidly increasing. However, immobilization on medical device scaffolds, drying, sterilization, and rehydration of biomolecules may alter the three-dimensional folding of the effector molecule and may lead to the loss of function. In this report, we describe a method that allows the monitoring of the three-dimensional structure of immobilized anti-Fas IgM on polyurethane, which may be used for the extracorporeal blood treatment to limit systemic inflammation in severely ill patients. We further report on

Biofunctional Surface Engineering
Edited by Martin Scholz

ISBN 978-981-4411-60-8 (Hardcover), 978-981-4411-61-5 (eBook)
www.panstanford.com

the stabilizing features of a nano-coating that efficiently protects immobilized proteins from stress-mediated damage.

7.1 Introduction

The implantation of metals or polymers into living tissues requires biocompatibility and effective functionality. Today, implantable materials combined with biological effector molecules are developed to improve the biocompatibility of the product, achieve a prolonged lifetime of the product, and promote specific physiological reactions within the host. The efforts to combine biological materials with implant materials for use in patients have been hampered because biologicals, such as immobilized effector proteins, are denatured after sterilization, thus requiring expensive and time-consuming aseptic production steps. We, therefore, used a nano-coating technology for the three-dimensional stabilization of immobilized proteins that preserves the function of biologic-device combination products during and after standard terminal sterilization (Tscheliessnig et al., 2012). The most common sterilization procedures for the production of medical devices are β- or γ-irradiation and ethylene oxide (EtO) gas sterilization. Each of these procedures occurs in conjunction with high energy transfer and thus leads to modified protein folding attributable to loading shifts, redistribution of charges within the protein, breakdown of hydrogen bonds, and eventually disruption of covalent bonds within the protein (Drake et al., 1957; Gianfreda and Scarfi, 1991; Kapoor and Priyadarsini, 2001). Especially with β- and γ-irradiation, the presence of oxygen and water facilitates the formation of destructive oxygen radicals (Garrison et al., 1962), which may lead to undesirable chain reactions within the protein for prolonged periods of time (e.g., during the storage of terminally sterilized material).

In the past, many efforts were made to identify ideal protein protectors. For example, the protective effects of sugars (e.g., trehalose and saccharose), sugar alcohols (e.g., mannitol), and proteins (e.g., albumin) are well known (Arakawa et al, 2007; Jain and Roy, 2009; Jorgensen et al., 2009). However, during freezing or lyophilization and reconstitution, sugars may result in unappreciated damage of the biomolecule (Han et al., 2007). Therefore, a sugar-free formulation, comprising small molecules such as amino acids in combination with glycyrrhizic acid, was used to stabilize and protect immobilized biomolecules.

This method presupposes that at least three prerequisites must be met to allow the irradiation of immobilized proteins without significant loss of function: (i) removal of water molecules, (ii) establishment of hydrogen bonds between co-solvent and protein, and (iii) avoidance of crystallization-mediated protein damage during dehydration/hydration. According to the concept of preferential exclusion (Timasheff et al., 1993; Arakawa et al., 2001), co-solvents that substitute for the water molecules, which normally constitute the hydrogen bonds in the hydrated form, were used in combination with glycosidic saponins (Fuchs et al., 2009). Glycyrrhizic acid, a member of glycosidic saponins, was selected because of its unique feature to form amorphous gels while chemically interacting with stabilizing amino acids. The amorphous nature of the dried films of the amino acid/glycyrrhizic acid solution on a suitable carrier material was shown by wide-angle X-ray diffraction (XRD). Thermal analysis of the frozen amino acid/glycyrrhizic acid solution by differential scanning calorimetry revealed two thermal transitions of the freeze-concentrated non-ice phase (T_g' is glass transitions of maximally freeze-concentrated phases): T_{g1}' at −60°C and T_{g2}' at −49°C, suggesting two different amorphous glass states in the frozen solution. The physical properties of the nano-coating enable the coating of any surface to reach homogenous thin films with variable thickness in the nanometer range (Tscheliessnig et al., 2012).

This saponin-mediated glassy state in conjunction with selected amino acids proved to be highly protective for the immobilized proteins, possibly because of the high numbers of hydroxyl groups present in the glycoside part of the saponin.

7.2 Nano-Coating

Figure 7.1 schematically illustrates the mode of function of the nano-coating that fulfils the three aforementioned prerequisites. The stabilizing solution comprises a specifically selected mixture of small molecules, such as amino acids, combined with saponin-type glycosides. The solution covers the medical device surface material, including the immobilized proteins. During careful drying and removal of water molecules, the small-molecule co-solutes subsequently interact with the protein, thereby maintaining its native conformation. At the end of the drying process, the glassy stabilizing and protective layer consists of a molecular film in the nanometer range that protects the functionality of the surface during sterilization by β- or γ-irradiation and EtO gas sterilization. After sterilization, the functionalized material can be applied to its intended use. Alternatively, because of the prolonged shelf life achieved by nano-coating, the materials can be used for long-term storage.

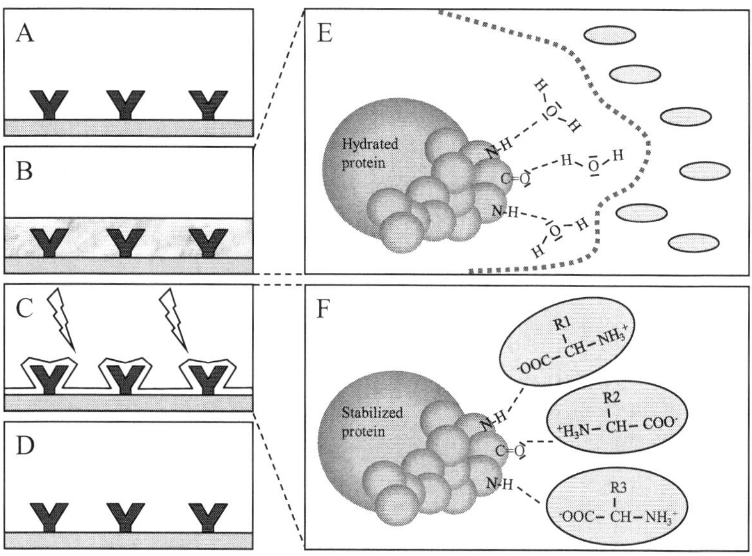

Figure 7.1 Fabrication process and mode of function of nano-coating. Schematic diagram of the procedure for protecting immobilized proteins during irradiation with IgG antibody as an example. The chemical interactions between protein, water, and co-solutes are depicted schematically. The relationship between compounds can be described by the interaction parameter ζ_3. Nano-coating compounds provide hydrogen bonds and substitute for water molecules. Reprinted from Tscheliessnig et al. (2012), with permission of Elsevier.

Protein stabilization by preferential exclusion depends on the concentration of the co-solute. The interaction parameter ζ_3 is a function of the molar concentration of the co-solute ($m_{\text{Co-solute}}$) and can be expressed mathematically by the following function (Arakawa et al., 2001):

$$\zeta_3 = \frac{\delta m_{\text{Co-Solute}}}{\delta m_{\text{Protein}}} = A_{\text{Co-Solute}} - (m_{\text{Co-Solute}} A_{\text{H}_2\text{O}})$$

Especially at high co-solute concentrations, the hydration term A_{H2O} has a significant impact so that ζ_3 may reach a negative value, indicating the preferential exclusion of the co-solute and protein stabilization.

Preferential exclusion requires sufficient amounts of water to be present at least locally. During drying, the concentration of the co-solute is increased, and the preferential exclusion effect is enhanced in the residual wet regions. The protein remains hydrated in its native form until the residual water molecules are removed, whereas hydrogen bonds are formed between the protein and the functional groups of the lyoprotectant (Timasheff, 2002; Auton et al., 2008; Shimizu and Smith, 2004).

The glassy state of the protecting (nano-coating) layer also helps to prevent undesirable microcrystal formation during freezing and drying. Although sugars are generally suitable as lyoprotectants because of their solubility and OH groups for hydrogen bonds, their rapid crystallization at higher concentrations is a clear disadvantage (Han et al., 2007). Given an initial molar ratio of 500:1 (sugar:protein), the ratio is further increased during the drying process. Therefore, crystallization occurs, which reduces the availability of sugar molecules and consequently their hydrogen-binding capacity. Surprisingly, we found that some members of the saponin group (e.g., glycyrrhizic acid) act as suitable lyoprotectants, possibly because of the presence of glycoside OH groups.

In contrast to saccharides, the saponin glycyrrhizic acid (Baltina, 2003), e.g., does not crystallize but rather forms an amorphous gel (glassy state), thereby providing the OH groups for forming hydrogen bonds until the protein is entirely dried.

Because of the high sensitivity to irradiation-induced damage, we used a highly complex and large (960 kD) IgM molecule as a model protein (anti-Fas IgM). The IgM was coupled to open porous polyurethane foam (PU-IgM$_{\text{Fas}}$) for the intended use in a medical device for extracorporeal immunotherapy. The antibody used here agonistically recognizes and stimulates Fas (CD95) (Scholz et al., 2005) on cell membranes without the need for additional cross-linkers because of the pentameric structure and presence of 10 Fas-specific paratopes on each IgM (Scholz et al., 2005; Peter et al., 2007;

Fadeel et al., 1998). The Fas/Fas ligand (FasL) system is a central regulatory component of the innate immune system that limits misdirected immune reactions by inducing apoptosis in immune cells (e.g., hyperactivated neutrophil granulocytes with autodestructive potential)(Scholz et al., 2005).

Covalent immobilization on biocompatible carriers was achieved by standard coupling chemistry, and the nano-coating procedure was performed by incubating the functionalized material with the protective solution for 1 h. After the drying step at room temperature, water molecules were almost completely removed to avoid the formation of oxygen radicals during sterilization or storage. The nano-coating layer was removed by a washing step to reconstitute the immobilized protein before use in biological systems. However, without rinsing, bodily fluids such as blood, plasma, or wound exudate will solubilize the stabilizers and reconstitute the protein.

7.3 Small-Angle X-ray Scattering

To demonstrate the protective effects of the nano-coating, the three-dimensional structure of the anti-Fas IgM immobilized on polyurethane was studied at the nanomolecular level by small-angle X-ray scattering (SAXS)(Glatter et al., 1982). IgM is considered self-similar and fractal. It displays a regular superstructure, according to an aggregate. Thus it is critical and described by a particular pair–pair correlation function (Chandler, 1987): $< \rho(\zeta')\rho(\zeta - \zeta') > = \gamma_R \zeta^{(3-D)}$.

Using SAXS, we accessed the scattering contrast, $I(Q)$, of the samples and mapped the characteristic spatial arrangement of anti-Fas IgM in the reciprocal space, $F\,(< \rho(\zeta')\rho(\zeta - \zeta') >)[Q]$. For a fractal system and for a small Q, the scattering contrast scales with $\log(I(Q)) = -D \log(Q) + \text{const.}$

According to Kotlarchyk and Chen (1983), we assumed that the scattering contrast $I(Q)$ for IgG may be given as the product of the protein form and the apparent protein structure factor.

$$I(Q) \propto P_{\mathbf{IgG}}(Q) \times S_{\mathbf{IgM}}(Q) \tag{7.1}$$

With $P_{\text{IgG}}(Q)$, we addressed the characteristic structure of an IgG that represents the five IgG-like substructures within the pentameric IgM, whereas with $S_{\text{IgM}}(Q)$, we mapped their particular arrangement.

The form factor $P_{\mathrm{IgG}}(Q)$ was reconstructed by the following function (Horejs et al., 2010):

$$P_{\mathbf{IgG}}(Q)=F(\rho_{\mathbf{IgG}}(\zeta))[Q]\approx\frac{1}{2\pi^{D}}\int_{0}^{\infty}duu^{D-1}\frac{1}{u^{2}+\kappa^{2}}\frac{J_{D/2-1}(Qu)}{(Qu)^{D/2-1}} \tag{7.2}$$

$$\approx\frac{1}{2\pi}^{D}\kappa^{D/2-1}\frac{K_{D/2-1}(Q\kappa)}{(Q\kappa)^{D/2-1}} \tag{7.3}$$

To reconstruct the IgM molecule (gray bead model in Fig. 7.2), we replaced the integral in Eq. 7.2 by a sum, and Eq. 7.2 formally obtains the fractal equivalent to Debye's formula (Debye, 1915).

For the untreated immobilized antibody on PU (PU-IgM$_{\mathrm{Fas}}$), the scattering contrast was too low with respect to the background signal of PU alone, and we calculated the relative change, $\Delta P(Q)$, of PU-IgM$_{\mathrm{Fas}}$ with nano-coating (PU-IgM$_{\mathrm{Fas}}$-NC), PU-IgM$_{\mathrm{Fas}}$, and PU-IgM$_{\mathrm{Fas}}$–NC after β-irradiation (*PU-IgM$_{\mathrm{Fas}}$, *PU-IgM$_{\mathrm{Fas}}$–NC) with respect to PU-IgM$_{\mathrm{Fas}}$.

We determined the structure of the IgM molecule. Specifically, the opening angle θ comprises the five IgG arms. We first observed that in the limit for low Q, the logarithm of the form factor is constant, and thus we can anticipate that in this limit the structure factor scales with $S_{\mathbf{IgM}}(Q) \approx Q^{-D}$ as $P(Q) \approx$ const. (see dashed lines in Fig. 7.2). The self-similarity of IgM and the relationship of the change in fractal dimension, D, with changes of the IgM structure are shown. The average size of the IgG arm is given by k, and its self-similar equivalent, at larger scale, is given by k_p. IgM and IgG structural models are given by green and gray bead models, respectively. In the upper panel, large red open circles correspond to background-corrected scattering intensities. Dashed lines indicate analytic form factors. The average size of an IgG arm resembles $\kappa \approx 4.0$–6.0 nm. Black lines give the full fit of SAXS data based on the gray IgG structural models and their mean forces. In the lower panel, small open connected circles indicate these corresponding mean forces.

In Fig. 7.2a, cattering intensities of dried samples *PU-IgM$_{\mathrm{Fas}}$, PU-IgM$_{\mathrm{Fas}}$–NC, and *PU-IgM$_{\mathrm{Fas}}$–NC and the relative change of the form factor DP(Q) are given with respect to the background and scattering intensity of PU-IgM$_{\mathrm{Fas}}$. The fractal dimension $D = 3$ and an anticipated green structural model are given. Mean forces hold a pronounced corrugation and are given as a multitude of kT (k is the Boltzmann constant and T the system temperature). In Fig. 7.2b, the sample

PU-IgM_{Fas} was rehydrated. The system's fractal dimension falls to D = 2.5. The corresponding angle θ increases, indicating a partially open IgM structural model (green bead model). The corrugation of corresponding mean force is decreased. As shown in Fig. 7.2c, The rehydrated samples PU-IgM_{Fas}–NC and *PU-IgM_{Fas}–NC exhibited a fractal dimension of D = 1.5. The corresponding angle θ supports a rather open IgM structural model (green bead model). Again, the corrugation of the corresponding mean force decreased.

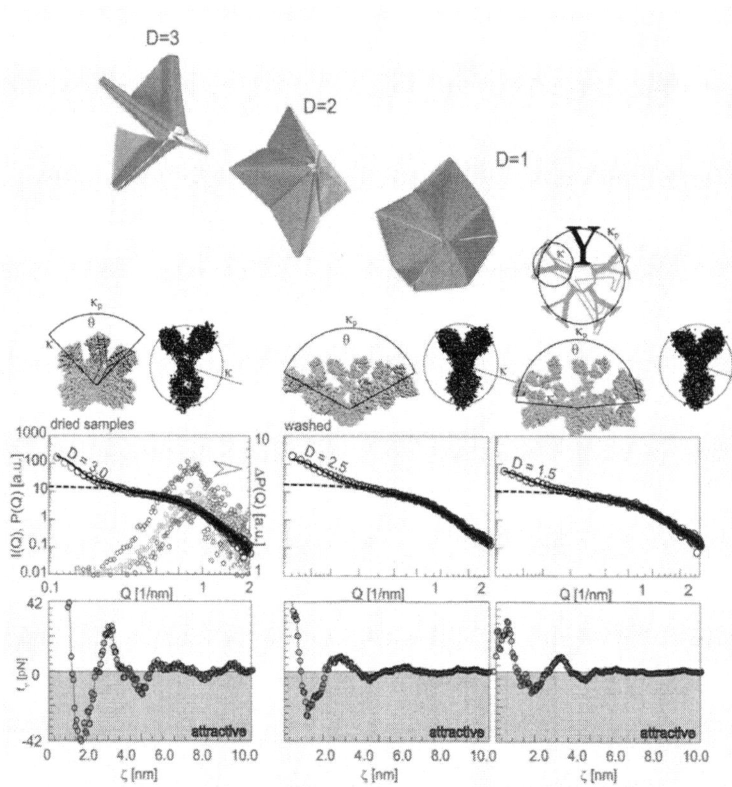

Figure 7.2 SAXS images of functionalized open porous polyurethane foam. Reprinted from Tscheliessnig et al. (2012), with permission of Elsevier.

We related the fractal dimension D to the particular opening angle θ (for detailed discussion, see below and Fig. 7.2). The radian measure is $\kappa\,\zeta_p = \theta \times \zeta$. Because the system under investigation has a fractal character, we needed to consider possible scale invariance, which in real space is given by $\rho(\zeta_p) = \lambda^{-\nu}\rho(\lambda^{\nu}\zeta)$ and in reciprocal space is given by $F[\rho(\zeta)](Q) = \lambda^{-2\nu} F[\rho(\zeta)](\lambda^{-\nu} Q)$.

We assumed that in the present case, $\nu = 1 - D/2$. We next assigned $\lambda = 4$, in which $D = 1$ gives an IgG chain angle of $\theta \approx 3.14(\pi)°$, $D = 2$ gives an angle of $\theta \approx 1.05(\pi/3)°$, and $D = 3$ gives an angle of $\theta \approx 0.51°$.

The self-similarity of the IgM molecule and the impact on the fractal dimension shall be motivated by the letter models in Fig. 7.2. With $D = 3$, the mean diameter of the IgG arm, κ, is smaller than the diameter κ_p. For $D = 2$, both radii are equivalent, and for $D = 1$, the equation $2\kappa = \kappa_p$ is applicable.

In a complementary approach, we calculated the mean forces to which an individual IgG arm is exposed. With the definition of the mean potential

$$S_{\mathbf{IgM}}(Q) = -F(-\int \beta\partial_{\zeta} w(\zeta)\exp(-\beta w(\zeta))d\zeta)[Q] \approx F(-\sum\nolimits_{\nu} f_{\nu}\delta(\zeta-\nu))[Q],$$

the fractal Fourier transformation (Vembu, 1961) gives the following:

$$S_{\mathbf{IgG}}(Q) = \sum_{\nu} f_{\nu} J_{D/2-1}(Q\nu)/(Q\nu)^{D/2-1} \qquad (7.4)$$

Therein, f_ν corresponds to the mean force.

The goal of nano-coated surfaces with immobilized proteins is to achieve stability of the proteins during sterilization procedures and storage. During these procedures, the nano-coating remains on the surface until further use. For the functional use of biologic-device combination products, the nano-coating will be washed away by an aqueous solution. Therefore, the SAXS characteristics for both washed and unwashed PU-IgM$_{\mathrm{Fas}}$-NC samples were studied. SAXS profiles of unwashed samples are shown in Fig. 7.2. Proteins are traced by their negative electronic contrast. We first investigated the dried samples, which resembled the product in its typical stored form.

The signals of the structure of bare samples (PU-IgM$_{\mathrm{Fas}}$) are at the lower limit of resolution. Therefore, we did not take the background-corrected signal to deduce a structure model but calculated and discussed the relative structural change if the samples were coated (PU-IgM$_{\mathrm{Fas}}$–NC), exposed to radiation (*PU-IgM$_{\mathrm{Fas}}$), or coated and subsequently exposed to radiation (*PU-IgM$_{\mathrm{Fas}}$–NC). The relative electronic contrast was negative. Dried PU-IgM$_{\mathrm{Fas}}$–NC samples had less electronic contrast than the untreated PU-IgM$_{\mathrm{Fas}}$ equivalents.

The greatest differences were found if untreated PU-IgM_{Fas} samples were compared with PU-IgM_{Fas}–NC (black open circles in Fig. 7.2). The coating decreased the scattering contrast for characteristic distances between ζ = 3 nm and ζ = 15 nm. These distances corresponded to the average extension of the IgM molecule and provided evidence that the IgM molecules were entirely coated.

When PU-IgM_{Fas} samples were compared with *PU-IgM_{Fas}, we again observed a significant decrease in electronic contrast, which was detectable between ζ = 3 nm and ζ = 12 nm. This difference, however, was less pronounced and much more localized within the characteristic size of the IgM molecule. This result may principally reflect the fact that radiation caused a faint conformational change or that radiation damaged the protein insofar as it broke bonds and thus decreased electronic contrast.

The next issue we addressed was whether nano-coating protects the IgM molecule. We compared PU-IgM_{Fas} with *PU-IgM_{Fas}–NC. The relative difference in electronic contrast is measurable but is low compared with the samples discussed so far and at the limit of detection. The cause of reduced electronic contrast is likely attributable to radiation-induced changes in protein conformation in conjunction with disruption of hydrogen bonds. However, the nano-coating lowered this effect to a small but detectable extent.

The PU-IgM_{Fas} samples were at the limit to be distinguishable from the scattering contrast of polyurethane foam, and we addressed the protein structure reconstruction of the samples *PU-IgM_{Fas}, PU-IgM_{Fas}–NC, and *PU-IgM_{Fas}–NC. All three samples showed comparable scattering profiles. Thus we deduced the structure and mean force from an average profile.

According to Eq. 7.3, we estimated the average size of an IgG arm to be $\kappa \approx 4.0 - 6.0$ nm (see dashed lines in Fig. 7.2). We next exchanged the integral in Eq. 7.2 by a sum and applied a Monte Carlo algorithm to reconstruct the molecule as depicted by the gray structural model in Fig. 7.2. The difference between the bead model and the SAXS scattering data is attributable to the structure factor. All dried systems had a common fractal dimension of $D = 3$. In terms of angles (θ), we anticipated that all dried samples had a common IgM superstructure with an angle θ and that the IgG arms comprise close to $\theta \approx 0.51°$ or $\theta \approx 29.22°$. The anticipated IgM structural model is given in Fig. 7.2 by the green bead model.

To reconstruct the entire SAXS signal, we determined the mean forces between the IgG arms. These are given at the bottom of Fig. 7.2. The high corrugation of the mean forces indicates a stabilized protein structure, which is collapsed. We related the high corrugation to the lack of a hydration shell in any of the dried samples.

After rehydration of the nano-coated and uncoated samples and reconstitution of the hydration shell, the scattering contrast for all samples was positive compared with the dried samples. Rehydrated PU-IgM_{Fas} samples have a fractal dimension of $D = 2.5$. According to our assumption, this indicates that the IgM superstructure comprises an increased angle (θ) caused by reimposing the hydration shell. We related these findings to the mean forces, which are given at the bottom of Fig. 7.2. For IgG molecules that are exposed to radiation, we clearly observed a decrease in the corrugation of these mean forces. Consequently, we anticipated that as the IgG molecules are less exposed to mean forces, the IgM protein can unfold. A related structural model is given by the green bead model in Fig. 7.2.

These effects are even more pronounced when *PU-IgM_{Fas}–NC is washed after radiation. A structural model for the IgG arms was calculated (gray bead model in Fig. 7.2). As the fractal dimension falls to $D = 1.5$, the angle can be expected to increase. We anticipated that coating favors rehydration of the protein. When we combined the structural model and the opening angle θ, we could reconstruct a structural model for the IgM molecule. This is given by the green bead model in Fig. 7.2. Again, we calculated the mean forces and found that the corrugation is lower than in the examples given in Fig. 7.2. These findings are consistent with the aforementioned interpretations. We anticipate that rehydration of the samples favors an open IgM structure.

7.4 Safety of Nano-Coating

Proving safety throughout the production process is mandatory for developing biologic-device combination products. An important question to answer is whether nano-coating may also protect against bacteria or viruses that might contaminate the medical device material during the production process. Therefore, the bioburden (ISO11137-1 and ISO11137-2) of functionalized and nano-coated polyurethane foams that were utilized for clinical evaluation was confirmed and validated according to the ISO11137 VD_{max} method (Tscheliessnig et al., 2012).

7.5 Functionality of Nano-Coating

As recently reported (Tscheliessnig et al., 2012), the functionality of the stabilized antibody on PU was clearly confirmed by antigen- and peptide-binding studies as well as apoptosis-inducing efficacy studies. For example, highly specific recombinant Fas antigen fragment (Schneider et al., 1997) and a recombinant 18mer Fas antigen peptide were used in these experiments. Moreover, the biological function of the agonistic anti-Fas antibody was shown to be maintained by using Fas-sensitive T-cells as a model and neutrophils from severely injured trauma patients.

In conclusion, the SAXS method is suitable for the monitoring of the three-dimensional folding of immobilized biomolecules on the surface of biofunctional medical devices. Our results described herein proved that the nano-coating technology enables the development of end-sterilized biofunctionalized materials without loss of function and safety. These findings are highly relevant because this technology may enable the easy and inexpensive production of biologic-device combination products by avoiding expensive clean-room processing (Shmulewitz et al., 2006; Ratner, 2007; Hupcey and Ekins, 2007; Masefield and Brinston, 2007; Brinston, 2008; Fireman, 2008; Woolston, 2009). The described nano-coating technology was presented herein with polyurethane as a possible carrier material and β-irradiation as an example of a standard sterilization procedure. However, nano-coating has already been successfully applied to other biocompatible materials used in medical devices and with γ-irradiation and EtO sterilization (Table 7.1). The currently discussed reduction of the standard irradiation dose of 25 kGy (Perkins et al., 1991), required for terminal sterilization of biologic-device combination products (ISO 11137-1:2006 and 11137-2:2006), may entail a higher risk of contamination. The features of the protective nano-coating allow terminal sterilization with currently existing irradiation standards and should be considered in ongoing discussions.

Table 7.1 Functional preservation of biomaterials after irradiation by nano-coating

Application	Biomaterial (carrier)	Biomolecule
Orthopedic and dental implants	Titanium	Bone morphogenic protein-2 Antimicrobial proteins
Cardiovascular stents	Steel	IgG antibodies
Wound dressings	Polyurethane Polyester Polyvinyl alcohol (PVA)	Proangiogenic growth factors Ascorbic acid
Catheters	Steel Gold Gold/Hydrogel combination Titanium alloys	IgG antibodies Antibody fragments
Extracorporeal blood treatment devices and circuit components	Polyurethane Polyester Polycarbonate	Anti-Fas IgM
Biofunctionalized micro- and nanobeads	Polyethylene Glass Silicon	IgG antibodies
Diagnostic devices	Silicon	IgG antibodies Circulating free DNA
Protein arrays	Polycarbonate Polystyrol Polytetrafluorethene Glass	Proteins range: 9–900 kDa
Formulation of therapeutic antibodies and biopharmaceuticals	Lyophilisates Microneedles	IgG and IgM antibodies
Vaccine generation and formulation	Lyophilisates	Viruses and viral antigens

Source: Reprinted from Tscheliessnig et al. (2012), with permission of Elsevier.

References

Arakawa T, Prestrelski SJ, Kenney WC, and Carpenter JF. 2001. Factors affecting short-term and long-term stabilities of proteins. *Adv Drug Deliv Rev*, **46**: 307–326.

Arakawa T, et al. 2007. Biotechnology applications of amino acids in protein purification and formulations. *Amino Acids*, **33**(4): 587–605.

Auton M, Bolen DW, and Rosgen J. 2008. Structural thermodynamics of protein preferential solvation: Osmolyte solvation of proteins, aminoacids, and peptides. *Proteins*, **73**(4): 802–813.

Baltina L. 2003. Chemical modification of glycyrrhizic acid as a route to new bioactive compounds for medicine. *Curr Med Chem*, **10**(2): 155–171.

Brinston R, Miller A, and Deeley C. 2008. Developments in radiation sterilization. *Med Device Technol*, **19**(2): 36–37.

Chandler D. 1987. *Introduction to Modern Statistical Mechanics*, Oxford University Press, USA, ISBN 0195042778.

Debye P. 1915. Zerstreuung von Röntgenstrahlen Annalen der. *Physik*, **46**: 809–823.

Drake MP, et al. 1957. Chemical effects of ionizing radiation on proteins.1,2 I. Effects of γ-radiation on the amino acid content of insulin. J Am Chem Soc, **79**(6): 1395–1401.

Fadeel B, Lindberg J, Achour A, and Chiodi F. 1998. A three-dimensional model of the Fas/Apo-1 molecule: Cross-reactivity of anti-Fas antibodies explained by structural mimicry of antigenic sites. *Int Immunol*, **10**(2): 131–140.

Fireman J. 2008. Modernizing sterilization standards: Re-evaluating current requirements could boost drug/device combinations. *Ortho Des Technol*, Nov-Dec.

Fuchs H, et al. 2009. Saponins as tool for improved targeted tumor therapies. *Curr Drug Targets*, **10**(2): 140–151.

Garrison WM, Jayko ME, and Bennett W. 1962. Radiation-induced oxidation of protein in aqueous solution. *J Radiat Res*, **16**: 483–502.

Gianfreda L and Scarfi MR. 1991. Enzyme stabilization: State of the art. *Mol Cell Biochem*, **100**(2): 97–128.

Glatter O and Kratky O. 1982. *Small-Angle X-Ray Scattering*, Academic Press, London, ISBN 0122862805.

Han Y, et al. 2007. Effects of sugar additives on protein stability of recombinant human serum albumin during lyophilization and storage. *Arch Pharm Res*, **30**(9): 1124–1131.

Horejs C, et al. 2010. S-layer protein characterization by SAXS and a fractal mean force concept: From protein structure to nano-disc assemblies. *J Chem Phys*, **133**(17): 175102. doi: 10.1063/1.3489682.

Hupcey MAZ and Ekins S. 2007. Improving the drug selection and development process for combination devices. *Drug Discov Today* **12**: 844–852.

ISO 11137-1:2006. Sterilization of health care products—Radiation—Part 1: Requirements for development, validation and routine control of a sterilization process for medical devices.

ISO 11137-2:2006. Sterilization of health care products—Radiation—Part 2: Establishing the sterilization dose.

Jain NK and Roy I. 2009. Effect of trehalose on protein structure. *Protein Sci*, **18**(1): 24–36.

Jorgensen L, et al. 2009. Recent trends in stabilizing peptides and proteins in pharmaceutical formulation—considerations in the choice of excipients. *Expert Opin Drug Deliv*, **6**(11): 1219–1230.

Kapoor S and Priyadarsini KI. 2001. Protection of radiation-induced protein damage by curcumin. *Biophys Chem*, **92**(1–2): 119–126.

Kotlarchyk M and Chen S-H. 1983. Analysis of small-angle neutron scattering spectra from polydisperse interacting colloids. *J Chem Phys*, **79**: 2461–2469.

Masefield J and Brinston R. 2007. Radiation sterilization of advanced drug-device combination products. *Med Device Tech*, **18**(2): 12–16.

Perkins SJ, Nealis AS, Sutton BJ, and Feinstein A. 1991. Solution structure of human and mouse immunoglobulin M by synchrotron X-ray scattering and molecular graphics modelling. A possible mechanism for complement activation. *J Mol Biol*, **221**: 1345–1366.

Peter ME, et al. 2007. The CD95 receptor: Apoptosis revisited. *Cell*, 129: 447–450.

Ratner M. 2007. Reality check for device-drug convergence. *Nat Biotechnol*, **25**: 157–159.

Schneider P, et al. 1997. Characterization of Fas (Apo-1, CD95)-Fas ligand interaction. *J Biol Chem*, **272**(30): 18827–18833.

Scholz M and Cinatl J. 2005. Fas/FasL interaction: A novel immune therapy approach with immobilized biologicals. *Med Res Rev*, **25**: 331–342.

Shimizu S and Smith DJ. 2004. Preferential hydration and the exclusion of co-solvents from protein surfaces. *J Chem Phys*, **121**(2): 1148–1154.

Shmulewitz A, Langer R, and Patton J. 2006. Convergence in biomedical technology. *Nat Biotechnol*, **24**: 277–281.

Timasheff SN. 1993. The control of protein stability and association by weak interactions with water: How do solvents affect these processes? *Annu Rev Biophys Biomol Struct*, **22**: 67–97.

Timasheff SN. 2002. Protein-solvent preferential interactions, protein hydration, and the modulation of biochemical reactions by solvent components. *Proc Natl Acad Sci USA*, **99**(15): 9721–9726.

Tscheliessnig R, et al. 2012. Nano-coating protects biofunctional materials. *Mater Today*, **15**(9): 394–404.

Vembu S. 1961. Fourier transformation of the n-dimensional radial delta function. *Q J Math*, **12**(1): 165–168.

Woolston J. 2009. Radiation processing: Adapting to a changing world. *Med Device Technol*, **20**(1): 14–17.

Chapter 8

Aptamers as Biomimetic Surface Coatings for Blood-Contacting Implants

Meltem Avci-Adali, Stefanie Krajewski, Nadja Perle, Nadja Wilhelm, Jan Niederländer, Heidi Stoll, Christian Schlensak, and Hans P. Wendel

Clinical Research Laboratory, Department of Thoracic, Cardiac and Vascular Surgery, University Hospital Tübingen, Calwerstr. 7/1, 72076 Tübingen, Germany

hans-peter.wendel@med.uni-tuebingen.de

This chapter introduces the approach to functionalize implants with aptamers. Aptamers are high-affinity RNA or DNA oligonucleotides, which, due to their spatial structure, can exhibit high affinity and specificity for a target molecule. This affinity can be 1000-fold higher when compared to antibodies. The generation of aptamers is performed by means of a combinatorial chemistry method called SELEX (Systematic Evolution of Ligands by Exponential Enrichment). It is based on the isolation of functional single-stranded nucleic acid ligands (ssDNA or RNA) from vast libraries of up to 10^{15} molecules. This review focuses on the efforts to catch endothelial progenitor cells out of the blood flow by means of aptamers on the vascular graft to develop endothelialized small-lumen vascular prostheses.

Biofunctional Surface Engineering
Edited by Martin Scholz

ISBN 978-981-4411-60-8 (Hardcover), 978-981-4411-61-5 (eBook)
www.panstanford.com

8.1 Introduction

The entire set of devices used clinically in intra- or extracorporeal applications are all made of technical materials such as polymers, metals, and alloys. Although these materials have excellent mechanical and physical properties, they were originally developed for industrial use and only secondarily for biomedical use (Yianni, 1992). All these materials are also associated with a more or less poor hemocompatibility, leading to a pathophysiological, traumatic shock-like response in the organism after blood contact (Wachtfogel et al., 1993; Hamsten, 1993; Colman et al., 1987).

During molecular interaction between a biomaterial surface and tissue or blood, a series of reactions take place that are crucial for the interface compatibility of the respective biomaterial. At first, plasma proteins are adsorbed nonspecifically to the artificial surface. These adsorbed proteins can function as signaling molecules after undergoing conformational changes and hence influence subsequent cellular colonization. Furthermore, the layer of adsorbed proteins builds a matrix for the adhesion of blood and tissue cells as well as for bacteria colonization. For these reasons, a variety of surface treatments have been developed to optimize the hemocompatibility of artificial surfaces (Wendel and Ziemer, 1999; Tanzi, 2005; Gunaydin, 2004a,b).

As also common in many other economic sectors, new and improved products displace old ones and consequently, for example, surface-coated oxygenation systems made their way to the market of extracorporeal circulation systems in recent years. In general, the whole amount of blood of a patient gets in contact with about 3 m^2 of foreign surface over a period of, sometimes, several hours during cardiopulmonary bypass surgery using the heart–lung machine. This contact causes a massive activation of humoral and cellular defense mechanisms against the supposedly pathogenic intruder of the human body leading to the instigation of various activation cascades.

Nowadays, many manufacturers offer only coated systems and have already withdrawn uncoated ones from the market. Despite numerous technical improvements a considerable activation of plasma proteins and corpuscular blood components still occurs. Heparin coating is certainly only the beginning to improve the biocompatibility of a biomaterial that comes into contact with blood or tissue. To further improve the surface properties of blood-contacting medical devices such as stents, oxygenators, etc., significantly more far-reaching knowledge about pathophysiologic immune responses is needed. Broad-based screening tests using DNA chips can be useful to investigate differential gene expression (Hoffmann et al., 2005). Such investigations may contribute to a better understanding of the defense mechanisms occurring during contact of blood with foreign unphysiological surfaces as well as to the development of completely new strategies for improving the biocompatibility of implants.

The optimum for rapid healing and long-term success of an implant, however, could be found in fast colonization by autologous cell populations specialized for the particular application. Until today, attempts are made using bioreactors to colonize materials with autologous cells prior to implantation. However, this process is currently still very labor intensive, little automated, hardly good manufacturing practice compliant, and therefore, clinically only feasible in exceptional cases. Current approaches are based on the development of simple and ready-to-use systems that can be used to attain good reproducibility and rapid cell growth.

A way to achieve this aim is the use of so-called capture molecules, which are applied to implants prior to bioreactor incubation. The respective capture molecules then lead to the binding of the desired cell population directly from biological materials such as apheresis product, bone marrow, fat, etc., to the implant surface.

Consequently, each patient could receive the required implant already colonized with autologous stem cells, which then differentiate to fully functional tissue, thereby generating an optimal physiological surface for the patient.

8.2 Aptamers

Aptamers are high-affinity RNA or DNA oligonucleotides, which, due to their spatial structure, can exhibit high affinity and specificity for a target molecule. This affinity can be up to 1000-fold higher when compared to antibodies. The generation of aptamers is performed by means of a combinatorial chemistry method called SELEX (Systematic Evolution of Ligands by Exponential Enrichment). It is based on the isolation of functional single-stranded nucleic acid ligands (ssDNA or RNA) from vast libraries of up to 10^{15} molecules.

Compared with other combinatorial libraries [phage display ($<10^{11}$ peptides), immune repertoire of the rat ($<10^{8}$ immunoglobulins)], the SELEX technology uses a startup library with such diversity that ligands against virtually any target structure should be available. Furthermore, once identified, aptamers with the highest affinity and specificity can be synthesized relatively easily (Brody, 2000; Gold, 1995; Blank et al., 2001).

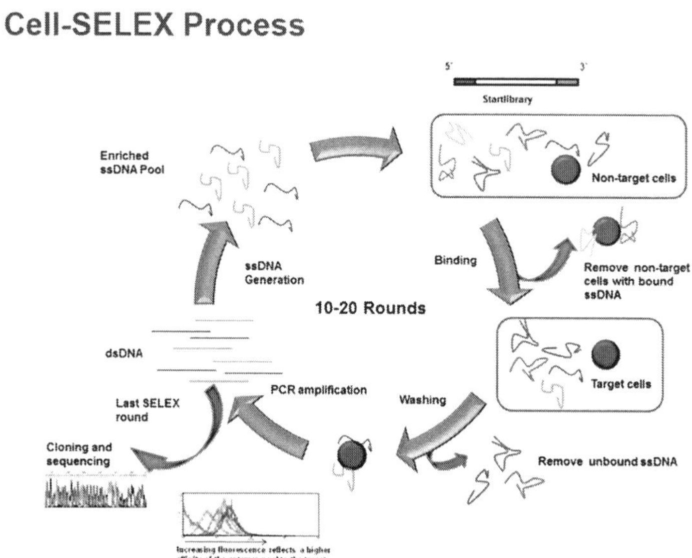

Figure 8.1 Schematic representation of the generation of aptamers using SELEX technology.

Moreover, the advantages of aptamers over antibodies are the ease of preparation, the high specificity and selectivity, and the long-term stability and sterilizability. In addition, ligands can be selected simultaneously against several membrane proteins, as described by Morris et al. for erythrocytes (Morris et al., 1998).

Aptamers can be used pharmacologically in many versatile ways: as specific inhibitors in, e.g., tumor treatment, as drugs directed against tropical parasites, and much more (Ireson and Kelland, 2006; Goringer et al., 2006). An aptamer-based drug has already been approved for clinical application by the Food and Drug Administration. This aptamer shows inhibitory activity against VEGF [trade name: Macugen (Pegaptanib: an acronym from the English

PEGylated aptamer inhibitor)] and is successfully applied against age-related macular degeneration (Tobin, 2006).

8.3 Execution of the SELEX Procedure

A synthetically produced and purified ssDNA library generally contains a central 30–nucleotide-long sequence of random base sequences, flanked by both 23- and 20-nucleotide-long primer hybridization sites (5′-GGG AGC TCA GAA TAA ACG CTC AA -30-nucleotide-TTC ATG GAC AGG CCC GGA TC-3′)(Morris et al., 1998). In the first step of the SELEX process, the complete library is incubated with the desired target cells, followed by the separation of binding and nonbinding nucleotides by centrifugation and washing steps. Afterward, the affine nucleotides are amplified via polymerase chain reaction and used for the next round of selection.

In the next SELEX round, already much less nucleotides compete for the target structures. To eliminate aptamers against general cell membrane structures, so-called counter selections can be performed using, e.g., blood cells. Since each nucleotide of the ssDNA library contains an FITC-18C-labeling, aptamer affinity can be evaluated by flow cytometry after each round of selection. Thereby, the number of SELEX rounds depends on the fluorescence enhancement. After the last selection, the obtained aptamers are isolated and analyzed for their affinity, specificity, and functionality with two de-convolution-SELEX steps. Those aptamers with the highest functionality can be sequenced and their base pair sequences compared to identify homologous families. Furthermore, their secondary structures can be calculated and the desired aptamers can now be produced synthetically for further experiments. To prolong their biological half-life, aptamers may be coupled to polyethylene glycol (PEG) at the 5′-end.

8.4 Coating Technology for Coupling of Aptamers to the Surface of Medical Devices

To immobilize aptamers on different foreign surfaces, treatment of the respective material is primarily required using plasma or reactive wet chemical processes. Thereby, functional groups can be produced by allowing a coating. To prevent immediate aptamer superposition by strong adherent proteins and blood cells, a hemocompatible layer needs to be built on the material surface first. In this regard, hydrogels on the basis of isophorone diisocyanates terminated star-PEG were found to be extremely beneficial (Hoffmann et al., 2006). Because of the high functionality of the star-shaped prepolymers, not all isocyanate groups can take part in the cross-linking reaction; hence, free amino groups in the star-PEG layers remain. These amino groups can be used for biological functionalization of the star-PEG layers (Groll et al., 2005a,b).

The modification of the aptamers at the 3′-end with a carboxyl group then allows the coupling to the amino groups of the star-PEGs. In Fig. 8.2, the individual modification steps are illustrated schematically.

8.5 The Holy Grail: Small-Diameter Artificial Vascular Prostheses

Atherosclerosis is a chronic inflammatory disease of the arterial vessel wall, which leads to a flat thickening of the intima (innermost layer of the arteries). Responsible for almost one-third of all deaths, it is the main cause of death in industrialized nations. Within the intima, the deposition of low-density lipoproteins causes the formation of a plaque consisting of lipids, inflammatory as well as immune cells (mainly macrophages and T-cells), collagen fibers, smooth muscle cells, fragments of dead cells, and calcium. Over time, the aggressive plaque expansion causes narrowing or even occlusion of the respective blood vessel.

Percutaneous transluminal angioplasty is one of the treatment methods to remove blockages in arteries. This method mostly uses a stent to keep the blood vessel open as long as possible. If the vessel is no longer functional, because of the massive atherosclerotic lesion in the clogged blood vessel, autologous bypass grafting is required. This is done by using the internal mammary artery or saphenous vein of the patient to redirect the blood flow around the blockage. However, due to inflammation and pathologic vascular changes caused by advanced atherosclerosis, many patients have no suitable autologous vessels. Moreover, it is often difficult to get a vessel with a sufficient length, which is however mandatory for an effective

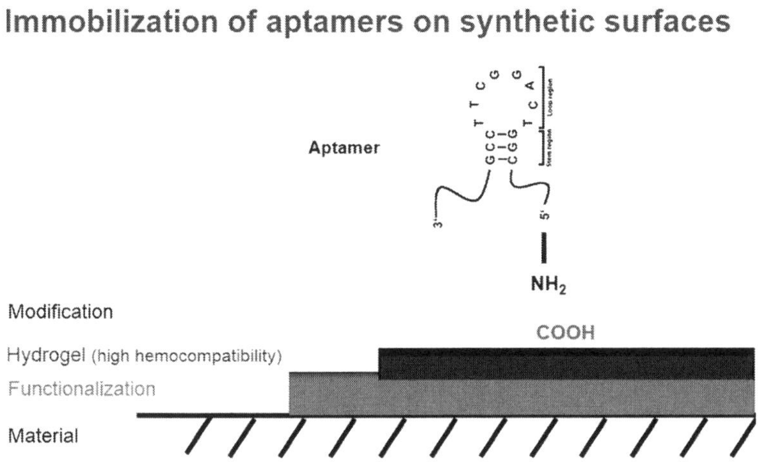

Figure 8.2 A+B: Methodological procedures to immobilize aptamers at the site of functionalized material surfaces (modified according to Hoffmann et al. 2006).

bypass. In such cases, the need for synthetic vascular grafts, which are currently made out of either polytetrafluoroethylene (ePTFE, Gore-Tex®) or polyethylene terephthalate (PET, Dacron®), is huge. Although prostheses with a large inner diameter have a long shelf life of several decades, prostheses with an inner diameter of less than 6 mm have, in contrast, a much higher stenosis rate. The thrombogenicity of a synthetic material or the intimal hyperplasia are mainly responsible for their long-term patency (Burkel, 1988).

Despite the enormous development of biomaterials and surface modifications in recent years, the native nonthrombogenic endothelium still represents the ideal surface for blood-contacting devices.

8.5.1 Endothelial Progenitor Cells: A Fascinating Alternative Source of Cells for Endothelialization of Vascular Prostheses

In 1997, Asahara et al., identified adult bone-marrow-derived endothelial progenitor cells (EPCs) in the blood circulation, which were able to obtain endothelial cell properties *in vitro*. Circulating EPCs are detected by their surface expression of the early surface markers CD34 (Asahara et al., 1997), CD133, and VEGFR-2 (Vascular Endothelial Growth Factor Receptor-2, KDR) (Miller-Kasprzak and Jagodzinski, 2007). Studies have shown that these cells were able to rebuild damaged blood vessels and restore the function of ischemic organs by vasculogenesis and angiogenesis *in vitro* (Hristov and Weber, 2003; Szmitko et al., 2006).

The presence of these precious stem cells in adults gives scientists the ability to generate an endothelium on a synthetic material. Indeed, efforts are made to colonize synthetic, blood-contacting implants with autologous endothelial cells prior to implantation (Klopsch and Steinhoff, 2012; Meinhart et al., 2001) to produce an autologous endothelium *in vitro*.

The Boston tissue-engineering research group of JE Mayer recently succeeded in the *in vitro* colonization of grafts with EPCs isolated from the circulating blood (Kaushal et al., 2001).However, this application requires surgical procedure in advance to obtain a vessel biopsy from the patient for the isolation of autologous endothelial cells to inoculate a prosthesis (Villalona et al., 2010). The isolated endothelial cells then grow *in vitro* until the required number of cells is reached. Thereafter, the prostheses are going to be seeded with these cells and cultured until confluent cell density. Finally, the *in vitro* endothelialized prosthesis is implanted in the patient. Due to this complex procedure, the endothelialization of prostheses is very time consuming and expensive and involves the risk of bacterial contamination making an application in clinical practice often not feasible.

Therefore, a further key step toward regenerative medicine is the targeted colonialization of implants *in vivo*, i.e., colonization directly after implantation in the human body. For this reasons, blood-contacting materials are coated with capture molecules such as peptides, proteins, antibodies, magnetic molecules, or aptamers, inducing the homing of EPCs to the implanted surfaces. After implantation, EPCs from the blood stream are directly attracted by the implanted surface and captured EPCs can then differentiate to fully functional endothelium at the desired location. In this way, the natural regeneration mechanism of the body is imitated, and an ideal surface with high biocompatibility is created (Fig. 8.3). The yet unknown "homing" factors that lead to a targeted accumulation of the EPCs at the damaged endothelium are mimicked by the immobilized capture molecules. With such functionalized artificial blood vessels, a novel autologous *in vivo* endothelialization might be performed, which opens up new treatment possibilities especially for small-lumen vascular grafts (<5 mm), such as coronary artery bypass and peripheral vessels. In addition, this technology could in principle be used for any other blood-contacting implant, i.e., heart valves, artificial hearts, artificial lungs, etc. (Fig. 8.4).

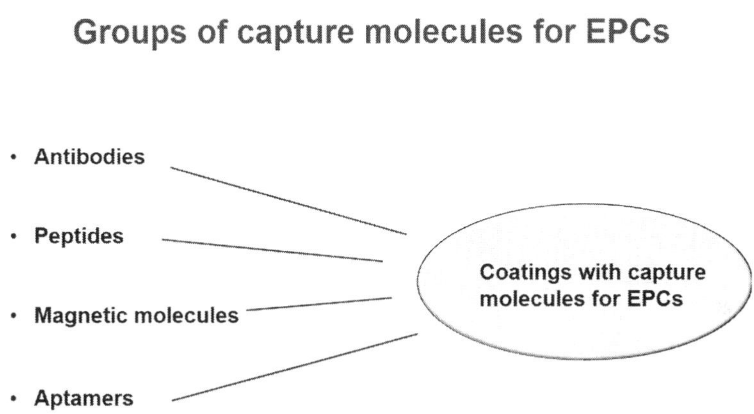

Figure 8.3 Capture molecules for EPCs.

To ensure successful homing of EPCs on implants, the surface should meet two requirements: The first requirement is the immobilization of highly specific receptor molecules, and the second is the prevention of nonspecific adhesion of other blood cells and serum proteins, which can quickly cover the immobilized capture molecules and thus prevent the capture of EPCs. Furthermore, the coatings may contain covalently immobilized growth factors such as VEGF and angiopoietin-1 (Chiu and Radisic, 2010) to support the differentiation of EPCs into endothelium cells as well as to maintain the survival and proliferation of these cells.

The recently developed *in vivo* endothelialization technology by a research group in Tokyo is based on the coating of stents with monoclonal antibodies against CD34. *In vitro* as well as animal studies demonstrate that a rapid cellular colonization of the stent surface takes place in circulating whole blood (Aoki et al., 2005; Ong et al., 2005). Nevertheless, the first clinical data were less satisfactory, which is not particularly surprising, since CD34+ cells only consist of a very small percentage of EPCs (Rotmanns et al., 2006). Comparable problems can probably also be expected in the case of stents coated with an integrin-binding cyclic Arg-Gly-Asp peptide (cRGD), because of its low specificity to EPC ligands (Blindt et al., 2006).

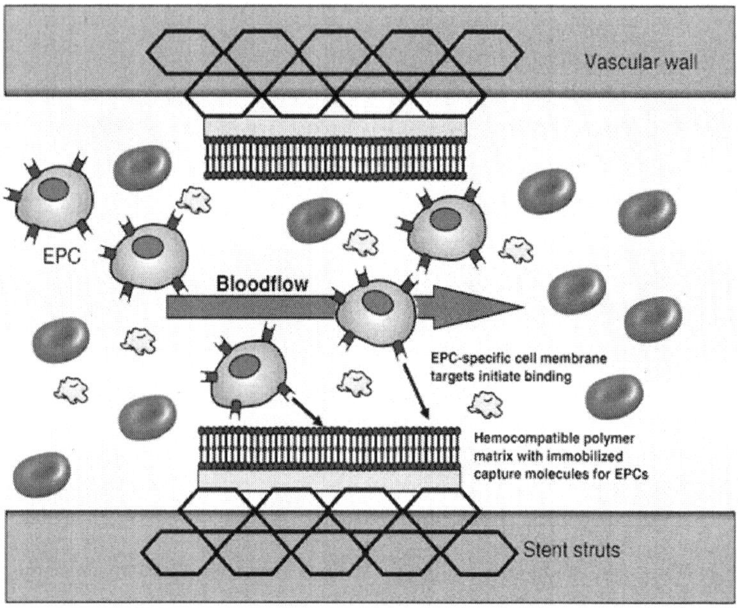

Figure 8.4 Stent coating with capture molecules for EPCs.

The EPC-capturing stent GenousTM (OrbusNeich Medical Technologies, Fort Lauderdale, USA), which is coated with anti-human CD34 monoclonal antibodies, is the first commercial biofunctional stent for *in vivo* endothelialization. The safety and feasibility of this stent have been shown by the single-center HEALING-FIM (Healthy Endothelial Accelerated Lining Inhibits Neointimal Growth-First In Man) study (Aoki et al., 2005). Thereafter, the efficacy of the GenousTM stent to prevent in-stent restenosis has been assessed (Silber, 2006; Duckers et al., 2007a,b). Furthermore, in the randomized single-center TRI-Stent Adjudication Study, the efficiency of the GenousTM stent was compared to a conventional drug-eluting stent (DES) (TAXUS®Liberté® Paclitaxel-Eluting Stent) in patients with *de novo* coronary lesions and a high risk for coronary restenosis (Beijk et al., 2010). The one-year results of this study showed that a subgroup of patients in the GenousTM stent group exhibited a significantly higher late lumen loss than in the TAXUS stent group. However, in comparison to four stent thromboses in the TAXUS stent group, no stent thrombosis could be observed in patients with a GenousTM stent implant.

Despite these promising results, the studies described above need to be considered critically, since CD34 is not only specific for EPCs, but also expressed on hematopoietic stem cells. Only 0.002% of the entire peripheral blood mononuclear cell population has been found positive for CD34 and only 0.4% ±0.2% of these CD34+ cells were actually EPCs (defined by additional expression of VEGFR-2 and CD133). This means that 99.6% of cells attracted by anti-CD34 antibodies are not EPCs and that a number of these cells have the ability to differentiate into pro-inflammatory cells. Thereby, the intimal hyperplasia, which is accompanied by the reduction of the prosthesis patency, can even be accelerated (Wendel et al., 2010).

Our working group currently works on the generation of aptamer-coated surfaces for small-lumen vascular prostheses using capture aptamers that directly bind to EPCs in the blood stream (Hoffmann et al., 2008). Using SELEX technology, we were able to generate DNA aptamers against CD31 (PECAM-1) positive EPCs derived from peripheral porcine blood. A few selected aptamers were then immobilized on polydimethylsiloxane and polytetrafluoroethylene surfaces by applying a hemocompatible reactive six-arm star-PEG coating (Hoffmann et al., 2006). As already mentioned, this antithrombogenic star-PEG coating inhibits undesirable protein adsorption and therefore prevents both covering of the immobilized capture molecules by serum proteins and significantly increases the specific binding of circulating EPCs onto the implants. Using a modified Chandler loop model, plates coated with immobilized aptamers or plates without aptamer as control were incubated with anticoagulated porcine whole blood. One of the aptamers generated was capable of capturing CD31 and CD144 (VE-cadherin) positive EPCs under flow conditions. During *in vitro* cell culture for 10 days, the cells exhibited endothelial cell properties. Hence, we demonstrated that respective aptamers are able to capture EPCs from the peripheral blood in a closed-loop model under flow conditions.

Further cell-SELEX experiments with the aim to generate specific aptamers against human EPCs are currently being conducted. Since the cell-SELEX technology requires viable cells as a target to generate cell-specific aptamers (Hoffmann et al., 2008), it is not necessary to know the molecular composition of the respective cell surface. However, it is important to perform SELEX experiments with defined and well-characterized EPC populations to avoid the loss of aptamers enriched by incubation with mature cells in the next rounds of selection. As cell-SELEX also has the potential to develop aptamers against unknown molecules, the selected aptamers can further be used for identification and detection of their target. In this way, new EPC-specific biomarkers can be discovered.

8.6 Conclusion

Now the time has come to realize what cardiologist Dr. Losordo has already postulated in 2003 (Losordo et al., 2003):

> "As cardiologists, vascular biologists and physicians, we must now consider an alternative to the 'antitumor' approach to restenosis prevention and seek to restore the normal biology of the vessel wall rather than perpetuate its disruption".

Rapid *in vivo* endothelialization of intravascular implants by capturing circulating autologous EPCs directly from the blood stream using biofunctionalized implanted materials is a fascinating concept to increase the hemocompatibility of blood-contacting materials. However, the success of this strategy is strongly influenced by the specificity and affinity of the EPC capture molecules. Although numerous procedures have already been developed to immobilize EPCs on synthetic materials, further studies are warranted to specify and optimize capture molecules for improved in vivo endothelialization before successful clinical applications can be performed.

References

Aoki J, Serruys PW, van Beusekom H, Ong AT, McFadden EP, Sianos G, van der Giessen WJ, Regar E, de Feyter PJ, Davis HR, Rowland S, and Kutryk MJ. 2005. Endothelial progenitor cell capture by stents coated with antibody against CD34: The HEALING-FIM (Healthy Endothelial Accelerated Lining Inhibits Neointimal Growth-First In Man) Registry. *J Am Coll Cardiol*, **45:** 1574–1579.

Asahara T, Murohara T, Sullivan A, Silver M, van der Zee RLiT, Witzenbichler B, Schatteman G, and Isner JM. 1997. Isolation of putative progenitor endothelial cells for angiogenesis. *Science*, **275:** 964–967.

Beijk MA, Klomp M, Verouden NJ, van GN, Koch KT, Henriques JP, Baan J, Vis MM, Scheunhage E, Piek JJ, Tijssen JG, and de Winter RJ. 2010. Genous endothelial progenitor cell capturing stent *vs.* the TaxusLiberte stent in patients with *de novo* coronary lesions with a high-risk of coronary restenosis: A randomized, single-centre, pilot study. *Eur Heart J*, **31:** 1055–1064.

Blank M, Weinschenk T, Priemer M, and Schluesener H. 2001. Systematic evolution of a DNA aptamer binding to rat brain tumor microvessels. Selective targeting of endothelial regulatory protein pigpen. *J Biol Chem*, **276:** 16464–16468.

Blindt R, Vogt F, Astafieva I, Fach C, Hristov M, Krott N, Seitz B, Kapurniotu A, Kwok C, Dewor M, Bosserhoff AK, Bernhagen J, Hanrath P, Hoffmann R, and Weber C. 2006. A novel drug-eluting stent coated with an integrin-binding cyclic Arg-Gly-Asp peptide inhibits neointimal hyperplasia by recruiting endothelial progenitor cells. *J Am Coll Cardiol*, **47:** 1786–1795.

Brody EN and Gold L. 2000. Aptamers as therapeutic and diagnostic agents. *J Biotechnol*, **74:** 5–13.

Burkel WE. 1988. The challenge of small diameter vascular grafts. *Med Prog Technol*, **14:** 165–175.

Chiu LL and Radisic M. 2010. Scaffolds with covalently immobilized VEGF and angiopoietin-1 for vascularization of engineered tissues. *Biomaterials*, **31:** 226–241.

Colman RW, Scott CF, Schmaier AH, Wachtfogel YT, Pixley RA, and Edmunds LH Jr. 1987. Initiation of blood coagulation at artificial surfaces. *Ann NY Acad Sci*, **516:** 253–267.

Duckers HJ, Silber S, de Winter R, den Heijer P, Rensing B, Rau M, Mudra H, Benit E, Verheye S, Wijns W, and Serruys PW. 2007a. Circulating endothelial progenitor cells predict angiographic and intravascular ultrasound outcome following percutaneous coronary interventions in the HEALING-II trial: Evaluation of an endothelial progenitor cell capturing stent. *EuroIntervention*, **3:** 67–75.

Duckers HJ, Soullie T, den Heijer P, Rensing B, de Winter RJ, Rau M, Mudra H, Silber S, Benit E, Verheye S, Wijns W, and Serruys PW. 2007b. Accelerated vascular repair following percutaneous coronary intervention by capture of endothelial progenitor cells promotes regression of neointimal growth at long term follow-up: Final results of the HEALING-II trial using an endothelial progenitor cell capturing stent (Genous R stent). *EuroIntervention*, **3**: 350–358.

Gold L. 1995. The SELEX process: A surprising source of therapeutic and diagnostic compounds. *Harvey Lect*, **91**: 47–57.

Goringer HU, Homann M, Zacharias M, and Adler A. 2006. RNA aptamers as potential pharmaceuticals against infections with African trypanosomes. *Handb Exp Pharmacol*, **173**: 375–393.

Groll J, Ameringer T, Spatz JP, and Moeller M. 2005b. Ultrathin coatings from isocyanate-terminated star-PEG prepolymers: Layer formation and characterization. *Langmuir*, **21**: 1991–1999.

Groll J, Haubensak W, Ameringer T, and Moeller M. 2005a. Ultrathin coatings from isocyanate terminated star-PEG prepolymers: Patterning of proteins on the layers. *Langmuir*, **21**: 3076–3083.

Gunaydin S. 2004a. Emerging technologies in biocompatible surface modifying additives: Quest for physiologic cardiopulmonary bypass. *Curr Med Chem Cardiovasc Hematol Agents*, **2**: 295–302.

Gunaydin S. 2004b. Clinical significance of coated extracorporeal circuits: A review of novel technologies. *Perfusion*, **19** (Suppl 1): S33–S41.

Hamsten A. 1993. The hemostatic system and coronary heart disease. *Thromb Res*, **70**: 1–38.

Hoffmann J, Groll J, Heuts J, Rong H, Klee D, Ziemer G, Moeller M, and Wendel HP. 2006. Blood cell and plasma protein repellent properties of star-PEG-modified surfaces. *J Biomater Sci Polym Ed*, **17**: 985–996.

Hoffmann J, Paul A, Harwardt M, Groll J, Reeswinkel T, Klee D, Moeller M, Fischer H, Walker T, Greiner T, Ziemer G, and Wendel HP. 2008. Immobilized DNA aptamers used as potent attractors for porcine endothelial precursor cells. *J Biomed Mater Res A*, **84**(3): 614–621.

Hoffmann J, Simon P, Zimmermann AK, Lemancyk M, Walter T, Beyer M, Hoffmeister HM, Ziemer G, and Wendel HP. 2005. Thrombospondin 1 as possible key factor in the hemocompatibility of endocoronary prostheses. *Biomaterials*, **26**(25): 5240–5250.

Hristov M, Erl W, and Weber PC. 2003. Endothelial progenitor cells: Mobilization, differentiation, and homing. *Arterioscler Thromb Vasc Biol*, **23**: 1185–1189.

Ireson CR and Kelland LR. 2006. Discovery and development of anticancer aptamers. *Mol Cancer Ther*, **5**: 2957–2962.

Kaushal S, Amiel GE, Guleserian KJ, Shapira OM, Perry T, Sutherland FW, Rabkin E, Moran AM, Schoen FJ, Atala A, Soker S, Bischoff J, and

Mayer JE. 2001. Functional small-diameter neovessels created using endothelial progenitor cells expanded *ex vivo*. *Nat Med*, **7:** 996–997.

Klopsch C and Steinhoff G. 2012. Tissue-engineered devices in cardiovascular surgery. *Eur Surg Res*, **49**(1): 44–52.

Losordo DW, Isner JM, and Diaz-Sandoval LJ. 2003. Endothelial recovery: The next target in restenosis prevention. *Circulation*, **107**(21): 2635–2637.

Meinhart JG, Deutsch M, Fischlein T, Howanietz N, Froschl A, and Zilla P. 2001. Clinical autologous *in vitro* endothelialization of 153 infrainguinale PTFE grafts. *Ann Thorac Surg*, **71:** S327–S331.

Miller-Kasprzak E and Jagodzinski PP. 2007. Endothelial progenitor cells as a new agent contributing to vascular repair. *Arch Immunol Ther Exp (Warsz)* **55:** 247–259.

Morris KN, Jensen KB, Julin CM, Weil M, and Gold L. 1998. High-affinity ligands from in vitro selection: Complex targets. *Proc Natl Acad Sci USA*, **95:** 2902–2907.

Ong AT, Aoki J, Kutryk MJ, and Serruys PW. 2005. How to accelerate the endothelialization of stents. *Arch Mal Coeur Vaiss*, **98:** 123–126.

Rotmanns JI, Heyligers JM, Stroes ES, and Pasterkamp G. 2006. Endothelial progenitor cell-seeded grafts: Rash and risky. *Can J Cardiol*, **22:** 1113–1116.

Silber S. 2006. Capturing circulating endothelial progenitor cells: A new concept tested in the HEALING studies. *Minerva Cardioangiol*, **54:** 1–3.

Szmitko PE, Kutryk MJ, Stewart DJ, Strauss MH, and Verma S. 2006. Endothelial progenitor cell-coated stents under scrutiny. *Can J Cardiol*, **22:** 1117–1119.

Tanzi MC. 2005. Bioactive technologies for hemocompatibility. *Expert Rev Med Devices*, **2:** 473–492.

Tobin KA. 2006. Macugen treatment for wet age-related macular degeneration. *Insight*, **31:** 11–14.

Villalona GA, Udelsman B, Duncan DR, McGillicuddy E, Sawh-Martinez R, Mirensky T, Hibino N, Painter C, Erickson B, Shinoka T, and Breuer C. 2010. Cell seeding techniques in vascular tissue engineering. *Tissue Eng Part B Rev*, **16:** 341–350.

Wachtfogel YT, DeLa Cadena R, and Colman RW. 1993. Structural biology, cellular interactions and pathophysiology of the contact system. *Thromb Res*, **72:** 1–21

Wendel HP and Ziemer G. 1999. Coating-techniques to improve the hemocompatibility of artificial surfaces used for extracorporeal circulation. *Eur J Cardiothorac Surg*, **16:** 342–350.

Wendel HP, Avci-Adali M, and Ziemer G. 2010. Endothelial progenitor cell capture stents— hype or hope? *Int J Cardiol*, **145**(1): 115–117.

Yianni YP. 1992. Biocompatible surfaces based upon biomembrane mimicry, in *Structural and Dynamic Properties of Lipids and Membranes* (Quinn PJ and Cherry RJ, eds), Portland Press Ltd., London, pp. 187–216.

Chapter 9

Microneedles and Nanopatches for Transdermal Vaccination

Andreas Muschaweck,[a] **Martin Scholz,**[b] **and Ulrike Protzer**[a]
[a]*Institute for Virology, TU-Munich, Germany*
[b]*LEUKOCARE AG, Am Klopferspitz 19, 82152 Martinsried/Munich, Germany*
Ulrike.Protzer@virologie.med.tum.de

This mini-review deals with microneedles and nanopatches, two innovative approaches to improve transdermal vaccination. Microneedles and nanopatches are expected to improve vaccination success, compliance, and cost reduction. A challenge to broadly establish this new strategy is the stabilization of the vaccines on the devices during sterilization and storage.

9.1 Vaccination via the Dermal Route

The skin contains a large number of Langerhans cells, which are important professional antigen-presenting cells. In addition to these cells, dendritic cells in the skin are essential for the formation of sufficient defense activity against infectious intruders. Dendritic

Biofunctional Surface Engineering
Edited by Martin Scholz

ISBN 978-981-4411-60-8 (Hardcover), 978-981-4411-61-5 (eBook)
www.panstanford.com

cells recognize foreign antigens and elicit highly efficient immune responses to counterattack transdermal infections. Therefore, intradermal vaccination and thus the pathogen-specific stimulation of dendritic cells are plausible approaches. The most prominent limitations of standard vaccination devices such as needle and syringe or patches for transdermal diffusion are summarized in the following paragraphs.

9.2 Limitations of Standard Vaccination Procedures

Intradermal immunization with vaccines in solution requires needle injection by medical personnel. It is often painful, time consuming and unreliable, as well as associated with needle injury and pathogen transmission (Kim et al., 2010). Accordingly, the compliance of the patients to be vaccinated is generally low. Moreover, the vaccination costs are very high due to the required high density of vaccine within the ampulla. A significant problem in the field of vaccination is the loss of vaccine activity during prolonged storage and transportation, especially in countries without secured cool chains.

9.3 Alternatives to Needles and Syringes

Dermal patches for transdermal diffusion of vaccines have been developed as an alternative to needles and syringes. However, the efficacy of these patches is limited by the low diffusion features of larger vaccines. Small molecules (<500 Da) may diffuse through the stratum corneum, the outer layer of the skin, but most of the vaccines are much larger (up to a million Da). The stratum corneum is, therefore, the natural barrier, which has to be overcome by the diffusion or penetration capability by vaccination procedures.

There are other approaches to deliver vaccines through the stratum corneum, such as electroporation (Prausnitz and Langer, 2008) or the use of biolistic microparticle delivery systems (Kendall et al., 2004). Those approaches are expensive and result in unappreciated painful irritations of the skin (Denet et al., 2004; Wallace et al., 2009; Zhou et al., 2008).

9.4 Microprojections for Transdermal Vaccination

The idea to apply antigens for transdermal vaccination by means of microneedles basically has been propagated by Mark Prausnitz and his group from the Georgia Institute of Technology, Atlanta (Prausnitz et al., 2009). Microneedles were developed as a hybrid medical device between vaccine patches and hypodermic needles to overcome the individual limitations of needles and patches (Gill and Prausnitz, 2007). Similar and alternative approaches such as nanopatches (Chen et al., 2011) were reported by the group around Kendall (Kendall et al., 2004). Examples of advantages of vaccination by means of microneedles or nanopatches, both based on coated microprojections for transdermal vaccine delivery, include (i) higher efficacy and compliance (minimal invasive), (ii) higher stability during prolonged storage and transport (especially in countries without guaranteed cool chain), and (iii) lower costs due to reduced amounts of required antigen per vaccination.

Microneedles may be composed of steel with projections having a length of about 700 μm (Fig. 9.1). The microneedle fabrication includes several steps such as laser cutting by infrared laser, as well as cleaning and bending with detergents and a razor blade, respectively. To make the tips sharp, microneedles can be electropolished by a method published by Gill and Prausnitz in 2007 (Gill and Prausnitz, 2007). A schematic diagram of an in-plane microneedle row-coating device is depicted in Fig. 9.2.

The nanopatches that have been recently propagated by the group of Kendall et al. comprise microprojections of silicon, sputter-coated with a thin layer (~100 nm) of gold. The density of the projections on these patches is >20.000/cm^2. Figure 9.3 shows a scanning electron microscopy image of microprojections. In comparison, the previously described microneedles consist of <321 projections/cm^2 (Chen et al., 2011). One of the key challenges for vaccine delivery to the skin by microprojections is coating the surface with vaccine (Chen et al., 2011). A method to enable homogenous vaccine coating of microprojections has been reported by the Kendall group. They used a solution comprising methylcellulose and a vaccine, which was distributed on the surface by means of a fast (~10 m/s) nitrogen gas-jet (Chen et al., 2009). A different approach is the dip coating and air drying of stainless steel microneedles. The coating solution also comprises methylcellulose (carboxymethylcellulose sodium salt) with trehalose or other stabilizers.

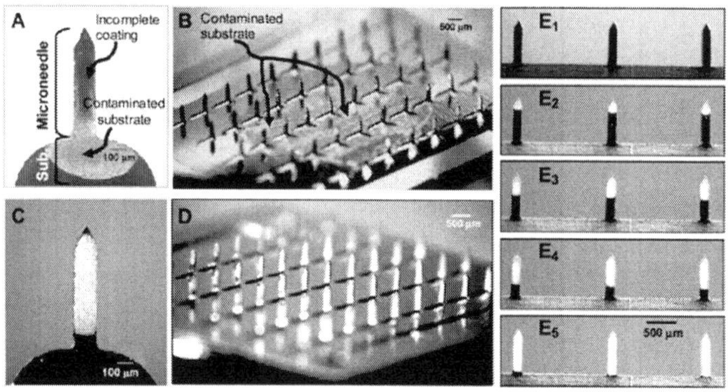

Figure 9.1 Examples of poor and good microneedle coatings via brightfield micrographs of vitamin B coated microneedles. Poor, nonuniform coatings with base-substrate contamination on: (A) a single microneedle and (B) a 50-microneedle out-of-plane array. Improved coating uniformity and elimination of base-substrate contamination after addition of coating-solution excipients and use of a micro-dip-coating device for (C) a single microneedle, (D) a 50-microneedle out-of-plane array, and (E) an in-plane microneedle row. Controlled length segment coverage at (E_1) uncoated, (E_2) 25% coated, (E_3) 50% coated, (E_4) 75% coated, and (E_5) 100% coated, demonstrating spatial control of the microneedle-coating process. Reprinted from Harvinder and Prausnitz (2007), with permission of Elsevier.

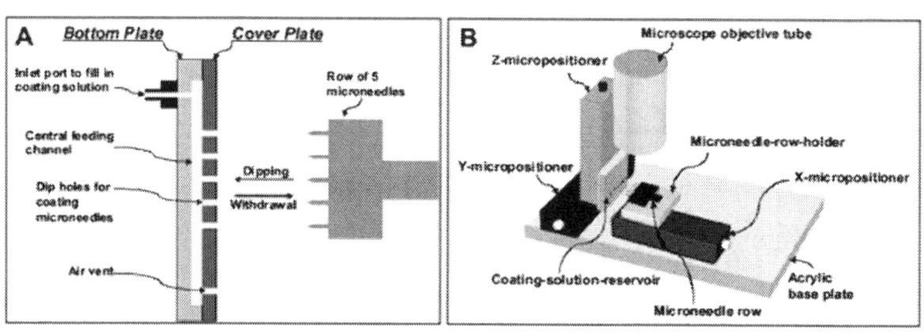

Figure 9.2 Schematic diagrams of in-plane microneedle row-coating device. (A) Cross-sectional view of the coating-solution reservoir showing the microneedles aligned with the dip holes. (B) Isometric projection of the entire device showing the *x*, *y*, and *z*-micropositioners used to align the microneedles with dip holes of the coating-solution reservoir. The cylindrical tube represents the stereo-microscope objective, which is used to view the microneedle alignment and coating process facilitating manual control. Reprinted from Harvinder and Prausnitz (2007), with permission of Elsevier.

A recently published review dealing with devices for intradermal vaccination (Kis et al., 2012) describes efforts to further improve the microneedle approach, For example, it has been suggested to generate microneedles consisting of biodegradable material such as polymers (e.g., polylactide) or sugar. Regarding the delivery of solid vaccine particles or vaccine-coated gold particles to the epidermal and dermal layers of the skin, the ballistic approach might be promising (Kis et al., 2012).

9.5 Feasibility of Transdermal Vaccination with Microprojections

The feasibility of the delivery approaches by using antigen-coated microprojections has been shown by several authors in animal models. For example, the distribution of antigens within the skin upon microneedle application had been tested in a cadaver porcine skin model (Gill and Prausnitz, 2007). The vaccination efficacy and long-lived protection was recently shown in a mouse model (Koutsonanos et al., 2012). This group evaluated the systemic recall and mucosal immune responses as well as the viral replication after challenge and showed that the hemagglutination inhibition tests as a measure for specific immune responses were two-fold higher

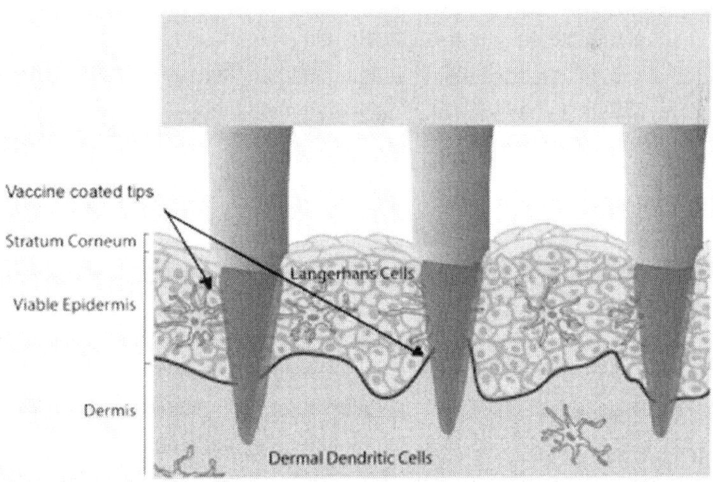

(a)

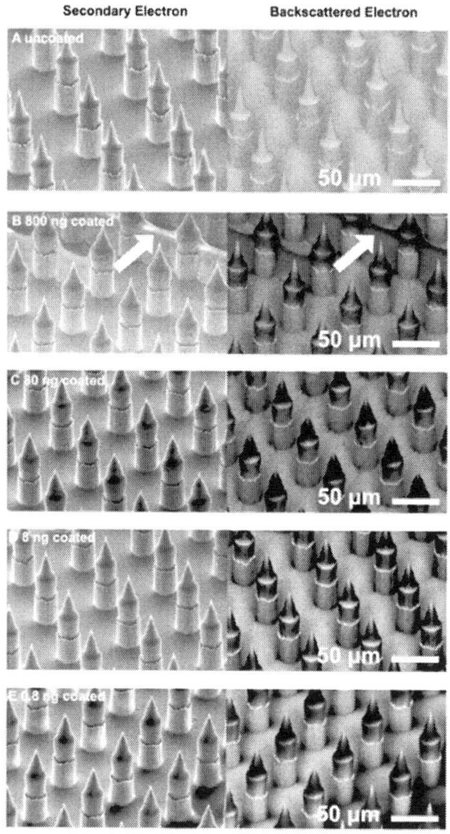

(b)

Figure 9.3 (a) The Nanopatch™ concept. A two-dimensional array of projections localizes dry-coated vaccines to layers of the skin rich in immune cells. Once the vaccine hydrates, it diffuses through the viable epidermis and dermis. (b) Representative scanning electron micrographs examining projection coating morphology in both secondary and backscattered electron modes. Secondary electron images show the surface morphology, while backscattered electron images show composition—with low atomic mass elements giving low signal—i.e., coated area appears dark in comparison with the uncoated Nanopatch™. Microprojections are coated at (b) 800 ng, (c) 80 ng, (d) 8 ng, and (e) 0.8 ng of HPV-16 protein per patch. While some bridging is occurring in the 800 ng group (panel b: white arrow), coating is seen on the tapered portion of projections in all dose groups. Reprinted from Corbett et al. (2010).

in the microneedle-immunized group than in the intramuscular immunized group. Along with this, the authors reported to find significantly elevated anti-inflammatory IL-10 in conjunction with reduced inflammation in the lungs. Interestingly, the longevity and efficacy of the microneedle approach were better than the intramuscular approach in challenged mice after a period of 36 weeks post-vaccination.

A preclinical study was done to show the feasibility of Bacillus Calmette-Guérin (BCG) vaccination by using microneedle patches (Hiraishi et al., 2011). The vaccine patches were fabricated by laser cutting and electropolishing (Gill and Prausnitz, 2007). BCG vaccine coating was done by dipping repeatedly into coating solution (carboxymethylcellulose sodium salt, Lutrol F-68 NF, trehalose dehydrate, and 3.75 mg/ml BCG vaccine) and then air dried at 25°C for 2 h. The BCG-coated microneedle vaccine patch was highly immunogenic in guinea pigs as shown by a strong antigen-specific lymphocyte proliferation and IFN-γ levels. A high frequency of proinflammatory cytokine (IFN-γ/TNF-α) expressing CD4+ cells was observed. In conclusion, the microneedle vaccine patch induced a robust cell-mediated immune response in both the lungs and the spleen of guinea pigs comparable to the traditional hypodermic needle-based intradermal BCG vaccination. The authors further conclude that the BCG-coated microneedle patch is a simpler, safer, and compliant vaccination that could facilitate increased coverage, especially in developing countries that lack adequate healthcare infrastructure.

9.6 Challenges of Microprojections for Transdermal Vaccination

The list of major challenges of the entire technology starts with the selection of biocompatible scaffold material that has to be approved to be safe and stable. It has been reported that the addition of trehalose to the vaccine formulation stabilized the vaccine and enhanced the protective effect upon microneedle delivery in the mouse skin (Kim et al., 2010; Quan et al., 2009). The production of defined microprojections in terms of the number of microprojections per cm^2 surface area, the amount of vaccine and homogenous distribution of vaccine on the microneedle or nanopatch, etc., ought to be standardized by the producer.

A major challenge, however, is the terminal sterilization of the end product, which is highly appreciated to circumvent expensive clean room production steps. Therefore, sterilization tests have been done with scaffold material coated with several lyophilized, spray-dried, and air-dried influenza A vaccines. The read out assay to monitor the activity of hemagglutinin as a major immunogenic part of the virus has been evaluated by the *in vitro* hemagglutinin activity test (HAT). This assay is based on the efficacy of hemagglutinin to aggregate red blood cells. The serial dilution of the antigen allows the determination of the titer and thus the functionality of the antigen. We systematically tested different stabilizing compositions in which the antigen was dissolved and dried by different methods. As an alternative approach, viral antigens were immobilized on metal scaffolds as a model for microneedles or patches and air dried. Terminal sterilization was done with irradiation at 25–40 kGy. After reconstituting the powders or eluting the sterilized antigens from the scaffolds, HAT assays were carried out to test the antigenic activity in a semiquantitative way. It could be shown that it is indeed possible to terminally sterilize both dried vaccines as powders and immobilized scaffolds without severe loss of antigenicity. As an example, representative data are shown in Fig. 9.4.

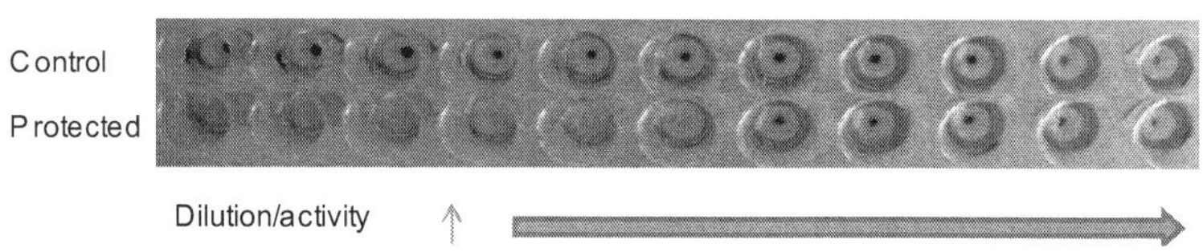

Figure 9.4 The activity of lyophilized/irradiated influenza A is higher in virus preparations with the protecting procedure as indicated by lattice formation (no visible red button) even at high dilutions of virus as compared with the lyophilized/irradiated but unprotected control.

9.7 Conclusion

Scaffolds for vaccines for the use of dried powder applications can be a feasible technology in not only transdermal application of vaccines but also in other application routes such as inhalation or oral application in the future. The major hurdles to bring these products to the patient seem to be solved by technical solutions, including the stabilization issues during storage, thermal stress, and irradiation stress.

References

Chen X, et al. 2009. Dry-coated microprojection array patches for targeted delivery of immunotherapeutics to the skin. *J Control Release*, **139:** 212–220.

Chen X, et al. 2011. Improving the reach of vaccines to low-resource regions, with a needle-free vaccine delivery device and long-term thermostabilization. *J Control Release*, **152:** 349–355.

Corbett HJ, Fernando GJP, Chen X, Frazer IH, Kendall MAF. 2010. Skin vaccination against cervical cancer associated human papillomavirus with a novel micro-projection array in a mouse model. *PLoS ONE*, **5**(10): e13460. doi: 10.371/journal.pone.0013460.

Denet AR, Vanbever R, and Preat V. 2004. Skin electroporation for transdermal and topical delivery. *Adv Drug Deliv Rev*, **56:** 659–674.

Gill HS and Prausnitz MR. 2007. Coated microneedles for transdermal delivery. *J Control Release*, **117:** 227–237.

Harvinder SG and Prausnitz MR. 2007. Coated microneedles for transdermal delivery. *J Control Release*, **117**: 227–237.

Hiraishi Y, et al. 2011. Bacillus Calmette-Guérin vaccination using a microneedle patch. *Vaccine*, **29**(14): 2626–2636.

Kendall M, Mitchell T, and Wrighton-Smith P. 2004. Intradermal ballistic delivery of microparticles into excised human skin for pharmaceutical applications. *J. Biomech*, **37:** 1733–1741.

Kim Y-C, et al. 2010. Formulation and coating of microneedles with inactivated influenza virus to improve vaccine stability and immunogenicity. *J Control Release*, **142:** 187–195.

Kis EE, Winter G, and Myschik J. 2012. Devices for intradermal vaccination. *Vaccine*, **30**(3): 523–538.

Koutsonanos DG., et al. 2012. Delivery of subunit influenza vaccine to skin with microneedles improves immunogenicity and long-lived protection. *Sci Rep*, **2:** 357–366.

Prausnitz MR and Langer R. 2008. Transdermal drug delivery. *Nat Biotechnol*, **26:** 1261–1268.

Prausnitz MR, Mikszta JA, Cormier M, and Andrianov AK. 2009. Microneedle-based vaccines. *Curr Top Microbiol Immunol*, **333**: 369–393.

Quan F-S, et al. 2009. Stabilization of influenza vaccine enhances protection by microneedle delivery in the mouse skin. *PLoS One*, **4**: e7152–7161.

Wallace M, et al. 2009. Tolerability of two sequential electroporation treatments using MedPulser DNA Delivery System (DDS) in healthy adults. *Mol Ther*, **17**: 922–928.

Zhou Y, et al. 2008. Electroporation at low voltages enables DNA vaccine to provide protection against a lethal H5N1 avian influenza virus challenge in mice. *Intervirology*, **51**: 241–246.

Chapter 10

Autoantibodies as Biomarkers for Disease Diagnosis

Angelika Lueking, Heike Göhler, and Peter Schulz-Knappe
Protagen AG, Otto-Hahn-Str. 15, 44227 Dortmund, Germany
angelika.lueking@protagen.com

New biomarkers with improved sensitivity and specificity are required to improve disease diagnosis and prognosis. Furthermore, to realize the concept of personalized medicine, new challenges of patient stratification and development of companion diagnostics need to be addressed. Consequently, biomarkers with diagnostic and prognostic value for cancer and autoimmune diseases will become more and more important. Autoantibodies are a class of analytes that have attracted attention over the last years. They are directed against certain human proteins and induced by immune system activity in response to disease processes, e.g., in neurodegenerative diseases, cancer, or classical autoimmune diseases.

Here we review the use of autoantibody/antigen interactions for diagnostic assays and drug development strategies, which overcomes the technical problems and limitations of other proteomic

Biofunctional Surface Engineering
Edited by Martin Scholz

ISBN 978-981-4411-60-8 (Hardcover), 978-981-4411-61-5 (eBook)
www.panstanford.com

markers found in the last decades. Different technology platforms are described enabling the discovery and validation of biomarkers as well as the development of diagnostic assays based on novel autoantibody/antigen interactions.

10.1 Autoantibodies as Biomarkers

Autoantibodies are a class of biomarkers suitable for risk assessment, screening, prognosis, disease stratification, and therapy monitoring. Autoantibodies, i.e., antibodies directed against certain human proteins, are induced by immune system activity in response to a disease process. Autoantibody production reflects the immune response to a continuous remodeling of cells or tissues caused by protein turnover and chronic disease processes. In this context, the immune system fails to properly distinguish between self and nonself, and attacks its own cells and tissues. However, in so-called autoimmune diseases, the autoantibodies present in blood are indicative for the clinical symptoms and the state of the disease. Prominent examples of autoimmune diseases are rheumatoid arthritis, multiple sclerosis, coeliac disease, diabetes mellitus type 1, systemic lupus erythematosus (SLE), Sjogren's syndrome, inflammatory bowel disease, and Hashimoto's thyroiditis.

Beyond classical autoimmune diseases, also in several cancer indications, the presence of autoantibodies has been shown and was correlated to the disease state. Autoantibodies against autologous tumor-associated antigens (TAAs) have been described (Anderson and LaBaer 2005). Most of them are altered, which renders them into an immunogenic form. They can be mutated (p53) (Soussi, 2000), overexpressed (NY-ESO-1) (Schubert et al., 2000), aberrantly degraded, or glycosylated (MUC-1) (von Mensdorff-Pouilly et al., 2000). Also aberrant localization as described for cyclin B1 may provoke an immune response (Suzuki et al., 2005). It is speculated that the humoral response against TAAs is triggered by aberrant tumor cell death due to defective apoptosis or necrosis leading to the release of intracellular modified proteins with immunogenic potential. Tumor cell death also releases proteases that would generate cryptic self-epitopes.

Historically, the immune system was separated into two branches: humoral immunity and cellular immunity. The protective function of humoral immunization could be found in cell-free bodily fluids or serum and is mediated by secreted antibodies produced by activated B-lymphocytes. In contrast, the cell-mediated immunity does not involve antibodies but requires the activation of macrophages, natural killer cells, antigen-specific cytotoxic T-lymphocytes, and the release of different cytokines in response to an antigen. However, both systems are linked together by the activation of naïve B-cells in a T-cell-dependent manner. During T-cell-dependent activation, an antigen-presenting cell such as a macrophage or dendritic cell has digested the immunogenic antigen to peptides and presents this processed antigen to a helper T-cell (T_h-cell), which is then primed to this antigen. When a B-cell processes and presents the same antigen to the primed T_h-cell, the T-cell secretes several cytokines, which trigger the B-cell to proliferation and differentiation into plasma cells.

Up to now it has been quite difficult and time consuming to identify reliable serum markers, especially proteins and peptides, for the diagnosis of a certain disease. A particularly important reason is that such diagnostic markers are present in patient samples often only in minute and highly variable concentrations and have a limited stability. In contrast to this, the use of autoantibodies as diagnostic markers has proven to be highly effective. Such antibodies can be detected by presenting their corresponding autoantigens in well-established assay formats, e.g., enzyme-linked immunosorbent assay, western blot, protein arrays, etc. A particular feature is their specific structure and high stability. They are present in serum or plasma in high concentrations and are not subjected to circadian rhythms or other short-term changes in physiological states. This means that sampling can occur any time because results are not influenced by the time of day of sampling or nutritional status. Due to their specificity and high affinity binding to their corresponding autoantigen, no enrichment or elaborated sample preparation is required. Enrichment occurs automatically during analysis by the binding of the autoantibodies to the autoantigen. Potentially, autoantibodies can also be used for the development of prognostic tests. Studies with SLE patients in the USA have shown that certain autoantibodies could be detected as long as 10 years prior to the onset of the disease (Arbuckle et al., 2003). This highlights that assessing the immune response by measuring autoantibodies is the most stable and efficient way of analyzing biomarkers for diagnostics.

Several autoantibodies are already established diagnostic markers (Table 10.1).

Table 10.1 Examples of established autoantibody biomarkers and their corresponding antigens

Antigen	Disease	Antibody Scaffold
SS-A	systemic lupus erythematosus	IgG
Ro-52	systemic lupus erythematosus	IgG
CCP	Rheumatoid Arthritis	IgG
SS-B	systemic lupus erythematosus	IgG
Sm	systemic lupus erythematosus	IgG
Scl-70	systemic sclerosis	IgG
Jo-1	polymyositis	IgG
SLA	autoimmune liver disease	IgG
LKM1	autoimmune liver disease	IgG
AMA M2	autoimmune liver disease	IgG
Sp100	autoimmune liver disease	IgG
gp210	autoimmune liver disease	IgG
LBR	autoimmune liver disease	IgG

As indicated in Table 10.1, several disease-specific antibodies are known and used in established diagnostic test systems. The presence of many of these antibodies is associated with more than one autoimmune disease. For example, the detection of Ro-52 is typical for neonatal lupus erythematodes, Sjogren's syndrome, and SLE. This shows that the detection of just one antibody will be insufficient for the diagnosis of a disease. On the contrary, 116 different target antigens have been described in the literature for SLE patients (Sherer et al., 2004). Thus the relatively small panel of target antigens/antibodies that are routinely measured does not probably assess the full heterogeneity of the disease. It is reasonable to assume that taking more disease-specific target antigens/antibodies into account will increase sensitivity and specificity of diagnosis.

Consequently, recent approaches measure a multitude of putative antibodies followed by data analysis using clustering or classification algorithms (Quintana et al., 2003; Li et al., 2007; Hueber et al., 2005). Due to cost effectiveness, the need for small sample volumes, and laborious procedures, the multiplex antigen array technology has become more and more accepted in this field (Robinson, 2006). This technology can be applied to improve diagnosis and used for the prediction of disease onset, classification of subjects into disease subgroups, as well as efficacy assessment of therapy regiments (Lueking and Cahill, 2006; Sharp and Utz, 2007).

10.2 Autoantibodies for Companion Diagnostics Enabling Personalized Medicine

Autoantibody signatures detected by blood screening can not only be useful for the diagnosis of a disease, but can also be used for patient stratification, i.e., divide patient populations into different groups, such as drug responders and nonresponders (Fig. 10.1). This is very desirable for the following reason: It is well established that for any disease not all patients respond equally well to a standard drug treatment. On the contrary, in many cases a significant proportion of patients will either not respond at all or even show adverse effects as a result of the drug treatment. Ineffective drug treatments put an enormous cost burden on pharmaceutical companies during drug development and the health care insurance providers. Therefore, in recent years both the scientific community as well as regulatory agencies (Food and Drug Administration, European Medicines Agency) started recommending the development of diagnostic markers, assays, and tools to establish so-called companion diagnostics. They should enable a more targeted therapy to either specifically select the eligible patient population for a standard treatment or define a specific dosing scheme based on a specific molecular patient profile. This approach provided a rational basis of personalized medicine.

A prominent example is the monoclonal IgG1-λ antibody belimumab (Benlysta; GlaxoSmithKline, UK), which binds to the soluble human BLyS there by inhibiting its biological activity. BLyS inhibits B-cell apoptosis and stimulates the differentiation of B-cells into immunoglobulin-producing plasma cells. In SLE, rheumatoid arthritis, and certain other autoimmune diseases, elevated levels of BLyS are believed to support the production of autoantibodies, which may contribute to the destruction of healthy tissue. It has been shown in a phase II dose-ranging study that belimumab was only effective in patients with serologically active SLE patients (Wallace et al., 2009). Subgroup analysis revealed that the clinical end points were successfully reached in this large subgroup. Therefore, only seropositive patients were enrolled in the subsequent clinical phase III, in which the effectiveness of belimumab was proven. In 2010, the Food and Drug Administration approved Benlysta as the first novel SLE treatment in about 50 years. Sales are estimated to reach the $1 billion blockbuster threshold rather soon (according to Datamonitor Product Profile SLE, June 2011). The yearly treatment costs are in the range of $30,000 per patient, illustrating the high potential for any SLE drug, although a small percentage of SLE patients are responding to the drug.

Therefore, autoantibodies in combination with their corresponding autoantigens have the potential to be used as companion diagnostics in this context, because they may enable classification of patients into different groups as indicated in Fig. 10.1.

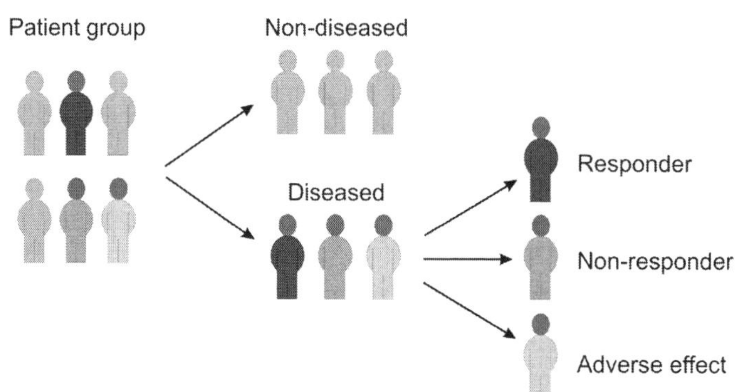

Figure 10.1 Use of biomarkers in diagnosis and personalized medicine. Diagnosis of a disease is based on the discriminative power of biomarker(s). Response or adverse effects of a patient to a drug can be predicted by biomarkers before or early during treatment.

10.3 Biomarker Discovery Strategies

The development of diagnostic markers comprises several phases from discovery to clinical assay development. Typically, the discovery process starts with high numbers of analytes tested against a low number of serum samples of cases and controls. Multiple rounds of verification and validation are carried out until the number of biomarkers is significantly decreased. Subsequently, four to ten biomarkers enter the phase of clinical assay development, whereas up to a few thousand samples are analyzed (Rifai et al, 2006).

Several techniques for autoantigen discovery are currently in use and encompass serological screening of cDNA expression libraries, phage display libraries, two-dimensional western blots, and different formats of protein arrays, such as planar or bead-based protein microarrays, peptide arrays, tissue arrays, and carbohydrates arrays.

The proteomics-based approach termed serological proteome analysis (SERPA9) combines two-dimensional electrophoresis, western blotting, and mass spectrometry (Klade et al., 2001). Proteins from tumor tissues or cell lines were separated by two-dimensional gel electrophoresis, transferred onto membranes, and incubated with serum samples from healthy people and patients. The autoantibody signatures were compared and patient-associated protein spots were analyzed by mass spectrometry. Although the time-consuming construction of cDNA libraries is avoided and post-translational modifications are accessible for the screening approach, this technology has the major drawbacks of low reproducibility, low automation grade, and low sample throughput.

In the phage display approach, a cDNA library is constructed using tumor tissue, a cancer cell line, or short synthetic DNA sequences leading to peptides or proteins displayed on the phage surface. Autoantibody screening in patient samples is done by a biopanning procedure involving succeeding rounds of immunoprecipitation and amplification/enrichment of autoantibody-binding phages. However, the analysis of large numbers of patient and control samples as well as the quantitative analysis of the identified antigens or peptide epitopes requires further techniques such as protein microarrays.

The serological analysis of tumor antigens by recombinant cDNA expression cloning (SEREX) applies a cDNA expression library obtained from autologous tumor tissue (Sahin et al, 1995). By SEREX, several TAAs have been identified in various types of cancers, including lung, liver, breast, ovarian, prostate, and renal cancers (Tan et al., 2009). Proteins derived from aberrant transcripts highly specific for tumor activity can be detected. However, a general bias toward antigens that are highly expressed in the tumor tissue is found. Since often these libraries are cloned in a λ gt11 system, SEREX is time consuming, labor intensive, not amenable for automation, and therefore not suitable for the analysis of large patient numbers.

Protagen applied the UNIarray® technology platform, which enables a systematic approach to autoantibody discovery in a unique way. The basis is founded in the availability of a large collection of recombinant human proteins. The company owns five tissue-specific recombinant human protein expression libraries (*Escherichia coli* expression, His-tag fusion proteins) enabling a high degree of automation in the downstream workflow. The largest library from human fetal brain represents >10,000 recombinant human protein expression products, i.e., potential autoantigens. Therefore, approximately 50% of the human genome can be currently accessed by the Protagen technology platform. More than 5,000 human-purified proteins are available for screening purposes. The interaction of autoantibodies from patient samples with these potential autoantigens can be detected very fast with a high efficiency. Applying a hypothesis-free strategy novel biomarker candidates can be identified and validated by miniaturized multiparameter assays such as planar or bead-based protein microarrays (Fig. 10.2). Using this approach, Protagen has identified (almost) exclusively novel, indication-specific sets of autoantigens in multiple sclerosis, rheumatoid arthritis, prostate cancer, and, in collaboration with academic partners, in Parkinson's disease, alopecia areata, dilated cardiomyopathy, and SLE (Lueking et al., 2005; Horn et al., 2006; Beyer et al., 2011; Massoner et al., 2011). In all indications studied so far, it became clear that for a precise diagnosis or differential diagnosis, multiple diagnostic marker panels will always be required.

An alternative strategy for the production of protein microarrays uses DNA as template immobilized onto a surface combined with an *in vitro* transcription and translation step. These approaches called nucleic-acid programmable protein array or DNA array to protein array (DAPA) (Sibani and LaBaer, 2011; He and Taussig, 2001) have the advantages that efforts for protein production can be circumvented and toxic proteins may be expressed *in vitro*. However, multiple process steps such as plasmid preparation, spotting of the DNA, and *in vitro* transcription and translation reactions are error prone and lead to considerable inter- and intra-batch differences, which may negatively affect the statistical and bioinformatical analysis.

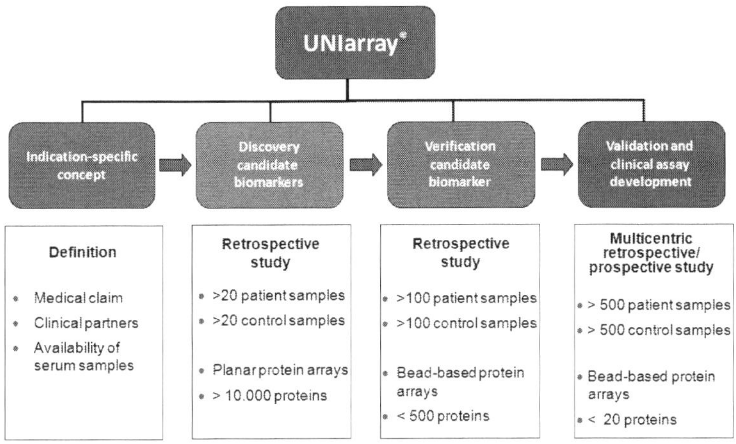

Figure 10.2 UNIarray® strategy shown as process chain for the discovery and validation of diagnostic relevant biomarkers based on antigen/autoantibody interactions.

Alternatively to recombinant proteins (derived from clonal expression and purification), the reverse phase protein microarray approach couples multidimensional liquid phase protein fractionation of localized and metastatic cancer tissue lysates to protein microarrays and subsequent antigen identification by mass spectrometry (Taylor et al., 2008). The analysis of the immunoreactive profile of these protein fractions is difficult, as each of the fractions consists of a number of different proteins and proteins may be represented by adjacent or different fractions. However, this platform enables the analysis of native antigens concerning post-translational modifications and presented linear and structural epitopes.

Tissue microarrays are not involved per se in biomarker discovery approaches but have a strong impact on the validation of discovered biomarkers. The analysis of miniaturized collections of arrayed tissues from pathologically evident tumor biopsies at the DNA, RNA, or protein level enables the linkage of molecular data with various tumor and patient data, such as clinicopathological information, survival, and treatment response.

Peptide microarrays represent overlapping epitopes of short amino acid sequences from selected (predefined) antigens pointing to a hypothesis-driven approach. Recently this was extended to a hypothesis-free strategy by applying several thousand oligo-N-substituted glycines as unnatural synthetic molecules (so-called peptoids) to discover ligands that bind antibodies in the serum of patients with Alzheimer's disease (Reddy et al., 2011). Due to the synthetic unnatural design of the peptoids, it is expected that artificial "mimotopes" are represented, which may allow binding of antibodies directed against glycostructures or citrullinated antigens. However, as these peptoids represent a collection of artificial molecular shapes, a direct link to the native antigen is missing.

Interactions between proteins and carbohydrates are essential for various biological processes as the carbohydrates contained in glycoproteins, glycolipids, and proteoglycans are involved in recognition processes such as cell adhesion, migration, and signaling. To profile such interactions, carbohydrate microarrays containing polysaccharides, natural glycoconjugates, and mono- and oligosaccharides coupled to carrier molecules have been developed and used for the detection of serum autoantibodies (Oyelaran and Gildersleeve, 2009). However, this technology is in its beginning and its impact on lead or therapeutic target discovery is, as yet, unclear.

Bead-based assays coupled with flow cytometry detection are a new and emerging technology platform in diagnostics allowing a high grade of multiplexing. The multiplex assay contains a set of different polystyrene beads, which can be differentiated by their different specific fluorescent color code. Each fluorescence-coded bead can be coupled to a specific target antigen following the quantitative determination of serum-contained autoantibodies by flow cytometry detection. The autoantibody–antigen interactions are measured with high accuracy and reproducibility at very high sensitivity.

10.4 Antigen/Autoantibody Interactions as Biomarker Candidates

The autoimmune profile of human covers a huge number of autoantibodies, which display an enormous resource to identify novel marker candidates for diagnostic purposes. With access to protein collections covering the human proteome and to protein array technology, the systematic exploration of alterations in autoimmune profiles triggered by the onset or progression of diseases is feasible.

First attempts using protein microarrays to characterize diagnostic relevant autoantibodies were carried out in the field of autoimmune diseases. For rheumatoid arthritis, patterns of differential antigen recognition were found to be associated with clinical subtype of rheumatoid arthritis. Autoreactivity directed against human cartilage gp39 and type II collagen was linked to less severe rheumatoid arthritis and against citrullinated epitopes to severe rheumatoid arthritis (Hueber et al., 2005). Using microarrays with a content of 70 autoantigens, Li and colleagues (Li et al., 2007) showed that serum samples of patients suffering from SLE and incomplete lupus erythematous displayed different autoimmune profiles.

Applying a strategy that uses thousands of antigens derived from a cDNA expression library to profile the humoral autoimmune repertoire, new putative autoantigens have been identified for different diseases such as dilated cardiomyopathy and alopecia areata (Lueking et al., 2005; Horn et al., 2006). Particularly, the two-step approach, including a discovery and a verification phase, resulted in the identification of eight antigen–autoantibody interactions depicting a highly disease-specific autoimmune response by alopecia areata.

In contrast to proteomic studies, a hypothesis-driven approach was carried out by Quintana and colleagues (Quintana et al., 2008) to identify biomarker candidates for multiple sclerosis. Thereby, microarrays were produced, which contained 64 lipids and 268 protein fragments covering 40 proteins associated with the central nervous system (CNS) or the heat-shock response. Serum samples of different subtypes of multiple sclerosis such as relapse-remitting multiple sclerosis (RRMS), secondary progressive multiple sclerosis, and primary progressive multiple sclerosis were analyzed. All three subtypes were characterized by unique patterns of reactivity to CNS, whereas autoantibodies against heat-shock proteins were only detected in RRMS serum samples. This suggested that autoantibody signature links pathologic subtypes of multiple sclerosis and appears to reflect immune processes in the CNS.

Cerebrospinal fluid (CSF) of multiple sclerosis patients is characterized by the presence of immunoglobulin. The immunoglobulin is detected as oligoclonal bands in CSF and support current diagnosis. However, a common identity of OCB reactivity is not yet known and could be of great value to develop a diagnostic test. In a study by Beyer and colleagues (Beyer et al., 2011), samples of OCB-positive CSF of 20 patients with RRMS were compared to CSF of sex- and age-matched controls using the UNIarray® technology platform of Protagen AG. Interestingly, the functional annotation of the top 100 identified antigens results in a strong linkage to diabetes and the insulin signaling pathway. It has been reported that the prevalence of type 2 diabetes was higher in multiple sclerosis patients, perhaps caused by muscle degradation due to neuron degeneration or use of high dose methylprednisolone pulse (Hussein and Reddy, 2006). Several investigators have found some metabolic disorders linking both diseases, such as abnormalities in fat, calcium, and vitamin D metabolism.

In the last two decades, protein arrays have also been used to investigate the autoimmune profile of cancer patients and identify TAAs. Most of the TAAs have been identified in a discovery approach but have not been further validated to develop a diagnostic test (Casiano et al., 2006). For ovarian cancer, protein microarrays were employed to screen 30 serum samples of cancer patients and controls, respectively. Ninety-four antigens were identified that exhibit enhanced reactivity from serum samples of cancer patients relative to control serum samples (Hudson et al., 2007). For validation, specific antibodies against identified antigens were subjected to tissue microarray and antibodies against Lamin A/C, SSRP1, and RALBP1 were recognized to produce a robust signature of cancer. However, the three antigens were prevalent not only in ovarian cancer but also in tissues of many types of cancer and a subset of healthy tissue. Therefore, the diagnostic value of the candidate tissue markers remains elusive.

In the study of Anderson and colleagues (Anderson et al., 2011) three subsequent rounds of screening approaches, including discovery and verification phases, were carried out to identify biomarker for the early detection of breast cancer. High-density custom protein arrays were used to analyze three cohorts of breast cancer case and control serum samples. In total, 285 serum samples were investigated and 28 TAAs were identified to react with autoantibodies arising with the onset of breast cancer. Using these antigens, the discrimination of cases and controls achieved an area under the curve value of 0.756. The study design and validation of identified TAAs indicate that these autoantibody biomarkers have a high potential to enter the development of a clinical-grade assay.

In the study by Massoner and colleagues (Massoner et al., 2011), the autoimmune profile of prostate cancer patients was investigated. Using the UNIarray® strategy (Fig. 10.2), 160 serum samples of patients diagnosed with prostate cancer or benign diseases as well as healthy control individuals were investigated to identify autoimmune profiles characteristic of each group. In the discovery screen, 408 proteins were identified as TAAs in serum samples of prostate cancer patients. In the validation screen, these 408 proteins were used to investigate whether the autoimmune profile of each group is discriminative and can be used by classification algorithms. After statistical analysis, 15 proteins were useful to yield an area under the curve value of 0.71, indicating a diverging autoimmune profile of prostate cancer and benign disease patients. Among these proteins, TTLL12 had been associated with prostate cancer, and six other proteins (RPIA, NOVA2, MAP2, HSPH1, RASSF7, and RBM15) had been described as relevant for other cancers. Thus autoantibodies in serum samples of prostate cancer patients are directed against known cancer-associated proteins and novel proteins and they are stable among different patients.

10.5 Diagnostic Assays Based on Antigen/Autoantibody Interactions

Following discovery, qualification, and verification, the successfully validated biomarker(s) is/are subjected to the development of a diagnostic assay. Currently in clinical laboratories, an increasing number of autoantibodies are measured employing a broad spectrum of techniques and methods. The main techniques involving functionalized surfaces for multiplexed measurements are line-blot immunoassays, bead-based assays with flow cytometry detection, and antigen microarrays.

As an example for line immunoblot assays, the recomLine ANA/ENA (Mikrogen, Martinsried, Germany) allows the multiplex analysis of 14 antigens (RNP68, RNPA, RNPC, SmB, SmD, SSA60, SSA52, SSB, PO, PCNA, CEN-B, Scl70, Jo-1, and histones) in a single procedure. With exception of histones, all antigens have a recombinant origin. Generally, line-blot assays are widely distributed and easy to use, but limited to a low number of analytes.

Currently, several companies supply commercial kits for the simultaneous measurement of different autoantibodies by bead-based assays. ENA/ANA analysis based on this technology platform is supplied, for example, by Inova Diagnostics (San Diego, USA), Bio-Rad (Hercules, USA), BMD (Marne la Vallie, France), and Zeus Scientific (Raritan, USA).

Antigen microarrays may contain up to a thousand proteins immobilized to the surface resulting in a high multiplex grade. Companies supplying commercial kits based on protein microarrays include Randox (Belfast, United Kingdom) and Thermo Fisher Scientific (Phadia, Uppsala, Sweden). SQI Diagnostics (Toronto, Canada) combines the microtiter format with the protein microarray technology by spotting antigen panels into each well of a microtiter plate. Different in vitro diagnostic products for the diagnosis of autoimmune diseases such as rheumatoid arthritis, SLE, or celiac disease are commercially available. However, the number of antigens is in the range of tens to hundred.

10.6 Conclusion

A large tool box is available for biomarker discovery. However, the reduction of a large panel of identified biomarkers to a small panel and transfer of these biomarker(s) to clinical test remain as a future challenge. The access to disease-specific reference serum samples and a pipeline with defined benchmark data for validation will help to develop clinically relevant biomarkers.

The hunt for innovative diagnostics and prognostic biomarkers as well as biomarkers indicating drug failure before therapies are applied gains an increasing scientific and commercial importance. It is anticipated that companion diagnostics will have a widespread use in the pharmaceutical market as they promise to make drug development faster and clinical trials smaller. As a consequence, the time to market for a drug is shorter, peak sales are higher, and patent protection is longer. Also existing drugs may more easily enter into new indications as shown for belimumab. As the use of such companion diagnostic assays can be integrated very early in clinical and even pre-clinical development, they can generate sales prior to achieving regulatory approval.

References

Anderson KS and LaBaer J. 2005. The sentinel within: Exploiting the immune system for cancer biomarkers. *J Proteome Res*, **4**(4): 1123–1133.

Anderson KS, Sibani S, Wallstrom G, Qiu J, Mendoza EA, Raphael J, et al. 2011. Protein microarray signature of autoantibody biomarkers for the early detection of breast cancer. *J Proteome Res*, **10**(1): 85–96.

Arbuckle MR, McClain MT, Rubertone MV, Scofield RH, Dennis GJ, James JA, et al. 2003. Development of autoantibodies before the clinical onset of systemic lupus erythematosus. *N Engl J Med*, **349**(16): 1526–1533.

Beyer NH, Lueking A, Kowald A, Frederiksen JL, and Heegaard NH. 2011. Investigation of autoantibody profiles for cerebrospinal fluid biomarker discovery in patients with relapsing-remitting multiple sclerosis. *J Neuroimmunol*, **242**(1–2): 26–32.

Casiano CA, Mediavilla-Varela M, and Tan EM. 2006. Tumor-associated antigen arrays for the serological diagnosis of cancer. *Mol Cell Proteomics*, **5**(10): 1745–1759.

He M and Taussig MJ. 2001. Single step generation of protein arrays from DNA by cell-free expression and in situ immobilisation (PISA method). *Nucleic Acids Res*, **29**(15): E73–73.

Horn S, Lueking A, Murphy D, Staudt A, Gutjahr C, Schulte K, et al. 2006. Profiling humoral autoimmune repertoire of dilated cardiomyopathy (DCM) patients and development of a disease-associated protein chip. *Proteomics*, **6**(2): 605–613.

Hudson ME, Pozdnyakova I, Haines K, Mor G, and Snyder M. 2007. Identification of differentially expressed proteins in ovarian cancer using high-density protein microarrays. *Proc Natl Acad Sci USA*, **104**(44): 17494–17499.

Hueber W, Kidd BA, Tomooka BH, Lee BJ, Bruce B, Fries JF, et al. 2005. Antigen microarray profiling of autoantibodies in rheumatoid arthritis. *Arthritis Rheum*, **52**(9): 2645–2655.

Hussein WI and Reddy SS. 2006. Prevalence of diabetes in patients with multiple sclerosis. *Diabetes Care*, **29**(8): 1984–1985.

Klade CS, Voss T, Krystek E, Ahorn H, Zatloukal K, Pummer K, et al. 2001. Identification of tumor antigens in renal cell carcinoma by serological proteome analysis. *Proteomics*, **1**(7): 890–898.

Li QZ, Zhou J, Wandstrat AE, Carr-Johnson F, Branch V, Karp DR, et al. 2007. Protein array autoantibody profiles for insights into systemic lupus erythematosus and incomplete lupus syndromes. *Clin Exp Immunol*, **147**(1): 60–70.

Lueking A and Cahill DJ. 2006. Protein biochips in the proteomic field, in *Proteomics in Drug Research* (Hamacher M, Marcus K, Stühler K, van Hall A, Warscheid B, and Meyer H E, eds), Wiley-VCH Verlag GmbH & Co. KGaA, Weinheim, FRG.

Lueking A, Huber O, Wirths C, Schulte K, Stieler KM, Blume-Peytavi U, et al. 2005. Profiling of alopecia areata autoantigens based on protein microarray technology. *Mol Cell Proteomics,* **4**(9): 1382–1390.

Massoner P, Lueking A, Goehler H, Hopfner A, Kowald A, Kugler KG, et al. 2011. Serum autoantibodies for discovery of prostate cancer specific biomarkers. *Prostate,* **72**(4): 427–436.

Oyelaran O and Gildersleeve JC. 2009. Glycan arrays: Recent advances and future challenges. *Curr Opin Chem Biol,* **13**(4): 406–413.

Quintana FJ, Farez MF, Viglietta V, Iglesias AH, Merbl Y, Izquierdo G, et al. 2008. Antigen microarrays identify unique serum autoantibody signatures in clinical and pathologic subtypes of multiple sclerosis. *Proc Natl Acad Sci USA,* **105**(48): 18889–18894.

Quintana FJ, Getz G, Hed G, Domany E, and Cohen IR. 2003. Cluster analysis of human autoantibody reactivities in health and in type 1 diabetes mellitus: A bio-informatic approach to immune complexity. *J Autoimmun,* **21**(1): 65–75.

Reddy MM, Wilson R, Wilson J, Connell S, Gocke A, Hynan L, et al. 2011. Identification of candidate IgG biomarkers for Alzheimer's disease via combinatorial library screening. *Cell,* **144**(1): 132–142.

Rifai N, Gillette MA, and Carr SA. 2006. Protein biomarker discovery and validation: The long and uncertain path to clinical utility. *Nat Biotechnol,* **24**(8): 971–983.

Robinson WH. 2006. Antigen arrays for antibody profiling. *Curr Opin Chem Biol,* **10**(1): 67–72.

Sahin U, Tureci O, Schmitt H, Cochlovius B, Johannes T, Schmits R, et al. 1995. Human neoplasms elicit multiple specific immune responses in the autologous host. *Proc Natl Acad Sci USA,* **92**(25): 11810–11813.

Schubert U, Anton LC, Gibbs J, Norbury CC, Yewdell JW, and Bennink JR. 2000. Rapid degradation of a large fraction of newly synthesized proteins by proteasomes. *Nature,* **404**(6779): 770–774.

Sharp V and Utz PJ. 2007. Technology insight: Can autoantibody profiling improve clinical practice? *Nat Clin Pract Rheumatol,* **3**(2): 96–103.

Sherer Y, Gorstein A, Fritzler MJ, and Shoenfeld Y. 2004. Autoantibody explosion in systemic lupus erythematosus: More than 100 different antibodies found in SLE patients. *Semin Arthritis Rheum*, **34**(2): 501–537.

Sibani S and LaBaer J. 2011. Immunoprofiling using NAPPA protein microarrays. *Methods Mol Biol*, **723**: 149–161.

Soussi T. 2000. p53 Antibodies in the sera of patients with various types of cancer: A review. *Cancer Res*, **60**(7): 1777–1788.

Suzuki H, Graziano DF, McKolanis J, and Finn OJ. 2005. T-cell-dependent antibody responses against aberrantly expressed cyclin B1 protein in patients with cancer and premalignant disease. *Clin Cancer Res*, **11**(4): 1521–1526.

Tan HT, Low J, Lim SG, and Chung MC. 2009. Serum autoantibodies as biomarkers for early cancer detection. *FEBS J*, **276**(23): 6880–6904.

Taylor BS, Pal M, Yu J, Laxman B, Kalyana-Sundaram S, Zhao R, et al. 2008. Humoral response profiling reveals pathways to prostate cancer progression. *Mol Cell Proteomics*, **7**(3): 600–611.

von Mensdorff-Pouilly S, Petrakou E, Kenemans P, van Uffelen K, Verstraeten AA, Snijdewint FG, et al. 2000. Reactivity of natural and induced human antibodies to MUC1 mucin with MUC1 peptides and n-acetylgalactosamine (GalNAc) peptides. *Int J Cancer*, **86**(5): 702–712.

Wallace DJ, Stohl W, Furie RA, Lisse JR, McKay JD, Merrill JT, et al. 2009. A phase II, randomized, double-blind, placebo-controlled, dose-ranging study of belimumab in patients with active systemic lupus erythematosus. *Arthritis Rheum*, **61**(9): 1168–1178.

Chapter 11

Biofunctionalized Wound Dressings for Advanced Wound Care

Martin Scholz
LEUKOCARE AG, Am Klopferspitz 19, 82152 Martinsried/Munich, Germany
martin.scholz@leukocare.com

The number of patients suffering from delayed wound healing and chronic wounds is rapidly increasing. This is partly due to the increasing number of diabetic patients worldwide. Diabetes is closely associated with chronic wounds. However, the underlying mechanisms are not fully understood. To help those patients with chronic wounds, current therapies are largely based on palliative strategies. Therefore, biofunctional "intelligent" wound dressings are urgently needed. This mini-review summarizes the state of the art in bioactive wound dressings and provides practical examples for bioengineered dressing materials.

Biofunctional Surface Engineering
Edited by Martin Scholz

ISBN 978-981-4411-60-8 (Hardcover), 978-981-4411-61-5 (eBook)
www.panstanford.com

11.1 Need for Biofunctional Wound Dressings

There are several experimental and clinical approaches to therapeutically improve impaired wound healing (Eming et al., 2004; Davidson et al., 2000; Hocking and Gibran 2010; Rizzi et al., 2010; Lansdown, 2006). A highly appreciated goal is to stimulate the development of granulation tissue and at the same time to improve or trigger angiogenic processes to increase the oxygen supply of the granulation tissue by newly formed blood vessels. However, pharmacologic approaches, e.g., the application of growth factors such as vascular endothelial growth factor (VEGF), to the wounds are discussed controversially (Roth et al., 2006; Przybylski, 2009; Li et al., 2005).

Some of the limitations of these approaches are as follows: (a) proteases within the wound fluid may degrade the growth factors; (b) the wound milieu and the biochemical interactions between the factors that are crucial for the granulation of the tissue are too complex and multifactorial, so that one single factor may not be sufficient; (c) the appreciated goal to achieve improved oxygenation by pro-angiogenic stimulation may be limited by the de novo synthesis of insufficient vessels due to the absence of other important cellular cofactors such as pericytes; (d) the application of strong pro-angiogenic factors or other growth factors carry the risk to support cancer development.

There is a clear clinical need and a tendency to develop wound-care products with integrated biological functionality. An example is the supplementation of wound dressings with silver, eliciting antimicrobial effects (Lansdown, 2006). Although silver particles target the bacterial load in the wounds, the impaired cellular cross talk that underlies delayed wound healing is not addressed. Currently, no biologic-device combination product exists that effectively stimulates pro-healing mechanisms in wounds.

We hypothesize that fibroblast stimulation in combination with distinct extrinsic induction of angiogenesis may be more effective than the application of single growth factors. Activated fibroblasts elicit many important functions for tissue remodeling and regeneration such as collagen production (Tuan et al., 1996), differentiation into myofibroblasts (Watsky et al., 2010), and the secretion of keratinocyte growth factor (Nolte et al., 2008).

11.2 Current Wound-Healing Procedures

There are several approaches to improve wound-healing processes in patients with delayed wound healing or chronic wounds. These approaches can be categorized as pharmaceutical agents, wound dressings, and medical devices. Wound dressings may comprise amorphous hydrogels, hydrocolloid dressings, alginate and composite dressings, transparent films, and silver dressings. In the following paragraphs, examples for some significant contributions to address delayed wound healing on the clinical stage are reviewed.

11.2.1 Negative Pressure Wound Therapy/Vacuum-Assisted Closure

The negative pressure is empirically found to support wound healing in several clinical settings, and the procedure is known as designated negative wound pressure therapy (NPWT). The branded term "vacuum-assisted closure (VAC)" is sometimes used when referring to NPWT. The approach has already been successfully evaluated during the last decades. However, the NPWT/VAC therapy requires expensive hardware such as pumps and circuits and clinical staff for the handling of the machine. The reason for the beneficial effects of NPWT/VAC is currently not exactly known. It is suggested that the mechanical stimulation of the wound and the negative pressure are directly associated with tissue granulation. Whether the physical tension mediated by the negative pressure might explain the clinical success alone remains speculative.

As a disadvantage, the negative pressure results in the growth of tissue within the foam and thus leads to complications and pain during dressing changes where the newly formed tissue is partially removed. Also, NPWT/VAC does not address the reduction of pathogens within the wound. The theory and practice of NPWT is reviewed by Schintler (2012) and, therefore, we refer to this publication.

11.2.2 Silver-Coated Wound Dressings

To address the reduction of pathogens, silver coating of dressings was established. Today, silver coatings are provided by many wound-dressing companies. However, the use of silver and the wound-healing promoting effects are discussed controversially. The reduction of bacterial load within the wound does not necessarily result in accelerated wound closure because underlying intercellular regulation mechanisms may be deregulated regardless of the contamination of wounds. In other words, bacterial load reduction is an important but not the only issue in advanced wound care.

From the regulatory point of view, for example, a wound dressing with a silver-coated material will be approved as a medical device as long as silver is not declared to elicit a pharmacologic effect in the wound. In this case, the silver coating may be rather declared to protect the dressing from bacterial contamination and thus is only an additive to the main intended use, namely, to cover the wound area and thus to avoid drying out and protect from further bacterial contamination. In contrast, a product with the declared intended use to deliver pharmaceutically active ingredients into the wound by elution or other technologies would probably not be approved as a medical device but as a pharmaceutical product. Companies that have experience in the approval of both medical devices and pharmaceutical products may have an advantage compared with companies with experience in either medical device or pharmaceutical approvals.

11.2.3 Growth Factor Eluting Dressing (Regranex)

A prominent example for an approach to accelerate wound healing by means of a growth factor is Regranex, a recombinant human platelet-derived growth factor (rhPDGF). Regranex was developed by Johnson & Johnson to treat neuropathic, chronic, diabetic ulcera. It has been shown that treatment of wounds with Regranex resulted in significantly accelerated healing (Embil et al. 2000). There is evidence that additional accelerated healing is achieved when a combination of Regranex with a collagen-oxidized regenerated cellulose dressing is used (Hollister and Li, 2007).

11.3 Possible Targets in Wound Healing and Phase-Specific Strategies

Physiological wound healing is achieved by an extremely complicated network of cellular interactions, which have to be considered differentially in each wound-healing phase. These different wound-healing phases and the basic science of wound healing are nicely summarized in a review by Broughton et al., (2006). In this review, the authors describe each wound-healing phase and the underlying cellular and physiological mechanisms in detail. From this understanding, it is clear that each wound-healing phase has its own specifications and thus needs specific and adequate treatment options.

In our present contribution, we only grossly summarize the different wound-healing phases by referring to the review of Broughton et al. (2006). During the first phase of wound healing, the control of bleeding is achieved by vasoconstriction and activation of the intrinsic part of the coagulation cascade. This is followed by inflammation, which is induced by activated platelets and released cytokines. The fibrin clot serves as a scaffold for invading cells, such as neutrophils, monocytes, fibroblasts, and endothelial cells. Hemostatic and platelet-derived factors have important functions in subsequent processes of wound healing.

About 48 to 96 h after injury, monocytes are attracted to the wound by several mediators and are transformed into macrophages. This activation is critical for the transition of the wound into the proliferative phase and for angiogenesis (by synthesizing VEGF and TNF-α). The clearing of the invading bacteria and cellular debris is achieved largely by neutrophils that release proteolytic enzymes for the digestion of bacteria and nonviable tissue. Neutrophils can also generate reactive oxygen free radicals to help sterilize the wound of bacteria.

The proliferative phase occurs approximately from day 4 to day 14 and includes epithelization, angiogenesis, and provisional matrix formation. Epithelial cells begin to proliferate and send out projections to re-establish a protective barrier against fluid losses and further bacterial invasion. Pro-inflammatory cytokines upregulate keratinocyte growth factor expression in fibroblasts, which in turn stimulate keratinocytes to migrate into the wound area, proliferate, and differentiate in the epidermis. Fibroblasts and endothelial cells are the predominant cells proliferating during this phase. Endothelial cells form new capillaries, a process which is regulated by a complex network of cytokines and growth factors. The secretion of cytokines and growth factors by the different involved cell types is also regulated by hypoxia, which triggers VEGF production and thus angiogenesis. Fibroblasts migrate into the wound site from the surrounding tissue upon stimulation mediated by cytokines and growth factors (PDGF, epidermal growth factor). Wound fibroblasts begin synthesizing collagen and transform into myofibroblasts for wound contraction. The provisional matrix consists of collagen type III, glycosaminoglycans, and fibronectin.

The maturation and remodeling phase occurs from day 8 through approximately one year. During this phase, the deposition of collagen in an organized and well-mannered network takes place. The initially formed matrix, which is mainly composed of fibrin and fibronectin, serves as a preliminary framework of the new matrix, which is stronger and organized. A central part in remodeling the matrix is mediated by matrix metalloproteases, which in turn are regulated by cytokines and growth factors. The contractility of the wound is conducted by myofibroblasts. The differentiation of fibroblasts into myofibroblasts is signaled by cell interaction with an alternatively spliced form of fibronectin that causes the fibroblast to increase its expression of α-smooth muscle actin (α-SMA) isotype, which is important for the cytoskeleton organization and contractility of the cell. The tension within the wound determines the amount of collagen production or apoptosis and thus the grade of contractility.

In conclusion, the differentiation of fibroblasts into myofibroblasts and the effector functions of these cells play a central role in the orchestration of wound healing. Therefore, myofibroblasts and the intercellular network around these cells should be considered a possible target in advanced wound care in more detail. There is evidence that the activity of fibroblasts in chronic wounds is downregulated. The stimulation of fibroblasts and myofibroblasts could, therefore, be an interesting therapeutic option in advanced wound care as outlined in the following paragraphs.

11.4 Stimulation of Myofibroblasts by Drug-Eluting Materials

As an early event during wound healing, dermal fibroblasts differentiate into myofibroblasts and start to migrate from the wound edge toward the center of the wound where they play a central role in the formation of a stable matrix and subsequently granulation tissue as a requirement for physiological tissue regeneration. Moreover, differentiated myofibroblasts largely orchestrate the complex interplay between different cell types such as platelets, macrophages, keratinocytes, endothelial cells, and immune cells within the wound. In chronic wounds, this interplay seems to be disturbed, resulting in deregulated clotting, inflammation, wound closure, and angiogenesis, respectively. Therefore, it is conceivable that therapeutic stimulation of dermal fibroblasts in wounds exhibiting delayed wound healing may catalyze the healing process. However, it has to be considered that overstimulation of fibroblast activity may be associated with inadequate wound healing, e.g., by fibrosis and scar formation. Therefore, when addressing this aspect, the controlled inactivation of fibroblasts within the later phase of wound healing has to be considered.

Figure 11.1 graphically depicts some of the known effector functions of dermal fibroblasts in the wound. The eluted drugs (here designated LC1 by the company LEUKOCARE as a place holder for any fibroblast-stimulating drug) diffuse into the wound during the early phase and stimulate the fibroblasts to differentiate and migrate. The differentiated fibroblasts secrete several cytokines and growth factors. For example, the keratinocyte growth factor stimulates keratinocytes to migrate and secrete other growth factors. Keratinocytes are essential for the closure of the wound. In addition, pro-angiogenic factors secreted by keratinocytes stimulate the endothelial cells to form new blood vessels, which is the prerequisite for sufficient oxygenation of the regenerating tissue and thus for efficient granulation.

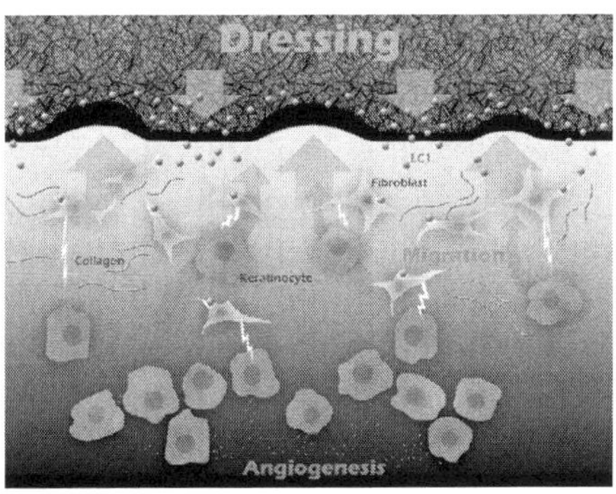

Figure 11.1 Proposed mechanisms elicited by a drug-eluting functionalized dressing material.

Drug-eluting dressings should have a prolonged elution profile that allows the release of relevant drug doses over a time period of more than four days. Mostly, wound dressings will be changed after three or four days. Moreover, the diffusion of the drugs is regulated by the stiffness of the regenerated tissue, and thus drugs will reach their targets more efficiently in the early phase of wound healing.

11.5 Fabrication of a Drug-Eluting Platform Device as an Example

As an example for a possible drug-eluting dressing material, a polymeric composition (LEUKOCARE AG, Munich, Germany) was developed, which comprises a combination of polyethylene terephthalate (PET; Sefar, Edling), polyurethane (PU; AdvanSource, Wilmington, USA), and polyvinyl alcohol (PVA, Sigma, Taufkirchen, Germany) layers forming a grid with 800 μm pore size that function as depots for the selected effector molecules. The grids were cut to fit for the standardized use in each experimental setting. As a model for drug elution, a stable form of ascorbic acid (Asc-2P) was used to load the drug-eluting polymer construct.

The PVA solution (14%) was produced by solving 2.8 g PVA in 20 ml distilled water at 85°C. When the PVA solution reached room temperature (while permanently stirred), it was mixed 1:1 (v/v) with an aqueous ascorbic acid solution (150 mg/ml). The PVA solution was used for the coating of PET grids. The grids were previously washed in ethanol and air dried. They were dipped into the PVA/Asc-2P solution and air dried overnight. A layer of Sefar-Nitex membranes (2 cm diameter) was prepared in a Petri dish. The tissue was overlaid with 200 μL PU/Asc-2P (PU: AdvanSource, Chronoflex C 80A) solution. The PVA/Asc-2P-coated PET grid was placed on the top and 200 μL PU/Asc-2P was used to overlay the grid. Finally, a second Sefar-Nitex tissue was placed on the top. The constructs were dried for 3 h at 37°C. The edges of the device were glued with a polyamide tissue (Sefar) and PU.

A list of different materials used during the selection process is provided in Table 11.1. The fabrication procedure is schematically shown in Fig. 11.2. The patch can be cut into pieces at any size. The material is flexible, and the edges of the layers with a thickness of 1 mm were sealed with polyamide tissue (Sefar) to stabilize the patch during mechanical stress.

Table 11.1 Materials tested for efficient drug release

Product	Source	Material	Physical Data	Drug Release
Monofile PP	Bückmann GmbH	Polypropylene	300 g/m^2 weight; 1000 μm pore size; 500 μm thread size; 44.5% pore area; 1020 μm thickness	Delayed (24 h) +
Saatifil PP 500	SAATItech	Polypropylene	180 g/m^2 weight; 500 μm pore size; 320 μm thread size; 36% pore area; 690 μm thickness	Delayed (24 h) +
PETEX 07-400/48	Sefar	Polyethylene terephthalate	400 μm pore size	Not delayed
PETEX 07-600/51	Sefar	Polyethylene terephthalate	600 μm pore size	Not delayed
PETEX 07-800/55	Sefar	Polyethylene terephthalate	800 μm pore size	Delayed +++
PROPYLTEX 05-1000/45	Sefar	Polypropylene	1000 μm pore size	Not delayed

(*Continued*)

Table 11.1 *(Continued)*

Product	Source	Material	Physical Data	Drug Release
PP-1000/45	Neolab	Polypropylene	Not specified	Not delayed
PA-1000/45	Neolab	Polyamid	Not specified	Not delayed
PES-1000/45	Neolab	Polyester	Not specified	Not delayed
Makrofilter 500	Novodirect GmbH	Nylon	500 μm pore size	Not delayed
Makrofilter 1000	Novodirect GmbH	Nylon	1000 μm pore size	Not delayed
Angimesh	Catgut	Polypropylene	56.3 g/m^2 weight; 155 μm thread size; 86.1% pore area	Not delayed (only slightly in combination with PU sealing)
Angimesh1	Catgut	Polypropylene	107 g/m^2 weight; 207.6 μm thread size; 68% pore area	Not delayed (only slightly in combination with PU sealing)
Angimesh9	Catgut	Polypropylene	127 g/m^2 weight; 198.5 μm thread size; 70,1 % pore area	Not delayed (only slightly in combination with PU sealing)

Product	Source	Material	Physical Data	Drug Release
OptileneMesh	BBRAUN	Polypropylene	60 g/m^2 weight	Not delayed (only slightly in combination with PU sealing but not in combination with polyvinyl alcohol; PVA)
OptileneMesh-Elastic	BBRAUN	Polypropylene	48 g/m^2 weight	Not delayed (only slightly in combination with PU or PU+PVA sealing)
OptileneMesh LP	BBRAUN	Polypropylene	36 g/m^2 weight	Not delayed (only slightly in combination with PU sealing but not in combination with PVA)
Sefar Nitex	Sefar	Polyamide	200 µm pore size; 39% pore area	Not delayed
Saatifil PP 980	SAATItech	Polypropylene	250 g/m^2 weight; 980 µm pore size; 490 µm thread size; 47% pore area; 960 µm thickness	Not delayed; material is instable

Source: Reprinted from Stumpf et al. (2011), with permission of John Wiley and Sons.

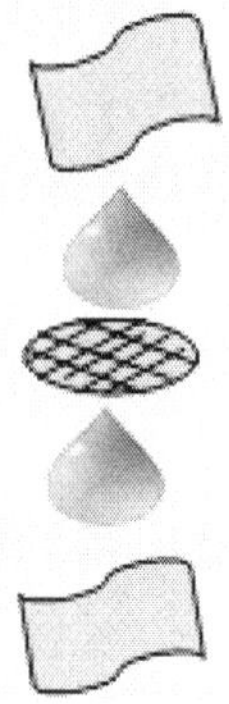

Figure 11.2 Construction of the drug-eluting grid comprising different polymers. Reprinted from Stumpf et al. (2011), with permission of John Wiley and Sons.

Defined pieces of these drug-eluting patches with different grid sizes were functionally evaluated *in vitro* and *in vivo* (Stumpf et al., 2011). In addition, the Asc-2P release kinetics was determined by means of the UV Nanorop method. In this read out, the attenuated and prolonged elution of Asc-2P in a millimolar range was more than 10 days when grids had a pore size of 800 μm. Prolonged presence of Asc-2P could also be detected in the wounds of pigs as a control in an animal study.

Interestingly, the Asc-2P-eluting patches induced collagen production and cell proliferation in dermal fibroblast cultures. Eluted Asc-2P concentrations were shown to have angiogenic potential in the tube formation assays *in vitro* and in the chorioallantoic membrane model *in vivo*. Other biomolecules such as PDGF, VEGF, and cytokines could also be efficiently eluted by the polymer composition as described above.

11.6 Stimulation of Myofibroblasts by Innovative Material Surfaces

Wound dressing materials may have fibroblast-stimulating properties by themselves. Based on the experience of many research groups dealing with the interaction of fibroblasts and keratinocytes, a three-dimensional cell culture model was proposed. Briefly, the contact of dermal fibroblasts with wound-dressing materials under culture conditions allows the microscopic analyses of cellular changes such as expression of cytoskeleton elements and migration behavior. The proposed model will be extended in a modular way, e.g., by fibroblast-keratinocyte co-cultures.

Similar approaches to understand the intercellular mechanisms between fibroblasts and keratinocytes have been intensively studied by several research groups. For example, Shephard et al. (2004) report that keratinocytes regulate the differentiation of fibroblasts into myofibroblasts in a biphasic event. In their setting, TGF-β and IL-1 play an important role, which is reminiscent of myofibroblast differentiation at early and later stages of wound healing (Shephard et al., 2004).

The differentiation of myofibroblasts and their functions is extremely complex on the cellular and molecular levels (Hinz, 2007). For example, there are proto-myofibroblasts, which further develop into "differentiated myofibroblasts" as indicated by the neoexpression of α-SMA. The incorporation of α-SMA into stress fibers significantly augments the contractile activity of fibroblastic cells, which is essential for the contractility of the wound and connective tissue remodeling (Hinz, 2007). The organized interplay between stress fibers, adhesion molecules, extracellular matrix, and physical tension within the wound is critical for the contractility of the wound (Hinz, 2007).

In vitro models that enable the monitoring of fibroblast differentiation under simulated stress conditions such as inflammation (Eming et al., 2007) are helpful to understand intercellular conditioning. Moreover, the impact of dressing materials or drug-eluting systems may be adequately studied in such *in vitro* systems.

11.7 Outlook

The future of wound dressings in advanced wound care will be determined by the efforts of companies to develop products with biologic functions, e.g., drug-device combinations such as drug-eluting dressings. The feasibility of drug-eluting materials has already been shown. In the light of personalized medicine, innovative and modular wound-dressing systems that address the intercellular cross talk in the wound environment may help the clinician to reduce or even avoid the suffering of the patient from delayed wound healing.

References

Broughton G, Janis JE, and Attinger CE. 2006. The basic science of wound healing. *Plast Reconstr Surg*, **117**(7 Suppl): 12S–34S.

Davidson JM, Krieg T, and Eming SA. 2000. Particle-mediated gene therapy of wounds. *Wound Repair Regen*, **8**: 452–459.

Embil JM, Papp K, Sibbald G, Tousignant J, Smiell JM, Wong B, and Lau CY. 2000. Recombinant human platelet-derived growth factor-BB (becaplermin) for healing chronic lower extremity diabetic ulcers: An open-label clinical evaluation of efficacy. *Wound Repair Regen*, **8**(3): 162–168.

Eming SA, Krieg T, and Davidson JM. 2004. Gene transfer in tissue repair: Status, challenges and future directions. *Expert Opin Biol Ther*, **4**: 1373–1386.

Eming SA, Krieg T, and Davidson JM. 2007. Inflammation in wound repair: Molecular and cellular mechanisms. *J Invest Dermatol*, **127**(3): 514–525.

Hinz B. 2007. Formation and function of the myofibroblast during tissue repair. *J Invest Dermatol*, **127**(3): 526–537.

Hocking AM and Gibran NS. 2010. Mesenchymal stem cells: Paracrine signaling and differentiation during cutaneous wound repair. *Exp Cell Res*, **316**: 2213–2219.

Hollister C and Li VW. 2007. Using angiogenesis in chronic wound care with becaplermin and oxidized regenerated cellulose/collagen. *Nurs Clin North Am*, **42**(3): 457–465.

Lansdown AB. 2006. Silver in health care: Antimicrobial effects and safety in use. *Curr Probl Dermatol*, **33**: 17–34.

Li WW, Talcott KE, Zhai AW, Kruger EA, and Li VW. 2005. The role of therapeutic angiogenesis in tissue repair and regeneration. *Adv Skin Wound Care*, **18**: 491–500.

Nolte SV, Xu W, Rennekampff HO, and Rodemann HP. 2008. Diversity of fibroblasts: A review on implications for skin tissue engineering. *Cells Tissues Organs*, **187**: 165–176.

Przybylski M. 2009. A review of the current research on the role of bFGF and VEGF in angiogenesis. *J Wound Care*, **18**: 516–519.

Rizzi SC, Upton Z, Bott K, and Dargaville TR. 2010. Recent advances in dermal wound healing: Biomedical device approaches. *Expert Rev Med Devices*, **7**: 143–154.

Roth D, Piekarek M, Paulsson M, Christ H, Bloch W, Krieg T, Davidson JM, and Eming SA. 2006. Plasmin modulates vascular endothelial growth factor-A-mediated angiogenesis during wound repair. *Am J Pathol,* **168**: 670–684.

Schintler MV. 2012. Negative pressure therapy: Theory and practice. *Diabetes Metab Res Rev,* 28 (Suppl 1): 72–77.

Shephard P, Martin G, Smola-Hess S, Brunner G, Krieg T, and Smola H. 2004. Myofibroblast differentiation is induced in keratinocyte-fibroblast co-cultures and is antagonistically regulated by endogenous transforming growth factor-beta and interleukin-1. *Am J Pathol,* **164**(6): 2055–2066.

Stumpf U, Michaelis M, Klassert D, Cinatl J, Altrichter J, Windolf J, Hergenröther J, Scholz M. 2011. Selection of pro-angiogenic ascorbate derivatives and their exploitation in a novel drug-releasing system for wound healing. *Wound Repair Regen,* **19**(5): 597–607.

Tuan TL, Song A, Chang S, Younai S, and Nimni ME. 1996. In vitro fibroplasia: Matrix contraction, cell growth, and collagen production of fibroblasts cultured in fibrin gels. *Exp Cell Res,* **223**: 127–134.

Watsky MA, Weber KT, Sun Y, and Postlethwaite A. 2010. New insights into the mechanism of fibroblast to myofibroblast transformation and associated pathologies. *Int Rev Cell Mol Biol,* **282**: 165–192.

Chapter 12

Circulating Tumor Cell: Trapping Devices

Frank A. W. Coumans, Sjoerd T. Ligthart, Joost Swennenhuis, and Leon W. M. M. Terstappen
Department of Medical Cell BioPhysics, MIRA institute, University of Twente, Carre Room C4437, Hallenweg 23, 7522 NH, Enschede, The Netherlands
l.w.m.m.terstappen@utwente.nl

The presence of tumor cells in the blood of carcinoma patients is associated with poor outcome and maybe used as a "liquid biopsy" to enable personalized treatment of cancer patients. Here we review the frequency of tumor cells in blood and its association with survival followed by the description of the enrichment and staining of circulating tumor cells (CTCs) and their identification and enumeration as performed by the CellSearch system. Challenges in the entrapment of the rare CTCs by immunomagnetic enrichment have been highlighted. For the identification of treatment targets on these CTCs, a large blood volume should be processed, requiring the development of new enrichment methods, we discuss a potential method employing biofunctionalized glass beads, which need to have a negligible specific adhesion.

Biofunctional Surface Engineering
Edited by Martin Scholz

ISBN 978-981-4411-60-8 (Hardcover), 978-981-4411-61-5 (eBook)
www.panstanford.com

12.1 Introduction

The increase in life expectancy since the early 20th century has been accompanied by a relative and absolute increase in people diagnosed with and treated for cancer. Death from cancer is or will soon be the primary cause of death in the developed world. The cause of death can mostly be attributed to the effects of metastasis rather than the primary tumor (Sporn, 1996). Tumor cells induce blood-vessel growth (angiogenesis) and may invade these blood vessels or the lymphatic system. After entering in the blood directly or through the lymphatic system, these cells are termed circulating tumor cells (CTCs). A majority of CTCs are destroyed by the reticuloendothelial system, but some escape, exit the blood stream, and form distant metastases. The ability to identify and characterize CTCs holds the promise of a liquid biopsy that can pave the way toward personalized care for cancer patients. The frequency of these CTCs is extremely rare and quite some technological challenges arise in the development of CTC-trapping devices. Here we will review the CellSearch platform, which is the first clinically validated platform for the detection of CTCs.

12.2 Frequency and Clinical Relevance of CTC

Circulating tumor cells are very rare cells in the blood of cancer patients and have previously only been observed in blood smears of patients with extensive metastatic disease (Carey et al., 1976; Engell, 1955; Gallivan and Lokich, 1984; Myerowitz *et al.*, 1977; Yam and Janckilla, 1987). The CellSearch system identifies CTCs in 7.5 ml of blood and has been extensively validated for patients with metastatic carcinoma (Allard *et al.*, 2004). Modeling of the CTC distribution in 7.5 ml of blood from patients with metastatic breast, colorectal, and prostate cancer was used to arrive at the CTC frequency distribution in all 5 L of blood (Coumans et al., 2011). Figure 12.1 depicts the cumulative probability in which CTCs can be detected as a function of blood volume in patients with metastatic carcinomas. The figure also shows the frequency of erythrocytes, platelets, and leukocytes in blood and highlights the difficulty of detecting CTCs in all patients. Ten CTCs per ml of blood can only be detected in ~20% of patients, 1 CTC per ml of blood in ~40% of patients, and 100 CTCs per liter of blood in ~80% of patients.

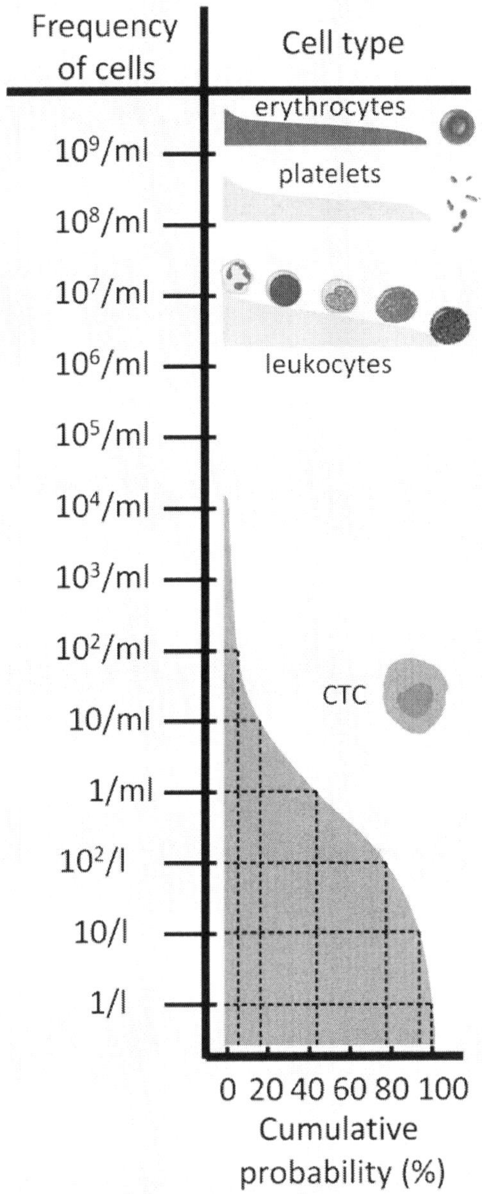

Figure 12.1 Frequency of erythrocytes, platelets, leukocytes, and circulating tumor cells in blood of metastatic carcinoma patients. Cumulative probability of finding at least one cell in a given sample volume is shown on the *x*-axis.

The CellSearch system detects CTCs that express both the epithelial cell adhesion molecule (EpCAM)(Herlyn et al., 1984; Momburg et al., 1987; Szala et al., 1990; Rao et al., 2005) and cytokeratin (CK) 8,18, or 19 (Rao et al., 2005; Franke et al., 1979; Moll et al., 1982; Barak et al., 2004). The reactivity of the antibodies used in the CellSearch system on the tumor tissue of breast cancer patients is shown in Table 12.1. Although expression was detected in the majority of breast cancer tissue samples, this does not imply that all the tumor cells in the tissue express these antigens and that these antigens are preserved during cell migration from tissue to blood. The CTC frequency may, therefore, be underestimated. While the impact of EpCAM+CK+DNA+CD45- CTCs on the outcome is well established, the relation between CTCs with alternative phenotypes and clinical outcome remains to be determined. Various technologies are currently being explored to identify CTCs by other means, which would further improve our understanding of CTCs (Griwatz et al., 1995; Vona et al., 2000; Nagrath et al., 2007; Alix-Panabieres et al., 2005; Gascoyne et al., 2009; Gleghorn et al., 2010; Kahn et al., 2004; Krivacic et al., 2004; Konigsberg et al., 2011; Tan et al., 2010). The CellSearch system may simply miss some EpCAM+, CK+ cells; however, enumeration of EpCAM+ CTCs in 100 μl of whole blood showed that the CTC yield can only be increased up to 6.5 fold (Coumans et al., 2011; Rao et al., 2005). The CTC definition used in the flow cytometric analysis is less strict, and a high false positive rate in the flow assay is the most likely explanation for the largest portion of this discrepancy. The definition of a CTC in the CellSearch system was set in as a series of preclinical studies and was used in system validation studies (Allard et al. 2004; Riethdorf et al., 2007) as well as in prospective multicenter studies for breast, colon, and prostate cancer (Cristofanilli et al., 2004; Cohen et al., 2008; de Bono et al., 2008). These studies showed that metastatic patients that had equal or more CTCs than a certain cut-off (five CTCs for breast and prostate cancer, three for colon cancer) had a significant lower probability of overall survival and thus a worse prognosis than the group that was below this cut-off. Re-analysis of prostate cancer data furthermore showed that a continuous relationship exists between the number of CTCs and survival (Coumans et al., 2011; Scher et al., 2009) and that fragments of tumor cells or tumor microparticles (TMPs)—CK-positive, CD45-negative objects that are <4 μm—are present at a much higher frequency and that their presence also indicates a worse prognosis (Coumans et al., 2010). Next to these three major types of carcinomas, CTCs were enumerated in patients suffering from lung cancer (Krebs et al., 2011; Tanaka et al., 2009), neuroendocrine tumors (Khan et al., 2011), gastric cancer (Matsusaka et al., 2010), bladder cancer (Rink et al., 2011), and ovarian cancer (Poveda et al., 2011).

Table 12.1 Immunohistochemical staining of monoclonal antibodies used in the CellSearch system on paraffin-embedded tissue sections and tissue microarrays of breast cancer patients

Antigen	Cytokeratin 8,18	Cytokeratin 19	EpCAM
Antibody	C11	A53	VU-1D9
Number of samples	280	272	282
Number of positive samples	273	272	278
Percentage of positive samples	97.5	100	98.6

The relation between CTCs and overall survival is illustrated in Fig. 12.2 by Kaplan–Meier plots for 296 metastatic breast and prostate cancer patients. For this analysis, CTCs were identified by an automated algorithm (Ligthart et al., 2011). Panel A shows the Kaplan–Meier plots of patients before the initiation of therapy. Patients with 0 CTC (N = 96, 32%, green line) had a median survival of 33.1 months; patients with 1–3 CTCs (N = 61, 21%, light blue line) had a median survival of 21.9 months; patients with 4–19 CTCs (N = 71, 24%, dark blue line) had a median survival of 15.8 months; and patients with >20 CTCs (N = 68, 23%, red line) had a median survival of only 9.5 months. Panel B shows the Kaplan-Meier plots of patients at first follow-up after the initiation of therapy. The number of patients with 0 CTC increased (N = 134, 45%) and had a median survival of 23.5 months. Patients with 1–3 CTCs also increased (N = 73, 25%) with a median survival of 21.3 months; patients with 4–19 CTCs decreased (N = 43, 15%) with a median survival of 10.6 months; and patients with >20 CTCs also decreased (N = 46, 16%) with an even shorter median survival 5.5 months. Panel C shows the Kaplan–Meier plots of patients subdivided by the changes in CTC counts upon treatment. CTCs remained above 20 in 58 of the 68

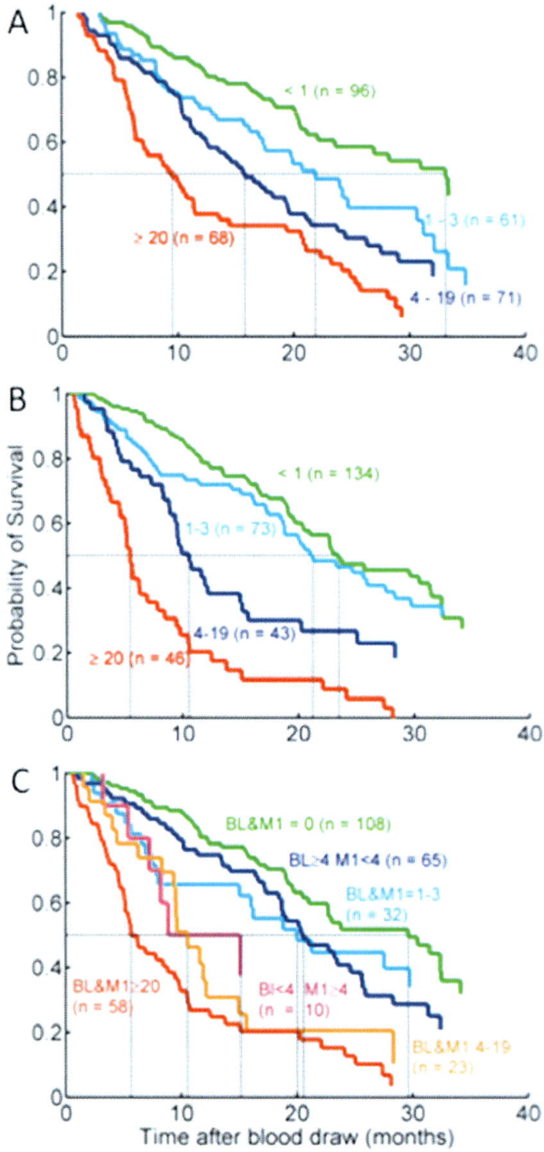

Figure 12.2 Circulating tumor cells (CTCs) and the probability of overall survival for 296 metastatic breast and prostate cancer patients. Panel A shows patients before therapy, Panel B shows the conditions 2–5 weeks after the initiation of therapy, Panel C shows changes in CTCs after the initiation of therapy.

patients with a median survival of 5.7 months (red line), indicating that therapy did not have a sufficiently beneficial effect. Survival also did not improve for those patients with lower (4–19 CTCs) but unchanged CTCs with a median survival of 10.6 months (orange line) or who gained CTCs during therapy with a median survival of 15.2 months (purple line). The 108 patients with 0 CTC (green line) before and after the initiation of therapy had a median survival of 29.6 months. Survival of the 65 patients with a CTC reduction (blue line) to below 4 clearly improved, and patients that remained with low counts (light blue line) did not significantly change. The low number of CTCs detected urges the need for the elimination of error in the assignments of CTCs as is achieved by the automation of the image analysis and also is strongly depended on the Poisson error. Patients in which no CTCs were detected in 7.5 ml of blood have metastatic disease, so the question arises whether this is a distinct group of patients, or CTCs are missed by the CellSearch system, or the volume of blood examined is simply too low. Extrapolation of the sample volume to 5 L of blood predicted that 99% of patients had at least 1 CTC before the initiation of therapy, which decreased to 97% after the first cycles of therapy. The survival chances of patients with EpCAM+ CK+ nucleated CTCs are reduced by 6.6 months for each tenfold CTC increase (Coumans et al., 2011). These results suggest that a technological leap is needed to identify CTCs in all patients with metastatic disease and likely in those patients with primary disease that are at risk for disease recurrence.

12.3 CTC Enrichment and Staining with the CellTracksAutoPrep

The CellTracksAutoPrep is an automated sample preparation device that is part of the CellSearch system. Blood is collected from a patient by venipuncture or from a venous port into a CellSave Preservative Tube™. These tubes contain EDTA as anticoagulant and a cellular preservative to avoid the degradation of the blood sample for up to 96 h while it is being transported to a facility where an AutoPrep system is present. Before placement on the AutoPrep, the blood is diluted, mixed by inversion, and centrifuged. The AutoPrep first detects the interface between plasma and blood and then aspirates and discards the plasma. Next ferrofluid conjugated to EpCAM is added as well as dilution and system buffers. The sample is placed between magnets, which causes the ferrofluid-labeled cells to travel to the area within the tube that has the highest magnetic gradient. After the magnetically labeled cells and the free ferrofluid are captured at the wall of the tube, the remaining blood is aspirated and discarded. Buffers are added and the magnetic separation is repeated. Next, fluorescent markers for DNA (4#,6-diamidino-2-phenylindole: DAPI), antibodies directed to CKs 8, 18, and 19 labeled to phycoerythrin (PE), and CD45 to allophycocyanin (APC) are added and the sample is left to incubate. After another magnetic separation step and more aspiration steps, the remaining 300 μl is transferred to the analysis cartridge, which is placed in a CellTracksMagNest™ cell presentation device (see Fig. 12.3).This MagNest consists of two magnets that create an upward magnetic force, pulling the ferrofluid-labeled cells to a cover slip within the cartridge. Simulated particle trajectories due to the magnetic field in the MagNest are shown in Fig. 12.4 (Tibbe et al., 2002), with the square box slightly underneath the magnets representing a cross section of the sample cartridge. As can be seen in Fig. 12.4, the magnets are designed in such a way that cells will move straight up; their distribution across the analysis surface is, therefore, homogeneous.

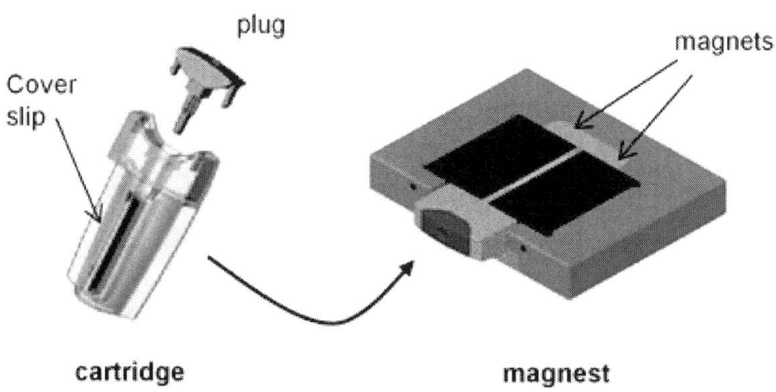

Figure 12.3 Analysis cartridge to which the enriched sample is transferred and MagNest in which cells are magnetically pulled to the cover slip.

12.4 Imaging and Enumeration of CTCs with CellTracks Analyzer

The CellTracks Analyzer is a semiautomated fluorescence microscope that is part of the CellSearch system. After the cells are settled, the MagNest is placed in the CellTracks Analyzer, a semiautomatic epifluorescence microscope. Employing a mercury arc lamp, a 10X/0.45NA objective, the whole cartridge is scanned at four fluorescence channels: channels for the detection of DNA-DAPI, CK-PE, and CD45-APC, and a fourth channel termed "FITC." This fourth channel may be used for control cells or an extra biomarker, but it is generally used to verify if objects are autofluorescent (and thus debris). Images are captured with a charge-coupled device camera with an effective pixel size of $0.65 \times 0.65\ \mu m^2$. When a scan is complete, the CellSearch software identifies objects that are positively stained for DNA and CK, and creates a thumbnail gallery showing these objects. Figure 12.5 shows an example of such a gallery. Next to the four fluorescence channels, an overlay of the DAPI and PE channels is shown. A trained reviewer must now distinguish CTCs from leukocytes and debris that were carried over during the enrichment procedure. The reviewers have a set of rules in determining whether an object is a CTC or not, which is shown in Fig. 12.6. These rules were set and tested by means of preclinical studies (Kagan et al., 2002; Moreno et al., 2001; Racila et al., 1998; Terstappen et al., 2000). By scoring the cells according to this set of rules, object A from Fig. 12.5 is a CTC next to a leukocyte. Object B are two bright CTCs close together that have some spill-over signal in the CD45-APC channel. Object C fails rule 2 (and also has questionable morphology), and object D fails rule 5. Although these examples are relatively straightforward, not all images are unambiguous, as is exemplified by the two objects in E and F. These seem to be small cells and are a bit speckled, suggesting that they are undergoing apoptosis (Larson et al., 2004). When shown to reviewers, it was found that these objects give rise to the highest inter-reviewer variability. The variability for the classification of CTCs between reviewers was reported to be between 4% and 31% (median 14%), and a variability of 7.5% between laboratories (Kraan et al., 2011). The rules for qualifying objects are mostly quantitative, because a reviewer cannot view the number of grey levels in the image easily. Reviewers may, therefore, be biased by the auto-scaling of these images, which is done purely for viewing purposes. If a bright object is located near a dim object, this dim object may be classified wrongly due to this effect.

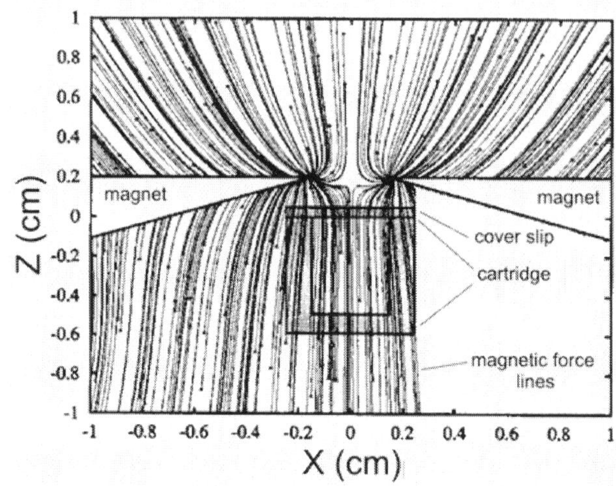

Figure 12.4 Simulation of magnetic particle trajectories inside the MagNest adapted from (Tibbe et al. 2002). Cells are pulled toward the cover slip inside the cartridge in a trajectory perpendicular to the cover slip. The force lines in the lower right part of the figure were erased for viewing purposes.

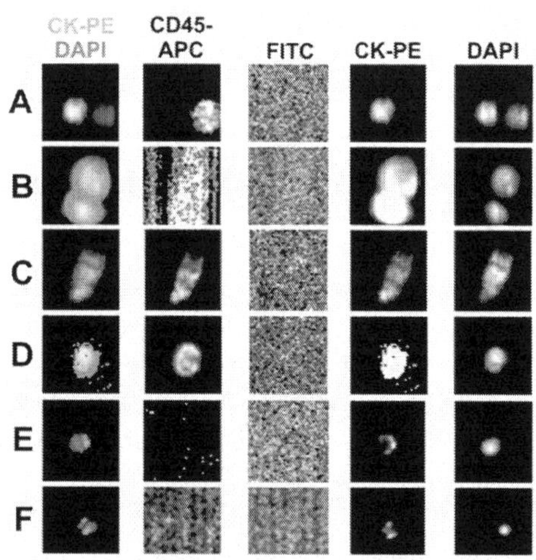

Figure 12.5 CellSearch thumbnail gallery. The CellSearch software presents all objects that are both positive for CK and DAPI. Panels A–D show examples of CTCs (A/B) and debris (C/D).

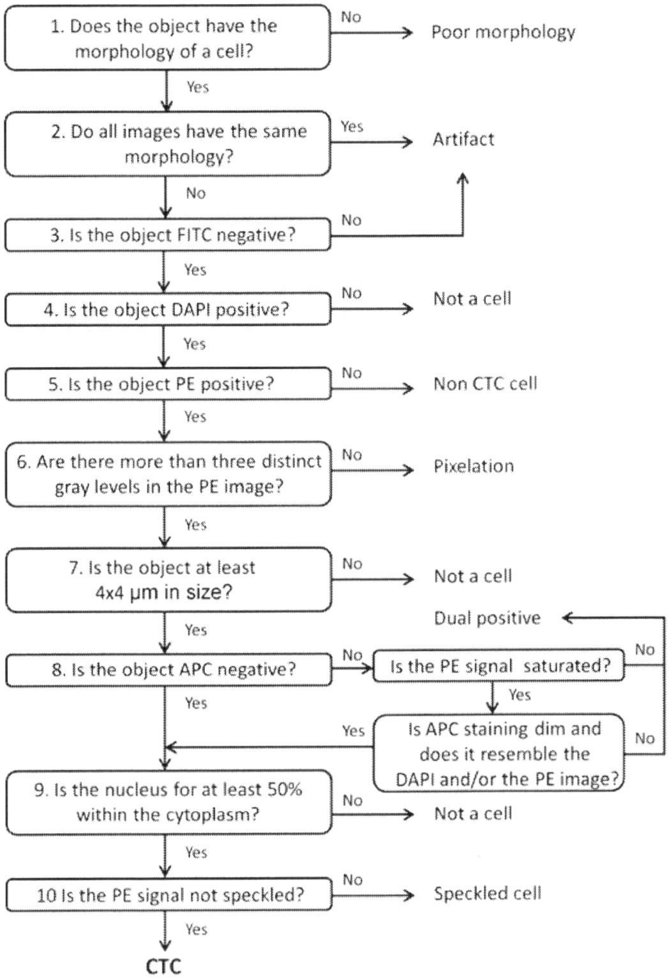

Figure 12.6 Decision tree showing how trained reviewers classify whether or not an object is a CTC.

12.5 Immunomagnetic Enrichment

For the enrichment of the rare CTCs, a high recovery of the CTCs and a low carryover of the blood cells are of utmost importance. In the CellSearch system, the choice was made to use immunomagnetic enrichment of CTCs. EpCAM was chosen as the antigen as it was expressed on the majority of breast cancer carcinomas (Table 12.1) and other carcinomas (Momburg et al., 1987); it was not expressed on cells of hematopoietic origin and was expressed at the cell surface. Cell surface markers do not need cell permeabilization, which is needed for intracellular antigens such as CK. The drawback of this approach is that CTCs not expressing the target antigen will be missed. As magnetic particles, the choice was made for ferrofluids with submicron-sized particles as they would not reduce the ability to visualize cells as much as μm sized magnetic particles. However, the ferrofluids need to have sufficient magnetic properties to be separated in an open magnetic field and avoid entrapment in mesh-like structures. This base ferrofluid is made by sonification of magnetite while adding BSA under controlled conditions to arrive at an average particle size of ~120 nm (Liberti et al., 1997). This ferrofluid consists of small clusters of Fe_3O_4 covered with bovine serum albumin (BSA) as illustrated in the electron micrographs in Fig. 12.7. The VU-1D9 monoclonal antibody directed against the EpCAM antigen is conjugated by standard coupling chemistry to the ferrofluid (Terstappen et al., 2008). Although this ferrofluid can be used to capture cells expressing the EpCAM antigen from blood, it was noted that the recovery of cells with a relatively low EpCAM expression was considerably less as compared to those expressing larger densities of the EpCAM antigen (Rao et al., 2005). To overcome this issue, a process called "controlled aggregation" was developed, which resulted in high cell recoveries along a larger range of antigen densities (Rao et al., 2005). To achieve this, the EpCAM ferrofluids are conjugated to desthiobiotin using *N*-hydroxysuccinimide-DL-desthiobiotin (Liberti et al., 2003). After the addition of EpCAM desthiobiotin ferrofluid to the blood, it will bind the EpCAM antigen at the cell surface (Fig. 12.8, panel A) upon the addition of a buffer containing streptavidin; more ferrofluids will bind to the cell surface (Fig. 12.8, panel B), thereby increasing the ability to separate the cells in a magnetic field and reduce the variability of cell recovery due to variations in antigen densities (Rao et al., 2005). After the enrichment has taken place, a buffer can be added containing biotin, which will replace the desthiobiotin in the streptavidin and release the additional ferrofluid from the cells (Fig. 12.8, panel C). Removal of the ferrofluid from the cells is needed to reduce the attenuation of fluorescence signals from the cells by ferrofluid. This increases the ability to visualize the cells and thus aids in their identification.

Aggregation of ferrofluid can also take place under the influence of plasma components in blood samples from some individuals. To reduce the influence of these factors, the blood samples are diluted and the plasma is aspirated and discarded by the CellTracksAutoPrep system. A ferrofluid that does not interact with plasma components is desirable because when the plasma gets discarded, the majority of tumor microparticles that are contained within the plasma fraction cannot be captured (Pawlowski et al., 2011; van der Pol et al., 2010).

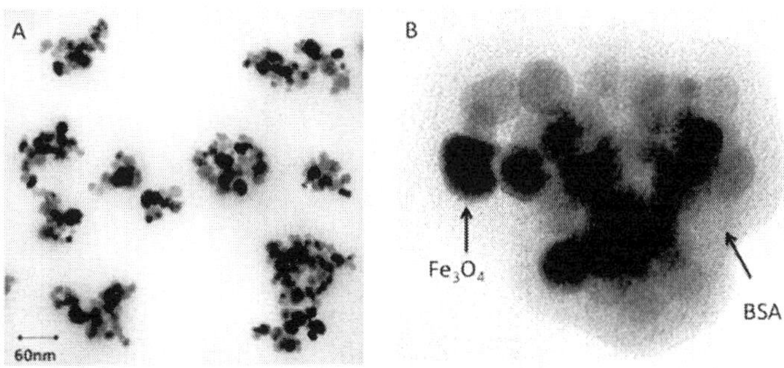

Figure 12.7 Ferrofluids visualized by electronic microscopy. Panel B shows particles imaged at higher resolution than panel A.

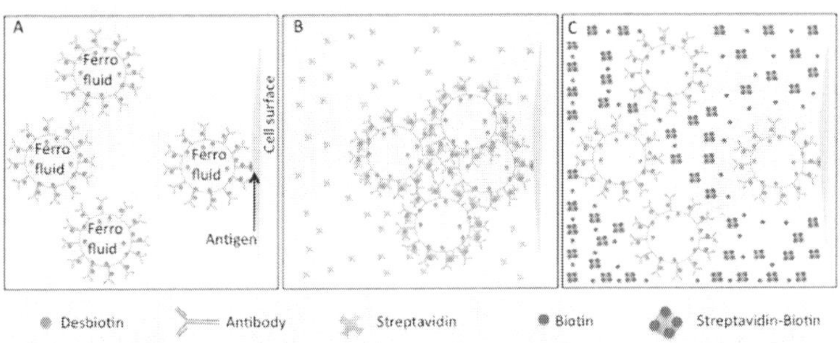

Figure 12.8 Transient increase in magnetic loading to improve the selection of CTCs with low EpCAM expression. Panel A shows EpCAM desthiobiotin ferrofluid binding EpCAM antigen at the cell surface. The majority of ferrofluid particles remain in suspension because the bound ferrofluids sterically hinder the binding sites. Panel B shows addition of streptavidin, recruiting unbound ferrofluids. This leads to an increase in magnetic cell loading. Panel C shows addition of unconjugated biotin, which replaces the desthiobiotin in the streptavidin linkers. This results in a release of the recruited ferrofluids.

12.6 Detection of Treatment Targets on CTCs

After the identification of CTCs, the presence of treatment targets on these CTCs can be assessed. Expression of these targets may be used to prescribe therapies directed against these targets. Expression of cell surface or intracellular treatment target antigens can be assessed by the addition of additional monoclonal antibodies labeled with fluorochromes not overlapping with the ones used for the identification of CTCs. Examples are the expression of Her-2 (Hayes et al., 2002; Riethdorf et al., 2010), uPAR (Meng et al., 2006), and IGF-1R (Karp et al., 2009; de Bono et al., 2007). The ability to revisit the CTCs in the CellSearch system provides the opportunity to examine gene expression by fluorescence in situ hybridization (Swennenhuis et al., 2009) and investigate amplification deletion and translocation of treatment-related genes such as HER2, PTEN, ERG, and AR (Attard et al., 2009; Meng, 2004). Alternative approaches are the examination of gene expression by multiplex PCR. For this approach, one can use an immunomagnetically enriched sample obtained after processing 7.5 ml whole blood by the CellTracksAutoPrep profile kit (Veridex, Raritan, NJ, USA). This typically results in a 900 μl sample volume containing ~1000 leukocytes and a varying number of CTCs. This material has been used successfully to detect the expression of numerous genes in CTCs by multiplex PCR (O'Hara, 2004; Smirnov, 2006; Sieuwerts et al., 2009).

The drawback of this approach is that only genes that have no or low expression in leukocytes can be examined (Smirnov, 2006; Kowalewska et al., 2006). A method that can deplete the residual leukocytes from a CTC-enriched sample could increase the number of genes that can be examined by PCR methods. One such approach is the depletion of leukocytes by a CD45 depletion column. A concept for a depletion column is shown in Fig. 12.9, panel A. The sample with leukocytes and CTCs is loaded onto the column, containing beads coated with the leukocyte-specific antibody CD45. Leukocytes will be retained by the column, while CTCs pass through for further processing. The composition of the coating is illustrated in panel B of Fig. 12.9. On a glass substrate, a layer of 3-aminopropyltriethoxysilane (APTES, Sigma Aldrich, St. Louis, USA) is formed. This layer covalently binds BSA-biotin molecules (Sigma Aldrich). Streptavidin (Thermo Fisher Scientific, Rockford, IL, USA) has four binding sites for biotin and is used as a linker between the BSA-biotin and biotinylated antibodies. When a cell expresses antigens to this antibody on the membrane, the cell can be captured. The construction of the depletion column is illustrated in panel C of Fig. 12.9. The container for the column consists of a 3 ml syringe barrel (BD, Franklin Lakes, NJ, USA). The substrate for the column consists of 210–300 μm soda lime glass beads (Sigma Aldrich); with maximum packing density, this leaves gaps large enough for cells to pass between the beads (>30 μm), while the coated surface area of a 2 ml column is approximately 113×10^3 mm^2. The beads are held in place on both ends by a nylon mesh (30 μm pore size, Spectrum Laboratories, Rancho Dominguez, CA, USA). The output flow rate of the column is controlled by squeezing a piece of flexible tubing (Tygon, Saint Gobain Plastics, Paris, France), which is connected to the output of the syringe. To test whether cells could indeed be efficiently passed through a column, the beads in the column depicted in Fig. 12.9 were coated with BSA. Leukocytes were obtained after the ammonium chloride lysing of whole blood and passed through the column at a flow rate of 0.85 mm/s in a volume of 1 ml at concentrations of 0.25×10^6, 1.00×10^6, 1.75×10^6, and 2.50×10^6 leukocytes/ml. Recovery was determined by centrifugation of the filtrate and re-suspending the cells in 0.1 ml. This sample was then stained with 8 μM Hoechst 33342 and enumerated on a counting chamber (Neubauer, Lauda-Königshofen, Germany). The results in Fig. 12.10 show a recovery of 92% minus an offset of 97,000 leukocytes. Inspection of the component parts of the functionalized column did not show any large accumulation of cells on the surface of the syringe barrel, nor on the mesh used to contain the beads. Inspection of the beads did not show many cells either, but due to the very large surface area of the beads, it is not possible to exclude the possibility that the lost cells could be found on the beads. Although a recovery of 92% is not that bad for rare event detection, it is not sufficient and especially the offset of 97,000 leukocytes is worrisome. To investigate cell capture on coated surfaces, a flow chamber was constructed. The bottom of the chamber was coated with two lanes of BSA-biotin, one lane of streptavidin, two lanes of mouse IgG monoclonal antibody specific for SKBR3 culture cells, and one blank as illustrated in panel A of Fig. 12.11. SKBR3 cells were flowed through the chamber, and the number of SKBR3 cells captured on each lane is shown at the bottom of panel A. The fields with antibody captured an average of 36 cells, while those without antibody captured an average of

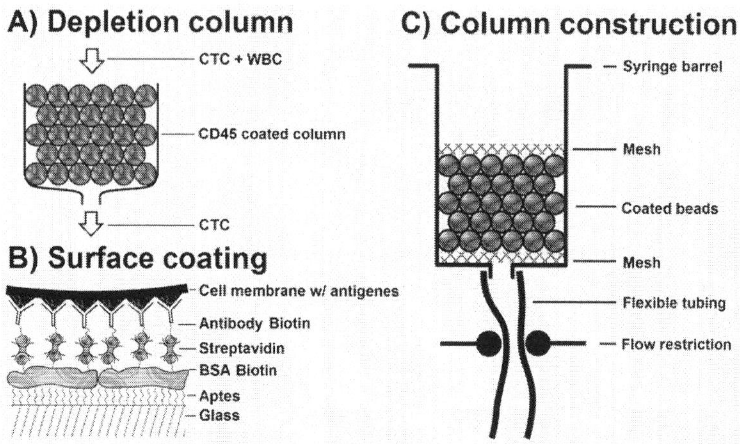

Figure 12.9 Design of a depletion column. Panel A shows the concept of cell depletion on a column. The sample containing CTCs and leukocytes is loaded onto the column, which is coated with CD45. The leukocytes are trapped while passing through the column, and CTCs pass through and can be captured for further processing. Panel B shows the different layers the antibody coating is constructed of. The substrate is glass. The glass is coated with silane (APTES) to which BSA-biotin is covalently bound. The streptavidin binds to the biotin, which in turn binds a biotinylated antibody. Cells expressing the membrane antigens to the antibody are directed and captured this way. Panel C shows the column construction. Antibody-coated beads are contained in between two layers of mesh and the barrel of a syringe to keep the column in place. The flow rate is controlled by squeezing a short length of flexible tubing connected to the outlet of the syringe barrel.

17 cells. The antibody-coated lanes do capture more cells than the lanes without antibody, but the nonspecific capture is too large. The use of BSA to reduce nonspecific adhesion is clearly not sufficient, and either the coating needs to be improved by eliminating the "nonspecific binding spots" or a different coating needs to be used that prevents cells from binding nonspecifically. In panel B of Fig. 12.11, the Poiseuille flow and the flow velocity profile within this chamber is illustrated. To study the effect of flow on the capture, biotinylated beads were flowed through a flow chamber of which all lanes were coated with streptavidin. A few fragments of a video of the biotinylated beads flowing through the chamber at a maximum

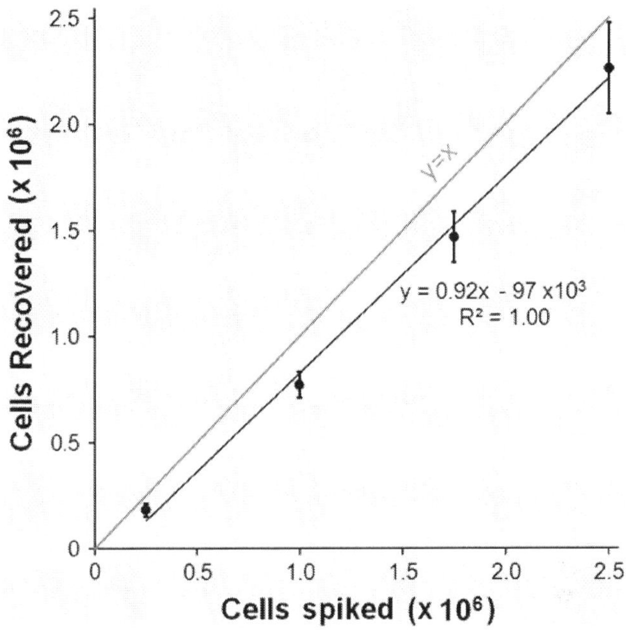

Figure 12.10 Leukocytes were passed through a column coated with BSA and their recovery was determined. Whiskers indicate one standard deviation Poisson error. A linear fit shows 92% recovery combined with a large offset of 97,000 cells lost per sample.

flow speed of 1.3 mm/s are shown in panel C of Fig. 12.11. The beads in the figure are labeled A–E. Bead A is decelerating, while bead B is accelerating. Bead C is attaching and did not move from the last position in the following 20 s, while bead D is already attached to the surface at the beginning of this movie fragment. Bead E has a higher speed (further from surface) and is, therefore, elongated and appears dimmer. While the beads at low speed manage to slow down and adhere to the surface, the fast beads appear to stay in the middle of the flow. This shows the importance of the flow profile of cells/beads passing a functionalized surface. Cells and beads in an aqueous media will have a low Reynolds number, giving rise to laminar flow, which prevents contact with the functionalized area. The design of a flow chamber thus needs to be such that a maximum number of collisions between cells and the functionalized surface are obtained.

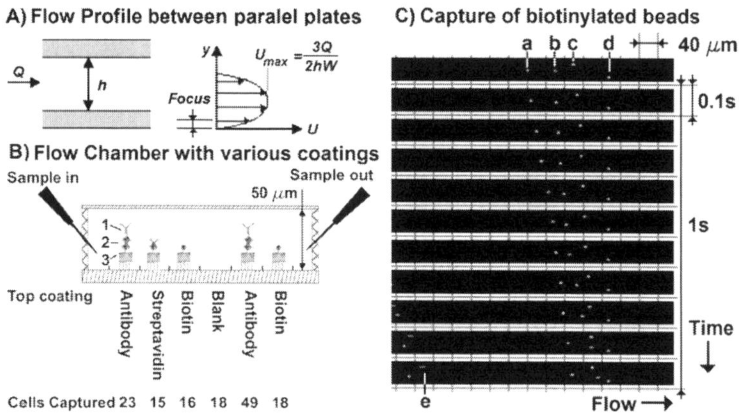

Figure 12.11 Capture of cells and beads in a flow chamber. Panel A shows a flow chamber with multiple coating regions; illustrations show which components are present on each area: BSA-biotin (1), streptavidin (2), and biotinylated antibody (3). Cells which should be captured by the antibody were flowed through. The number of captured cells for each region is shown below the diagram. Panel B shows the Poiseuille flow between two parallel plates and the flow velocity (U) profile between the plates. The depth of focus of the microscope is shown on the right of the profile. Panel C shows a series of images taken of 1 μm biotinylated beads moving through a streptavidin-coated flow chamber. Beads of interest are labeled with letters A–E.

References

Alix-Panabieres C, Brouillet JP, Fabbro M, Yssel H, Rousset T, Maudelonde T, Choquet-Kastylevsky G, and Vendrell JP. 2005. Characterization and enumeration of cells secreting tumor markers in the peripheral blood of breast cancer patients. *J Immunol Methods*, **299**(1–2): 177–188.

Allard WJ, Matera J, Miller MC, Repollet M, Connelly MC, Rao C, Tibbe AG, Uhr JW, and Terstappen LW. 2004. Tumor cells circulate in the peripheral blood of all major carcinomas but not in healthy subjects or patients with nonmalignant diseases. *Clin Cancer Res* **10**(20): 6897–6904.

Attard G, et al. 2009. Characterization of ERG, AR and PTEN gene status in circulating tumor cells from patients with castration-resistant prostate cancer. *Cancer Res*, **69**(7): 2912–2918.

Barak V, Goike H, Panaretakis KW, and Einarsson R. 2004. Clinical utility of cytokeratins as tumor markers. *Clin Biochem*, **37**(7): 529–540.

Carey RW, Taft PD, Bennett JM, and Kaufman S. 1976. Carcinocythemia (carcinoma cell leukemia). An acute leukemia-like picture due to metastatic carcinoma cells. *Am J Med*, **60**(2): 273–278.

Cohen SJ, et al. 2008. Relationship of circulating tumor cells to tumor response, progression-free survival, and overall survival in patients with metastatic colorectal cancer. *J Clin Oncol*, **26**(19): 3213–3221.

Coumans FAW, Doggen CJM, Attard G, de Bono JS, and Terstappen LWMM. 2010. All circulating EpCAM+CK+CD45- objects predict overall survival in castration-resistant prostate cancer. *Ann Oncol*, **21**(9): 1851–1857.

Coumans FAW, Ligthart ST, Uhr J, and Terstappen LWMM. 2012. Challenges in the enumeration and phenotyping of CTC. *Clin Can Res*, **18:** 5711–5718.

Cristofanilli M, et al. 2004. Circulating tumor cells, disease progression, and survival in metastatic breast cancer. *N Engl J Med*, **351**(8): 781–791.

de Bono JS, et al. 2007. Potential applications for circulating tumor cells expressing the insulin-like growth factor-I receptor. *Clin Cancer Res*, **13**(12): 3611–3616.

de Bono JS, Scher HI, Montgomery RB, Parker C, Miller MC, Tissing H, Doyle GV, Terstappen LWMM, Pienta KJ, and Raghavan D. 2008. Circulating tumor cells predict survival benefit from treatment in metastatic castration-resistant prostate cancer. *Clin Cancer Res*, **14**(19): 6302–6309.

Engell HC. 1955. Cancer cells in the circulating blood: A clinical study on the occurrence of cancer cells in the peripheral blood and in venous blood draining the tumour area at operation. *Acta Chir Scand Suppl*, **201**: 1–70.

Franke WW, Schmid E, Osborn M, and Weber K. 1979. Intermediate-sized filaments of human endothelial cells. *J Cell Biol*, **81**(3): 570–580.

Gallivan MV and Lokich JJ. 1984. Carcinocythemia (carcinoma cell leukemia): Report of two cases with English literature review. *Ann Ny Acad Sci*, **53**(5): 1100–1102.

Gascoyne PR, Noshari J, Anderson TJ, and Becker FF. 2009. Isolation of rare cells from cell mixtures by dielectrophoresis. *Electrophoresis*, **30**(8): 1388–1398.

Gleghorn JP, Pratt ED, Denning D, Liu H, Bander NH, Tagawa ST, Nanus DM, Giannakakou PA, and Kirby BJ. 2010. Capture of circulating tumor cells from whole blood of prostate cancer patients using geometrically enhanced differential immunocapture (GEDI) and a prostate-specific antibody. *Lab Chip*, **10**(1): 27–29.

Griwatz C, Brandt B, Assmann G, and Zanker KS. 1995. An immunological enrichment method for epithelial cells from peripheral blood. *J Immunol Methods*, **183**(2): 251–265.

Hayes DF, et al. 2002. Monitoring expression of HER-2 on circulating epithelial cells in patients with advanced breast cancer. *Int J Oncol*, **21**(5): 1111–1117.

Herlyn D, Herlyn M, Ross AH, Ernst C, Atkinson B, and Koprowski H. 1984. Efficient selection of human tumor growth-inhibiting monoclonal antibodies. *J Immunol Methods*, **73**(1): 157–167.

Kagan M, et al. 2002. A sample preparation and analysis system for identification of circulating tumor cells. *J Clin Ligand Assay*, **25**(1): 104–110.

Kahn HJ, Presta A, Yang LY, Blondal J, Trudeau M, Lickley L, Holloway C, McCready DR, Maclean D, and Marks A. 2004. Enumeration of circulating tumor cells in the blood of breast cancer patients after filtration enrichment: Correlation with disease stage. *Breast Cancer Res Tr*, **86**(3): 237–247.

Karp DD, et al. 2009. Safety, pharmacokinetics, and pharmacodynamics of the insulin-like growth factor type 1 receptor inhibitor figitumumab (CP-751,871) in combination with paclitaxel and carboplatin. *J Thorac Oncol*, **4**(11): 1397–1403.

Khan MS, Tsigani T, Rashid M, Rabouhans JS, Yu D, Luong TV, Caplin M, and Meyer T. 2011. Circulating tumor cells and EpCAM expression in neuroendocrine tumors. *Clin Cancer Res*, **17**(2): 337–345.

Konigsberg R, Obermayr E, Bises G, Pfeiler G, Gneist M, Wrba F, de Santis M, Zeillinger R, Hudec M, and Dittrich C. 2011. Detection of EpCAM positive and negative circulating tumor cells in metastatic breast cancer patients. *Acta Oncol*, **50**(5): 700–710.

Kowalewska M, Chechlinska M, Markowicz S, Kober P, and Nowak R. 2006. The relevance of RT-PCR detection of disseminated tumour cells is hampered by the expression of markers regarded as tumour-specific in activated lymphocytes. *Eur J Cancer*, **42**(16): 2671–2674.

Kraan J, et al. 2011. External quality assurance of circulating tumor cell enumeration using the CellSearch system: A feasibility study. *Cytometry Part B, Clin Cytometry*, **80**(2): 112–118.

Krebs MG, et al. 2011. Evaluation and prognostic significance of circulating tumor cells in patients with non-small-cell lung cancer. *J Clin Oncol*, **29**(12): 1556–1563.

Krivacic RT, et al. 2004. A rare-cell detector for cancer. *Proc Natl Acad Sci USA*, **101**(29): 10501–10504.

Larson CJ, Moreno JG, Pienta KJ, Gross S, Repollet M, O'Hara SM, Russell T, and Terstappen LWMM. 2004. Apoptosis of circulating tumor cells in prostate cancer patients. *Cytometry*, **62A**(1): 46–53.

Liberti PA, Rao GC, and Chiarappa JN. 1997. Methods for the manufacture of magnetically responsive particles. *Immunivest Corporation (Wilmington, DE)*. US patent No 5,698,271.

Liberti PA, Rao GC, and Terstappen LWMM. 2003. Increased separation efficiency via controlled aggregation of magnetic nanoparticles. *Immunivest Corporation (Wilmington, DE)*. US Patent No. 6,620,627 B1 & 6,551,843 B1.

Ligthart ST, Coumans FAW, Attard G, Mulick Cassidy A, de Bono JS, and Terstappen LWMM. 2011. Unbiased and automated identification of a circulating tumour cell definition that associates with overall survival. *PLoS One*, **6**(11): e27419.

Matsusaka S, Chin K, Ogura M, Suenaga M, Shinozaki E, Mishima Y, Terui Y, Mizunuma N, and Hatake K. 2010. Circulating tumor cells as a surrogate marker for determining response to chemotherapy in patients with advanced gastric cancer. *Cancer Sci*, **101**(4): 1067–1071.

Meng S, et al. 2006. uPAR and HER-2 gene status in individual breast cancer cells from blood and tissues. *Proc Natl Acad Sci USA*, **103**(46): 17361–17365.

Meng S. 2004. HER-2 gene amplification can be acquired as breast cancer progresses. *Proc Nat Acad Sci USA*, **101**(25): 9393–9398.

Moll R, Franke WW, Schiller DL, Geiger B, and Krepler R. 1982. The catalog of human cytokeratins: Patterns of expression in normal epithelia, tumors and cultured cells. *Cell*, **31**(1): 11–24.

Momburg F, Moldenhauer G, Hammerling GJ, and Moller P. 1987. Immunohistochemical study of the expression of a Mr 34,000 human epithelium-specific surface glycoprotein in normal and malignant tissues. *Cancer Res*, **47**(11): 2883–2891.

Moreno JG, O'Hara SM, Gross S, Doyle G, Fritsche H, Gomella LG, and Terstappen LW. 2001. Changes in circulating carcinoma cells in patients with metastatic prostate cancer correlate with disease status. *Urology*, **58**(3): 386–392.

Myerowitz RL, Edwards PA, and Sartiano GP. 1977. Carcinocythemia (carcinoma cell leukemia) due to metastatic carcinoma of the breast: Report of a case. *Ann Ny Acad Sci*, **40**(6): 3107–3111.

Nagrath S, et al. 2007. Isolation of rare circulating tumour cells in cancer patients by microchip technology. *Nature*, **450**(7173): 1235–1239.

O'Hara SM. 2004. Multigene reverse transcription-PCR profiling of circulating tumor cells in hormone-refractory prostate cancer. *Clin Chem*, **50**(5): 826–835.

Pawlowski T, Akhavan R, Tasinato A, Millis M, Kojima Y, Zhong JS, and Kuslich C. 2011. Expression of MIR-497 in circulating microvesicles is a potential biomarker for the early detection of NSCLC. *J Thorac Oncol*, **6**(6): S1079–S1080.

Poveda A, Kaye SB, McCormack R, Wang S, Parekh T, Ricci D, Lebedinsky CA, Tercero JC, Zintl P, and Monk BJ. 2011. Circulating tumor cells predict progression free survival and overall survival in patients with relapsed/recurrent advanced ovarian cancer. *Gynecologic oncology*, **122**(3): 567–572.

Racila E, Euhus D, Weiss AJ, Rao C, McConnell J, Terstappen L, and Uhr JW. 1998. Detection and characterization of carcinoma cells in the blood. *Proc Natl Acad Sci USA*, **95**(8): 4589–4594.

Rao CG, Chianese D, Doyle GV, Miller MC, Russell T, Sanders RA Jr, and Terstappen LW. 2005. Expression of epithelial cell adhesion molecule in carcinoma cells present in blood and primary and metastatic tumors. *Int J Oncol*, **27**(1): 49–57.

Riethdorf S, et al. 2007. Detection of circulating tumor cells in peripheral blood of patients with metastatic breast cancer: A validation study of the CellSearch system. *Clin Cancer Res*, **13**(3): 920–928.

Riethdorf S, et al. 2010. Detection and HER-2 expression of circulating tumor cells: Prospective monitoring in breast cancer patients treated in the neoadjuvant GeparQuattro trial. *Clin Cancer Res*, **16**(9): 2634–2645.

Rink M, Chun FK, Minner S, Friedrich M, Mauermann O, Heinzer H, Huland H, Fisch M, Pantel K, and Riethdorf S. 2011. Detection of circulating tumour cells in peripheral blood of patients with advanced non-metastatic bladder cancer. *BJU Int*, **107**(10): 1668–1675.

Scher HI, Jia XY, de Bono JS, Fleisher M, Pienta KJ, Raghavan D, and Heller G. 2009. Circulating tumour cells as prognostic markers in progressive, castration-resistant prostate cancer: A reanalysis of IMMC38 trial data. *Lancet Oncol*, **10**(3): 233–239.

Sieuwerts AM, Kraan J, Bolt J, van der Spoel P, Elstrodt F, Schutte M, Martens JW, Gratama JW, Sleijfer S, and Foekens JA. 2009. Anti-epithelial cell adhesion molecule antibodies and the detection of circulating normal-like breast tumor cells. *J Natl Cancer Inst*, **101**(1): 61–66.

Smirnov DA. 2006. Global gene expression profiling of circulating endothelial cells in patients with metastatic carcinomas. *Cancer Res*, **66**(6): 2918–2922.

Sporn MB. 1996. The war on cancer. *Lancet*, **347**(9012): 1377–1381.

Swennenhuis JF, Tibbe AGJ, Levink R, Sipkema RCJ, and Terstappen LWMM. 2009. Characterization of circulating tumor cells by fluorescence in situ hybridization. *Cytometry Part A*, **75A**(6): 520–527.

Szala S, Froehlich M, Scollon M, Kasai Y, Steplewski Z, Koprowski H, and Linnenbach AJ. 1990. Molecular cloning of cDNA for the carcinoma-associated antigen GA733-2. *Proc Natl Acad Sci USA*, **87**(9): 3542–3546.

Tan SJ, Lakshmi RL, Chen P, Lim WT, Yobas L, and Lim CT. 2010. Versatile label free biochip for the detection of circulating tumor cells from peripheral blood in cancer patients. *Biosens Bioelectron*, **26**(4): 1701–1705.

Tanaka F, et al. 2009. Circulating tumor cell as a diagnostic marker in primary lung cancer. *Clin Cancer Res*, **15**(22): 6980–6986.

Terstappen LW, Rao C, Gross S, and Weiss AJ. 2000. Peripheral blood tumor cell load reflects the clinical activity of the disease in patients with carcinoma of the breast. *Int J Oncol*, **17**(3): 573–578.

Terstappen LWMM, Rao GC, Uhr JW, Racila EV, and Liberti P A. 2008. Methods and reagents for the rapid and efficient isolation of circulating cancer cells. *Immunivest Corporation (Wilmington, DE)*. US Patent No 7,332,288 & 6,645,731 B2.

Tibbe AGJ, de Grooth BG, Greve J, Dolan GJ, Rao C, and Terstappen LWMM. 2002. Magnetic field design for selecting and aligning immunomagnetic labeled cells. *Cytometry*, **47**(3): 163–172.

van der Pol E, Hoekstra AG, Sturk A, Otto C, van Leeuwen TG, and Nieuwland R. 2010. Optical and non-optical methods for detection and characterization of microparticles and exosomes. *J Thromb Haemostasis*, **8**(12): 2596–2607.

Vona G, et al. 2000. Isolation by size of epithelial tumor cells: A new method for the immunomorphological and molecular characterization of circulating tumor cells. *Am J Pathol*, **156**(1): 57–63.

Yam LT and Janckilla AJ. 1987. Immunocytodiagnosis of carcinocythemia in disseminated breast cancer. *Acta Cytol*, **31**(1): 68–72.

Chapter 13

Evidence Generation for Medical Devices: The Case of Cemented Joint Replacement Surgery in Arthroplasty Registries

Antonis Kontekakis,[a] Mareike Berghaus,[a] Sebastian Gaiser,[b] and Klaus-Dieter Kühn[c]

[a]*Heraeus Medical GmbH,*
Philipp Reis Strasse 8/13, 61273 Wehrheim, Germany
[b]*St Jude Medical, Coordination Center BVBA,*
Da Vincilaan 11, Box 1, 1935 Zaventem, Belgium
[c]*Department of Orthopaedic Surgery, Medical University of Graz,*
Auenbruggerplatz 5, 8036 Graz, Austria
Klaus.kuehn@medunigraz.at

13.1 Evidence-Based Medicine

Evidence-based medicine has had significant influence on the decision of how health care professionals treated patients in the past decade. The idea of evidence-based medicine is to combine individual clinical expertise with results of high quality external research (Sackett et al., 1996; Rosenberg and Donald, 1995), whereby randomized clinical trials are seen as the gold standard for the evaluation of health care interventions (Concate et al., 2000). When it comes to medical

Biofunctional Surface Engineering
Edited by Martin Scholz

ISBN 978-981-4411-60-8 (Hardcover), 978-981-4411-61-5 (eBook)
www.panstanford.com

devices, however, RCTs are often not feasible or would be overly burdensome. Issues like ongoing modifications, user characteristics, learning curve and prolonged follow-up are discussed elsewhere (Sorenson et al., 2011; Drummond et al., 2009). Registries can be one way to generate evidence and overcome the challenges that are predetermined in clinical trials.

We qualitatively assessed the effectiveness of various aspects of cemented arthroplasty to demonstrate that registry data can provide invaluable information in generating evidence for medical devices.

13.2 What Is an Arthroplasty Registry?

Arthroplasty registries (ARs) are prospective cohort studies designed to evaluate the long-term outcomes of total joint arthroplasty (Gorenoi et al., 2009; Gliklich and Dreyer, 2007). They ensure the standardized documentation of all primary and revision operations from defined areas in a central database. All implants are followed up until they are revised or the patient dies or emigrates from the targeted region (Robertsson, 2007; Labek and Böhler, 2005). Many European countries (Swedish Knee Register, 2011; Norwegian Register, 2010; Danish Knee Register, 2010, National Joint Registry, 2012) as well as Australia (Graves et al., 2004) and New Zealand (New Zealand Registry, 2011) have implemented comprehensive and fully working national registries. Besides that, several regional ARs exist, for example in Spain (Catalonia) (Serra-Sutton et al., 2009) or Italy (Emilia Romagna) (R.I.P.O, 2010; Stea et al., 2009). The USA (Smith et al., 2012), Germany (Gorenoi et al., 2009) and Japan (Akiyama et al., 2012) are among the countries that currently set up arthroplasty registries. Some ARs only collect data for specific joints while others include implants for all types of arthroplasties. Most commonly total hip arthroplasty (THA) and total knee arthroplasty (TKA) are included in ARs (Gorenoi et al., 2009). Table 13.1 provides a list of joint replacement registers with country, joint and founding year.

Table 13.1 List of national arthroplasty registries (Berghaus, 2013)

Country	Founding year	Joint	Source
National			
Sweden	1975	Knee	Swedish Knee Register (2011)
Sweden	1979	Hip	Swedish Hip Register (2010)

Country	Founding year	Joint	Source
Finland	1980	Hip, knee, shoulder, elbow, ankle, metacarpophalangeal joint	Puolakka et al. (2001)
Norway	1987	Hip, knee, shoulder, elbow, ankle, metacarpophalangeal joint	Norwegian Register (2010)
Sweden	1993	Ankle	Henricson et al. (2007)
Denmark	1995	Hip	Danish Hip Register (2010)
Scotland	1996	Shoulder	Sharma and Dreghorn (2006)
Denmark	1997	Knee	Danish Knee Register (2010)
Hungary	1998	Hip, knee	Gorenoi et al. (2009)
Sweden	1999	Shoulder, elbow	Rasmussen et al. (2012b)
Australia	1999	Hip, knee, shoulder, elbow, ankle, metacarpophalangeal joint	Australian Joint Replacement Registry (2011)
New Zealand	1999	Hip, knee, shoulder, elbow, ankle, metacarpophalangeal joint	New Zealand Registry (2011)
Romania	2001	Hip, knee	Romanian Register (2012)
Canada	2001	Hip, knee	Canadian Registry (2009)
England & Wales	2003	Hip, knee, ankle	National Joint Registry (2012)
Slovakia	2003	Hip, knee	Necas and Katina (2011)
Denmark	2004	shoulder	Rasmussen et al. (2012a)
France	2006	Hip	SoFCOT Register (2011)
Scotland	2008	Hip, knee	Scottish Arthroplasty Project (2010)
Portugal	2009	Hip, knee, shoulder, elbow, spine, forefoot and foot, hand and wrist	Portuguese Register (2012)

13.3 What Data Are Captured within an Arthroplasty Register?

For an AR focused on long-term outcomes, revision is the most common endpoint. The International Society of Arthroplasty Registries (ISAR) defined a minimum dataset (Table 13.2) for such registries. It includes information on the implanted prostheses, the patient, the performed operation, the hospital and surgeon (Robertsson, 2007). In order to assess long-term results unique patient and surgeon identifiers need to be established. Blinded codes can help avoid conflicts with data protection laws (EAR, 2009).

Table 13.2 The ISAR Minimum Data Set (ISAR 2007)

Data	Collected
Prosthesis	Catalogue number Lot number
Patient	National identity number Full name, age, gender Address Operative hospital patient identifier
Surgery	Date Operation side Diagnosis Primary or Revision Reason for Revision
Hospital	Identity number or name and address
Surgeon	Name or code number

In addition to revision as endpoint, a few large registries recently started to collect patient-reported outcome measures (PROMs) to assess the results of total joint arthroplasty (TJA) (National Joint Registry, 2012; Swedish Hip Register, 2010). PROMs are used to incorporate a more patient centered perspective, as the sole absence of revision does not necessarily indicate a satisfying result. Patients may be, for example, reluctant to additional surgery or too ill to undergo revision despite an unsatisfying outcome of primary arthroplasty (Goodfellow et al., 2010; Söderman et al., 2000; Labek et al., 2011). Common patient-reported outcomes in TJA are functional status (e.g., Oxford hip and knee score) (Dawson et al., 1996; Dawson et al., 1998), experienced pain (e.g., visual pain scales) (Downie et al., 1978) or health related quality of life (e.g., EQ-5D) (EuroQol Group, 1990). The patient interviews to obtain the required information are conducted before and at predefined times after surgery. The Swedish Hip Arthroplasty Register for example, uses the EQ-5D index as health related quality of life measure as well as visual analogue scales for pain and patients satisfaction and the Charnley class categorization (Rolfson et al., 2011). The National Joint Registry (NJR) for England and Wales also uses, among others, the EQ-5D (Baker et al., 2012).

13.4 Methods

In order to evaluate the results of arthroplasty registries on the comparative effectiveness of cemented fixation, antibiotic-loaded bone cement (ALBC) and different types and brands of cement, we searched the databases Medline, Embase, and the Cochrane Library. The search terms "cement," "uncemented," and "cementless," were combined with "knee arthroplasty," "hip arthroplasty," "antibiotic," "type," and "brand." In addition the recent reports of the national joint registries published in English were identified by searching Google for "arthroplasty registry" and "joint replacement registry." Subsequently, those reports were screened for evaluations on the outcome of cemented TJA. All publications, which were not based on the data of national arthroplasty registries or did not contain comparative evaluations, were excluded. It should be noted that the evidence presented below can only be one aspect in the choice of how to treat a specific patient. This decision must always be made by the surgeon and the patient based on the circumstances of each case.

13.5 Cemented Total Knee Arthroplasty in Arthroplasty Registries

The National Joint Registry of England and Wales (NJR) reported data with a follow-up of 8 years on 448,925 knees. The lowest revision rates were identified in cemented TKA with 2.82%, followed by hybrid knees with 2.95%, and uncemented implants with 3.69% (Fig. 13.1) (National Joint Registry, 2011). In Sweden, the use of uncemented and hybrid prostheses for knee arthroplasty was nearly completely stopped after the registry revealed inferior results of those systems. For the period of 1985 to 1994, when the use of cementless implants was still common, the registry found a 1.5 times higher risk of revision (Swedish Knee Register, 2011). The national arthroplasty registry of New Zealand also showed that cemented TKA has the lowest failure rate. The revision rate per 100 component years was 0.55 for fully cemented implants, compared to 0.82 for uncemented and 0.65 for hybrid fixation (New Zealand Registry, 2011). The Australian registry however could not find any differences in survival between the fixation techniques (Australian Joint Replacement Registry, 2011).

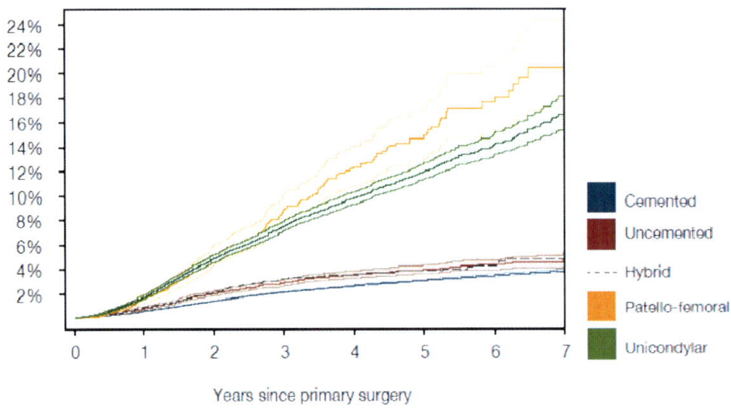

Figure 13.1 Risk of revision following primary knee replacement by prosthesis type (cumulative hazard with 95% confidence interval) (National Joint Registry 2011).

One published study based on data of the Danish Knee Arthroplasty Registry observed uncemented implants to have a higher risk for revision (RR = 1.48) compared to cemented knees, whereas hybrid prostheses showed a lower risk for revision (RR = 0.84). Furnes et al. published another study on information collected by the Norwegian registry. They did not find any differences in revision rates between cemented, uncemented and hybrid fixation. It should be noted, though, that their evaluation of uncemented and hybrid knees was based on small numbers (Furnes et al., 2002). The main reason for the often reported higher risk of revision in uncemented systems seems to be the inferior results of the tibia component (Pedersen et al., 2012). This can be explained by the tendency of uncemented tibia components to migrate during the first 3–12 months after surgery. In consequence, the risk of early aseptic loosening seems to be increased (Bohm et al., 2012a).

Registry data indicate that cementing both components is the gold standard for TKA and leads to a superior survival rate of implants.

13.6 Cemented Total Hip Arthroplasty in Arthroplasty Registries

The largest registry in the world, the NJR, evaluated the survival of 414,985 hips with a follow-up of 8 years. The lowest revision rate, 2.29%, was identified for cemented hips, compared to 2.95% for hybrid hips and 5.10% for uncemented prostheses (National Joint Registry, 2012). The Australian registry revealed slightly different results. The best survival at a follow-up of 10 years were observed with hybrid fixation (94.7%), followed by cemented (93.8%) and cementless (93.2%) anchoring of the implants. These results varied in different age groups. Cemented and hybrid fixation lead to the lowest revision rates in patients over 75 years. In lower age bands cementless and hybrid fixation performed better (Australian Joint Replacement Registry, 2011).

Several research articles from the Norwegian and Swedish Arthroplasty Registry, based on data collected before 2000, found significantly lower revision rates in cemented THA (Havelin et al., 1995a; Havelin et al., 2000; Furnes et al., 2001; Malchau et al., 2002; Herberts and Malchau, 2000). A more recent publication by Hailer et al., analyzing arthroplasties from 1992 to 2007, also found the revision-free 10-year survival of cemented THA was superior to that of cementless hip arthroplasty (85% vs. 94%). Cemented implants performed better over all age groups and all indications. It should be noted that this difference was not significant any more when only the 5 most common cementless systems were considered in the analysis. Evaluation of the single components revealed that the higher revision rates of uncemented systems seemed to be related to inferior results of cementless cups. Uncemented stems however may perform slightly better than cemented ones (Hailer et al., 2010). Another evaluation of Swedish data, published in the latest annual report of the registry, could not detect any clear differences in outcome between both fixation methods. Evaluation of components and age groups revealed a 2.5 times higher risk of revision for cemented stems in men below 50 years. Men and women above 70 years, on the other hand, had a substantially lower risk for revision (0.39 for men and 0.23 for women) when cement was used for anchoring the stem. Cemented cups performed significantly better than cementless acetabular components. The authors noted, though, that comparability of both groups is limited due to demographic differences (Swedish Hip Register, 2010).

Hooper et al. assessed the outcome of different fixation techniques with New Zealand registry data from the period of 1999 to 2006. They found that cemented THAs had an overall lower revision rate per 100 component years (0.49) than uncemented (0.84) and hybrid (0.66) hips. Their work confirms the findings in Swedish evaluation regarding the varying results among different age groups. In patients older than 65 years, cemented fixation showed a significantly lower rate of revision than cementless and hybrid anchoring. In patients below 55 years cementless implants showed better results (Hooper et al., 2009). The recent report of the New Zealand Joint Replacement Registry denoted similar outcomes. Cementless hips had a significantly higher revision rate than cemented implants, except in the age band under 55 years. Cemented prostheses performed best in patients above 75 years. The lowest revision rate in the general population was achieved with hybrid fixation (New Zealand Registry, 2011).

Two evaluations of Finnish registry data performed by Eskelinen et al. and Mäkelä et al. found uncemented stems to have a better long-term survival in patients with osteoarthritis below 55 years of age (Eskelinen et al., 2005; Mäkelä et al., 2011). When survival of both components was considered, cemented and uncemented fixation methods had again similar revision rates. This outcome was related to the unsatisfying results of uncemented cups (Eskelinen et al., 2006; Mäkelä et al., 2011; Eskelinen et al., 2005). Older uncemented systems, implanted in the period from 1987–1996, showed overall inferior results than the cemented reference group (Mäkelä et al., 2011). Another study from Finland evaluated primary total hip arthroplasty for patients with primary osteoarthritis older than 55 years. The overall survival of the cemented reference system was higher than its cementless comparators, again due to problems with uncemented cup designs (Mäkelä et al., 2008). Ongino et al. evaluated the revision rates in patient of 80 years and older based on Finnish registry data. The different anchoring techniques showed fairly similar results. The risk of revision for cemented stems however was 0.4 compared to cementless ones (Ogino et al., 2008).

Revisions in cemented and uncemented implants generally tend to occur at different stages after surgery and also vary regarding their cause. Early revision appears to be more common in uncemented systems (Australian Joint Replacement Registry, 2011). The main reason for this effect seems to be an increased risk of periprosthetic fracture with uncemented stems and osteolysis in the first period after surgery (Hailer et al., 2010; National Joint Registry, 2012). After the ingrowth of the bone, some of the uncemented hip systems achieve comparable or even better results than cemented implants (Hooper et al., 2009; Australian Registry, 2011, Hailer et al., 2010). This pattern seems to confirm the general believe that cement leads to better stability immediately after surgery. Uncemented implants on the other hand are more susceptible to failure in the initial stage but provide well long-term fixation after integration into the host bone (Willert and Buchhorn, 1999).

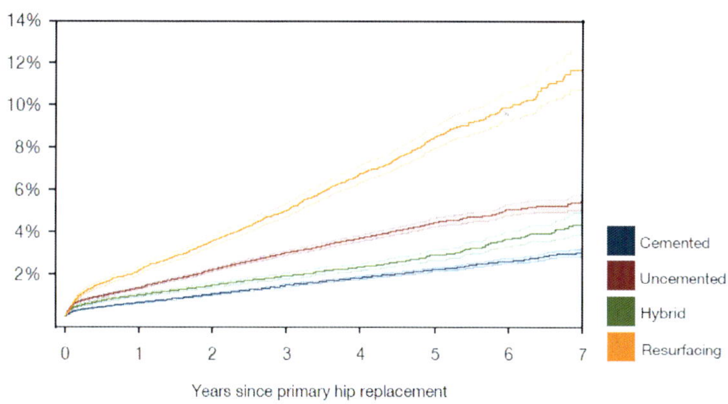

Figure 13.2 Risk of revision following primary hip replacement surgery by prosthesis type (cumulative hazard with 95% CI) (National Joint Registry 2011).

Arthroplasty registries suggest that cemented fixation has comparable or even better results in all age groups, except the band below 55 years. Cementing should always be considered an option in older patients. Especially people above 75 seem to profit highly from anchoring the implants with bone cement. Several registries indicate that the increased rate of failure of some uncemented implants is often related to the acetabular components.

13.7 Economic Remark

Despite the similar or even better outcomes of cemented THA in most cases there is clear trend towards uncemented fixation across all age groups in the majority of countries. This trend was referred to as the "cement paradox" (Kjaersgaard-Andersen, 2011). The development towards more uncemented fixation is particularly surprising as cemented implants are significantly less costly than uncemented prosthesis. The difference easily sums up to several hundred Euros per procedure (Griffiths et al., 2012; Unnanuntana, 2009).

Table 13.3 Exemplary calculation for a UK hospital

Implant costs cemented THA	Implant costs uncemented THA
Stem: £680	Stem: £915
Cup: £285	Cup: £511
Cement, mixing, lavage: £140	Liner: £150
Total (cemented): approx. £1.105	**Total (uncemented): approx. £1.576**

Source: Adapted from Griffiths et al. 2012.

13.8 Antibiotic-Loaded Bone Cement in Arthroplasty Registries

13.8.1 Hip

Antibiotics are commonly added to cement to prevent the occurrence of periprosthetic infections (Joseph et al., 2003; Buchholz et al., 1984; Parvizi et al., 2008). Espehaug et al. analyzed Norwegian Arthroplasty Registry data, in the period from 1987 to 1995, on about 11,000 THAs regarding the effectiveness of antibiotic prophylaxis in total hip arthroplasty. They found the lowest rate of septic revisions in patients who received a combination of systemic antibiotics and

ALBC. If the same systemic protocol was administered with plain cement, a 4.3 times increased risk for septic revision was observed. Moreover a reduction in the rate of aseptic revisions was found when ALBC was used instead of plain cement (Espehaug et al., 1997). These results were confirmed by a more recent evaluation from 2003, which was also based on Norwegian registry data. The authors identified a 1.4 times increased revision rate for all reasons in the group who received only systemic antibiotic prophylaxis compared to the combined regime. The risks for septic and aseptic revision were increased by 1.8 and 1.3 respectively (Engesaeter et al., 2003). Earlier research from Norway analyzing the effectiveness of ALBC in combination with the Charnley prosthesis could confirm the positive effect on revision rate (Havelin et al., 1995b). The effect of antibiotic-loaded bone cement on aseptic revision seems to be related to low-grade infections that are not adequately diagnosed (Moojen et al., 2010; Maathuis et al., 2005).

Persson et al. analyzed the incidence of deep infection in 148,359 THAs, with a follow-up of 5 years, collected by the Swedish registry. They found a reduction of the infection rate with ALBC independent from other measures, like ultra clean environment or systemic antibiotics. Depending on the prophylactic methods applied simultaneously, in some cases the decrease of deep sepsis was over 50% (Persson et al., 1999). It should be noted that recently a trend towards higher rates of infection was observed in THA. Registry data indicate that this development is particularly pronounced in uncemented hip arthroplasty. Antibiotic-loaded bone cement can be one answer to this thread, as registry data prove its effectiveness in preventing deep sepsis.

13.8.2 Knee

Namba et al. analyzed the infection rates in 22.880 primary knee arthroplasties. 8.9% of the total knee arthroplasties were performed with ALBC. They identified lower survival rates in the group treated with antibiotic cement. However, the authors did not adjusted for any risk factors and the outcome may therefore be heavily biased. The results of a Canadian registry study also indicate that ALBC did not influence the rate of deep infection. Although there was no reduction in septic revisions, the number of aseptic implant failures was twice as high in the group of TKAs that received plain cement (Bohm et al.,

2012b). In contrast, a large Finnish register study including 43.149 patients found the combination of systemic and local antibiotics leads to the lowest rate of revision for infection. The adjusted hazard ratio for infection was 2.10 when plain cement was used for fixation in total knee arthroplasty (Jämsen et al., 2009).

Despite the conflicting evidence, several authors recommend the routine use of antibiotic cement in total knee arthroplasty as prophylaxis to minimize the danger of periprosthetic infection and its devastating consequences (Srivastav et al., 2009; Dunbar, 2009; O'Connor and MacDonald, 2011). It should be noted that the effect of ALBC measured by registries is a synthesis of the results of different types of cement with various antibiotics. However, some antibiotics may be less effective against the common germs in periprosthetic infection. Furthermore, it needs to be considered that cements differ in their elution rate (Zimmerli et al., 2004; Trampuz and Zimmerli, 2006; Brien et al., 2003; Torrado et al., 2001; Dall et al., 2007). Some bone cements may therefore be better suited than others to prevent infection in TJA.

13.9 Different Types and Brands of Bone Cement in Arthroplasty Registries

Havelin et al. evaluated comparative effectiveness of different types and brands of cement in context of the survival of 8579 Charnley hip prostheses. The authors specified three types of cement: low-viscosity, high viscosity, and Boneloc, which was based on a new formulation and cannot be classified into the prenamed categories. While viscosity had little effect on the survival of the acetabular component, high viscosity cement resulted in significantly lower revision rates of the femoral component. Regarding cement brand, there were again no differences in outcome for the cup. The best result for the fixation of the stem was achieved when Palacos R+G was used (Havelin et al., 1995b) (Table 13.4).

A more recent study by Espehaug et al., based on the information of 17,323 Charnley prostheses also collected by the Norwegian registry, again analyzed the effect of cement brands on outcome in THA. Endpoint was failure due to aseptic loosening either of the acetabular or the femoral component. Statistically significant differences in survival of the implant for different types of cement

Table 13.4 Cumulative survival in regard to cement brand (Havelin et al., 1995b)

Brand	Number of hips	Number of revisions	Cumulative 5.5 years survival	95% Confidence interval
CMW 1	2309	34	97.4	96.3 to 98.4
CMW 3	1193	38	94.1	92.1 to 96.2
Simplex	435	3	98.3	96.2 to 100
Palacos	1037	10	98.0	96.4 to 99.6
Palacos R+G	2775	19	98.7	98.1 to 99.4

were found for both parts, but were more pronounced for the femoral component. The best survival rates of plain cements were observed with Palacos R. The overall best results were achieved when Palacos R+G was used to fixate both parts of the implants (Espehaug et al., 2002).

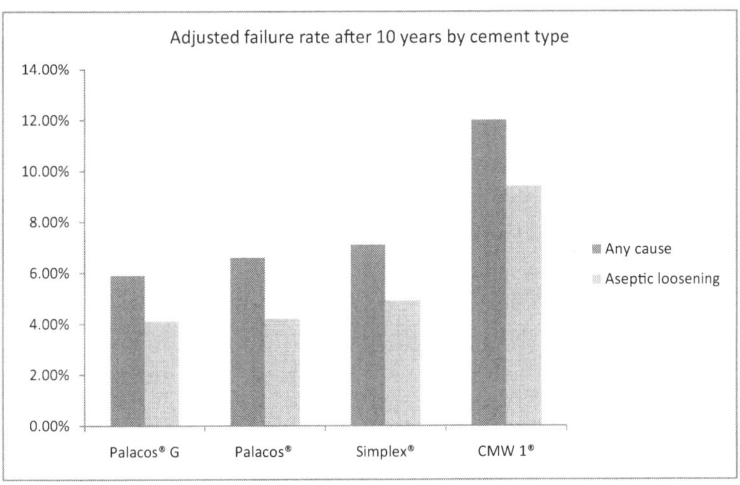

Figure 13.3 Revision rates of different cement brands (based on Espehaug et al. 2002).

Another publication from 2000, based on the Swedish Hip Registry, assessed the risk of revision in regard to cement brand with a multivariate Poisson model. The authors reported revisions for all reasons and aseptic loosening as endpoints. Again, the best result was achieved when Palacos R+G was used for fixation (Malchau et al., 2000).

Several studies indicate there is considerable variation regarding mechanical properties and stability of different cements (Kuehn et al., 2005). Therefore it is surprising so little research regarding the effect of cement on clinical outcome, especially on the results of TKA, was conducted.

Table 13.5 Estimated risk for revision is shown for the different cement brands reported to the register

	Aseptic loosening and arthrosis		All revisions—all diagnoses	
Variable	Risk ratio	95% confidence limits	Risk ratio	95% confidence limits
Palacos	0.53	0.46–0.61	0.51	0.45–0.57
Palacos Gentamycin	0.52	0.46–0.59	0.49	0.44–0.54
Simplex	0.65	0.59–0.72	0.60	0.55–0.66
CMW	0.66	0.52–0.84	0.73	0.56–0.94

Note: The risk ratio for Sulfix® is nominator (Malchau et al. 2000).

13.10 How Do Registry Data Compare to the Information Provided by Clinical Trials?

Registry data provide complementary information to the evidence gathered in clinical trials. Trials are designed to determine causality with respect to outcome. As such, researchers aim to limit the number of confounding factors, in order to minimize a potential bias (Pocock, 1983; Friedman et al., 1998). In trials that are evaluating new endoprostheses the study design determines, among others, patient characteristics, trial site, the surgeons involved as well as the type of prostheses and surgical approach (Graves, 2010). While a careful design grants high internal validity, the same results are not necessarily observed when a technology passes into general use (Horton, 2000). Clinical reality will inevitably vary from the trial setting (Rothwell, 2005). For example patient characteristics may differ and surgeons may be less trained or use different approaches or different combinations of products. The observations in clinical trials are normally limited to a predefined period of time. Resource constraints do not allow increasing the duration of trials indefinitely. Therefore, the follow-up might not always be sufficient to evaluate long-term outcomes (Graves, 2010). Moreover, differences in outcomes between technologies are usually small. For obtaining a statistical significant result in a controlled study, for instance, over 13.000 patients would be required to detect a one percent difference in revision rates between two implants after 10 years in the population (Labek et al., 2011).

Registries on the other hand do not try to establish causality. They are built as ongoing long-term monitoring tools for the outcome of joint arthroplasty. To improve the results of TJA it is not necessary to know exactly why there is a difference (Graves, 2010). It is, however, possible to perform statistical analyses to assess whether and, if so, which factors captured by the AR contribute to a specific outcome. Nevertheless, it should be noted that comparative effectiveness research based on registry data must be interpreted cautiously. Various factors, such as patient characteristics or surgeon experience, may influence the outcome. University hospitals, for example, tend to have worse results because of often more complicated initial cases (Labek et al., 2011). If the factors are known, the outcome can be adjusted for those aspects (Ranstam and Robertsson, 2010). However it can never be excluded that unknown confounding factors could bias the results.

In arthroplasty the comparability of the fixation techniques is often questioned in THA, as different techniques tend to be used in different age groups. Registries try to overcome this challenge with statistical methods like stratification and/or risk adjustment, yet the results need to be interpreted cautiously (Berger et al. 200). Other variables that might influence the outcome, like activity level or certain comorbidities, may not be captured by the registry and not reflected adequately in age (Rosenbaum, 1991). Another source of bias can be the surgeons' experience with a specific technique in certain countries (Hooper et al., 2009) The Scandinavian registries for example might be skewed towards more cemented fixation, Australia towards more uncemented (Swedish Hip Registry, 2010; Norwegian Arthroplasty Register, 2010; Australian Joint Replacement Registry, 2011). In some countries however, like the

UK or New Zealand, all fixation techniques were used fairly common and with at least some overlaps, in most age groups (NJR, 2012; New Zealand Joint Registry, 2011). This allows comparability to at least some extent. Nevertheless, it always needs to be considered that previous research might not reflect the latest developments in implant technique.

13.11 Conclusion

The case of cemented joint replacement surgery demonstrates that arthroplasty registries can be an invaluable tool for generating evidence on medical devices. By implementing registries several countries were able to improve the outcomes of TJA substantially (Herberts and Malchau, 2000; Robertsson et al., 2012) Sweden for example could reduce its revision burden from 18% in 1979 to 6.4% in 2001 (Malchau et al., 2002). Declining revision rates not only benefit the patients but may help to avoid unnecessary costs to health care systems in times of scarce resources (Luo et al., 2012). Recently, researchers compared the outcome of implants in clinical trials and registry datasets. They found significantly lower revision rates in trials, especially when the cases were published by the inventors of an implant. The authors of the study concluded that registry data provide better information to surgeons for making day-to-day decisions in the operating room (Labek et al., 2009). Evidence created by registries can therefore be an important step towards providing the optimal care for patients (Sackett et al., 1996; Rosenberg and Donald, 1995).

References

Akiyama H, Hoshino A, Iida H, Shindo H et al. A pilot project for the Japan Arthroplasty Register. *J Orthop Sci*, 2012, 17: 358–369.

Australian Orthopaedic Association National Joint Replacement Registry, Hip and Knee Arthroplasty. Annual Report 2011.

Baker PN, Petheram T, Jameson SS, Avery PJ, Reed MR, Gregg PJ, Deehan DJ. Comparison of patient-reported outcome measures following total und unicondylar knee replacement. *J Bone Joint Surg Br*, 2012, 94-B: 919–927.

Berger ML, Mamdani M, Atkins D, Johnson ML. Good research practices for comparative effectiveness research: defining, reporting and interpreting nonrandomized studies of treatment effects using secondary data sources: The ISPOR Good Research Practices for Retrospective Database Analysis Task Force Report—Part I, 2009.

Berghaus M. Masterthesis, Funding of Registers using the Example of Arthroplasty Registries, FAU Erlangen-Nürnberg 2013.

Bohm ER, Gu J, Zhu N, et al. The addition of antibiotics to cement does not appear to lower the risk of early revision in knee replacement surgery. Paper #133. Presented at the American Academy of Orthopaedic Surgeons. Annual Meeting. Feb. 7–11. San Francisco, 2012a.

Bohm ER, Slobodian I, Turgeon TR, Petrak M. Cemented vs. uncemented Fixation in Total Knee Arthroplasty. In *Evidence-Based Orthopedics* (Bhandari M, ed), BMJ Books Wiley-Blackwell, 2012b.

Brien WW, Salvati EA, Klein R, Brause B, Stern S. Antibiotic impregnated bone cement in total hip arthroplasty. An in vivo comparison of the elution properties of tobramycin and vancomycin. *Clin Orthop Relat Res* 1993, 296: 242–248.

Buchholz HW, Elson RA, Heinert K. Antibiotic-loaded acrylic cement: current concepts. *Clin Orthop Relat Res* 1984, (190): 96–108.

Canadian Joint Replacement Registry, Hip and Knee Replacements in Canada, 2008–2009 Annual Report, Canadian Institute for Health Information. 2009.

Concato J, Shah N, Horwitz RI. Randomized, controlled trials, observational studies, and the hierarchy of research designs. *N Engl J Med* 2000, 342 (25): 1887–1892.

Dall GF, Simpson PMS, Breusch SJ. In vitro comparison of Refobacin-Palacos R with Refobacin Bone Cement and Palacos R+G. *Acta Orthopaedica*, 2007, 78 (3): 404–411.

Danish Hip Arthroplasty Register. About the registry: www.dhr.dk/About%20registry.htm (17.09.2012).

Danish Knee Arthroplasty Register. Annual Report 2010.

Dawson J, Fitzpatrick R, Carr A, Murray D. Questionnaire on the perceptions of patients about total hip replacement. *Bone Joint Surg Br* 1996, 78-B (2): 185–190.

Dawson J, Fitzpatrick R, Murray D, Carr A. Questionnaire on the perceptions of patients about total knee replacement. *Bone Joint Surg Br* 1998, 80-B (1): 63–69.

Downie WW, Leatham PA, Rhind VM, Wright V, Branco JA, Anderson JA. Studies with pain rating scales. *Ann Rheumatic Dis* 1978, 37: 378–381.

Drummond M, Griffin A, Tarricone R. Economic evaluation for devices and drugs—same or different? *Value Health* 2009, 12 (4): 402–404.

Dunbar MJ. Antibiotic bone cements: Their use in routine primary total joint arthroplasty is justified. *Orthopedics*, 2009, 32(9).

EAR European Arthroplasty Register: Handbook for the development and operation of an outcome register for medical devices, published at the EFFORT Congress 2009 by Gerold Labek on the behalf of the European Arthroplasty Register, 2009.

Engesaeter LB, Espehaug B, Lie SA, Furnes O, Havelin LI. Does cement increase the risk of infection in primary total hip arthroplasty? Revision rates in 56,275 cemented and uncemented primary THAs followed for 0–16 years in the Norwegian Arthroplasty Register. *Acta Orthop* 2006, 77(3): 351–358.

Engesaeter LB, Lie SA, Espehaug B, Furnes O, Vollset SE, Havelin LI. Antibiotic prophylaxis in total hip arthroplasty: effects of antibiotic prophylaxis systemically and in bone cement on the revision rate of 22,170 primary hip replacements followed 0–14 years in the Norwegian Arthroplasty Register. *Acta Orthop Scand* 2003, 74(6): 644–651.

Eskelinen A, Remes V, Helenius I, Pulkkinen P, Nevalainen J, Paavolainen P. Total hip arthroplasty for primary osteoarthrosis in younger patients in the Finnish arthroplasty register. 4,661 primary replacements followed for 0–22 years. *Acta Orthop* 2005, 76(1): 28–41.

Eskelinen A, Remes V, Helenius I, Pulkkinen P, Nevalainen J, Paavolainen P. Uncemented total hip arthroplasty for primary osteoarthritis in young patients: a mid-to long-term follow-up study from the Finnish Arthroplasty Register. *Acta Orthop* 2006, 77(1): 57–70.

Espehaug B, Engesaeter LB, Vollset SE, Havelin LI, Langeland N. Antibiotic prophylaxis in total hip arthroplasty. Review of 10,905 primary cemented total hip replacements reported to the Norwegian Arthroplasty Register, 1987 to 1995. *J Bone Joint Surg Br* 1997, 79(4): 590–595.

Espehaug B, Furnes O, Havelin LI, Engesaeter LB, Vollset SE. The type of cement and failure of total hip replacements. *J Bone Joint Surg Br* 2002, 84(6): 832–838.

EuroQol Group, The. EuroQol: A new facility for the measurement of health-related quality of life. *Health Policy* 1990, 16: 199–208.

Friedman LM, Furberg CD, DeMets DL. *Fundamentals of Clinical Trials.* 3rd ed. New York: Springer 1998.

Furnes O, Espehaug B, Lie SA, Vollset SE, Engesaeter LB, Havelin LI. Early failures among 7,174 primary total knee replacements: a follow-up study from the Norwegian Arthroplasty Register 1994–2000. *Acta Orthop Scand* 2002, 73(2): 117–129.

Furnes O, Lie SA, Espehaug B, Vollset SE, Engesaeter LB, Havelin LI. Hip disease and the prognosis of total hip replacements. A review of 53,698 primary total hip replacements reported to the Norwegian Arthroplasty Register 1987–99. *J Bone Joint Surg Br* 2001, 83(4): 579–586.

Gliklich RE, Dreyer NA, eds. Registries for Evaluating Patient Outcomes: A User's Guide (Prepared by Outcome DEcIDE Center [Outcome Sciences, Inc. dba Outcome] under Contract No. HHSA29020050035ITO1.) AHRQ Publication No. 07-EHCoo1-1. Rockville, MD: Agency for Healthcare Research and Quality. April 2007.

Gorenoi V, Schönermark MP, Hagen A. Gelenkendoprothesenregister für Deutschland, HTA-Bericht 92: Schriftenreihe Health Technology Assessment (HTA) in der Bundesrepublik Deutschland, DIMDI 2009.

Gorenoi V, Schönermark MP, Hagen A. Arthroplasty Register for Germany; HTA-Kurzfassung; GMS Health Technology Assessment 2009, vol. 5.

Goodfellow JW, O'Connor JJ, Murray DW. A critique of revision rate as an outcome measure. *J Bone Joint Surg Br* 2010, 92-B: 1628–1631.

Graves SE, Davidson D, Ingerson L, Ryan P, Griffith EC, McDermott BFJ, McElroy HJ, Pratt NL. The Australian Orthopaedic Association National Joint Replacement Registry, *MJA* 2004, 180: S31–S34.

Graves SE. The value of arthroplasty registry data. *Acta Orthop* 2010, 81(1): 8–9.

Griffiths EJ, Stevenson D, Porteous MJ. Cost savings of using a cemented total hip replacement: An analysis of the National Joint Registry data. *J Bone Joint Surg Br* 2012, 94(8): 1032–1035.

Hailer NP, Garellick G, Kärrholm J. Uncemented and cemented primary total hip arthroplasty in the Swedish Hip Arthroplasty Register. *Acta Orthop* 2010, 81(1): 34–41.

Havelin LI, Engesaeter LB, Espehaug B, Furnes O, Lie SA, Vollset SE. The Norwegian Arthroplasty Register: 11 years and 73,000 arthroplasties. *Acta Orthop Scand* 2000, 71(4): 337–353.

Havelin LI, Espehaug B, Vollset SE, Engesaeter LB. Early aseptic loosening of uncemented femoral components in primary total hip replacement. A review based on the Norwegian Arthroplasty Register. *J Bone Joint Surg Br* 1995a, 77(1): 11–17.

Havelin L I, Engesaeter L B, Espehaug B, Vollset S E. The effect of cement type on early revision of 8,579 primary Charnley prostheses. The Norwegian Arthroplasty Register. *J Bone Joint Surg Am* 1995b, 77(10): 1543–1550.

Henricson A, Skoog A, Carlsson A. The Swedish Ankle Arthroplasty Register: An analysis of 531 arthroplasties between 1993 and 2005. *Acta Orthop* 2007, 78 (5): 569–574.

Herberts P, Malchau H. Long-term registration has improved the quality of hip replacement: A review of the Swedish THR Register comparing 160,000 cases. *Acta Orthop Scand* 2000, 71 (2): 111–121.

Hooper GJ, Rothwell AG, Stringer M, Frampton C. Revision following cemented and uncemented primary total hip replacement: A seven-year analysis from the New Zealand Joint Registry. *J Bone Joint Surg Br* 2009, 91(4): 451–458.

Horton R. Common sense and figures: The rhetoric of validity in medicine (Bradford Hill Memorial Lecture 1999). *Stat Med* 2000, 19(23): 3149–3164.

International Society of Arthroplasty Registries, Mission, aims and objectives; February 2007 http://www.isarhome.org/statements (20.09.2012).

Jämsen E, Huhtala H, Puolakka T, Moilanen T. Risk factors for infection after knee arthroplasty. A register-based analysis of 43,149 cases. *J Bone Joint Surg Am* 2009, 91(1): 38–47.

Joseph TN, Chen AL, Di Cesare PE. Use of antibiotic-impregnated cement in total joint arthroplasty, *J Am Acad Orthop Surg* 2003, 11 (1): 38–47.

Kjærsgaard-Andersen P. What is wrong with the cemented total hip? *Orthop Today Eur* 2011, 14 (1).

Kuehn KD, Ege W, Gopp U. Acrylic bone cements: Composition and properties. *Orthop Clin North Am* 2005, 36(1): 17–28.

Labek G, Frischhut S, Heubl M, et al. Selection and publication bias in orthopaedic literature. Paper #F473. Presented at the 10th EFORT Congress. June 3–6, 2009. Vienna.

Labek G, Böhler N. Endoprothesenregister: Organisation, Ergebnisse und Limits. *Fortbildung Orthopädie, Traumatologie* 2005, 11 (7), 156–165.

Labek G, Janda W, Agreiter M, Schuh R, Böhler N. Organisation, data evaluation, interpretation and effect of arthroplasty register data on the outcome in terms of revision rate in total hip arthroplasty. *International Orthopaedics* (SICOT) 2011, 35, 157–163.

Labek G, Thaler M, Janda W, Agreiter M, Stöckl B. Revision rates after total joint replacement: Cumulative results from worldwide joint register datasets. *J Bone Joint Surg Br* 2011, 93(3): 293–297.

Luo R, Brekke A, Noble PC. The financial impact of joint registries in identifying poorly performing implants. *J Arthroplasty* 2012, 27 (8 Suppl): 66–71.

Maathuis PG, Neut D, Busscher HJ, van der Mei HC, van Horn JR. Perioperative contamination in primary total hip arthroplasty. *Clin Orthop Relat Res* 2005, 433: 136–139.

Mäkelä K, Eskelinen A, Pulkkinen P, Paavolainen P, Remes V. Cemented total hip replacement for primary osteoarthritis in patients aged 55 years or older: Results of the 12 most common cemented implants followed for 25 years in the Finnish Arthroplasty Register. *J Bone Joint Surg Br* 2008, 90(12): 1562–1569.

Mäkelä KT, Eskelinen E, Pulkkinen P, Paavolainen P, Remes V. Results of 3,668 primary total hip replacements for primary osteoarthritis in patients under the age of 55 years. *Acta Orthop* 2011, 82(5): 521–529.

Malchau H, Herberts P, Eisler T, Garellick G, Söderman P. The Swedish Total Hip Replacement Register. *J Bone Joint Surg* 2002, 84-A, Suppl 2.

Malchau H, Herberts P, Söderman P, Odén A. Update and validation of results from the Swedish National Hip Arthroplasty Register 1979–1998. Presented at the 67th Annual Meeting of the American Academy of Orthopaedic Surgeons, March 15–19, 2000, Orlando, USA.

Moojen DJ, van Hellemondt G, Vogely HC, Burger BJ, Walenkamp GH, Tulp NJ, Schreurs BW, de Meulemeester FR, Schot CS, van de Pol I, Fujishiro T, Schouls LM, Bauer TW, Dhert WJ. Incidence of low-grade infection in aseptic loosening of total hip arthroplasty. *Acta Orthop* 2010, 81(6): 667–673.

National Joint Registry for England and Wales, 8th Annual report 2011.

National Joint Registry for England and Wales, 9th Annual Report 2012.

Necas L, Katina S. Slovakian Arthroplasty Register: Review of the annual report of the Slovakian Arthroplasty Register 2010. *Acta Chir Orthop Traum Cech* 2011, 78.

New Zealand Orthopaedic Association. The New Zealand Joint Registry: Twelve year report, January 1999 to December 2010.

Norwegian Arthroplasty Register. Annual Report June 2010.

O'Connor PA, MacDonald SJ. Antibiotic Cement in Total Knee Arthroplasty. In *Evidence-Based Orthopedics* (Bhandari M, ed), BMJ Books Wiley-Blackwell, 2012.

Ogino D, Kawaji H, Konttinen L, Lehto M, Rantanen P, Malmivaara A, Konttinen YT, Salo J. Total hip replacement in patients eighty years of age and older. *J Bone Joint Surg Am* 2008, 90(9): 1884–1890.

Parvizi J, Saleh KJ, Ragland PS, Pour AE, Mont MA. Efficacy of antibiotic-impregnated cement in total hip replacement. *Acta Orthop* 2008, 79 (3): 335–342.

Pedersen AB, Mehnert F, Odgaard A, Schrøder HM. Existing data sources for clinical epidemiology: The Danish Knee Arthroplasty Register. *Clin Epidemiol* 2012, 4: 125–135. Epub 2012 May 7.

Persson U, Persson M, Malchau H. The economics of preventing revisions in total hip replacement. *Acta Orthop Scand* 1999, 70(2): 163–169.

Pocock SJ. *Clinical Trials: A Practical Approach*. Chichester: John Wiley, 1983.

Portuguese Arthroplasty Register. www.rpa.spot.pt (17.09.2012).

Puolakka TJS, Pajamäki KJJ, Halonen PJ, Pulkkinen PO et al. The Finnish Arthroplasty Register: Report of the hip register. *Acta Orthop Scand* 2001, 72 (5): 433–441.

Ranstam J, Robertsson O. Statistical analysis of arthroplasty register data. *Acta Orthop* 2010, 81(1): 10–14.

Rasmussen JV, Jakobsen J, Brorson S, Olsen BS: The Danish Shoulder Arthroplasty Registry: Clinical outcome and short-term survival of 2,137 primary shoulder replacements. *Acta Orthopaedica* 2012, 83 (2): 171–173.

Rasmussen JV, Olsen BS, Fevang BTS, Furnes O, Skytta ET, et al. A review of national shoulder and elbow joint replacement registries. *J Shoulder Elbow Surg* 2012, 1–8.

Robertsson O: Knee arthroplasty registers. *J Bone Joint Surg Br* 2007, 89-B: 1–4.

Robertsson O, Bizjajeva S, Fenstadt AM, Furnes O, Lidgren L, et al. Knee arthroplasty in Denmark, Norway and Sweden: A pilot study from the Nordic Arthroplasty Register Association. *Acta Orthopaedica* 2010, 81 (1): 82–89.

Rolfson O, Kärrholm J, Dahlberg LE, Garellick G. Patient-reported outcomes in the Swedish Hip Arthroplasty Register: Result of a nationwide prospective observational study. *J Bone Joint Surg Br* 2011, 93-B: 867–875.

Romanian Arthroplasty Register. About RAR, www.rne.ro/?lang=en (17.09.2012).

Rosenbaum PR. Discussing hidden bias in observational studies. *Ann Intern Med* 1991, 115(11): 901–905.

Rosenberg W, Donald A. Evidence based medicine: An approach to clinical problem-solving *BMJ* 1995, 310: 1122–1126.

Rothwell PM. External validity of randomised controlled trials: "to whom do the results of this trial apply?". *Lancet* 2005, 365(9453): 82–93.

Sackett DL, Rosenberg WM, Gray JA, Haynes RB, Richardson WS. Evidence based medicine: What it is and what it isn't. *BMJ* 1996, 312: 71–72.

Scottish Arthroplasty Project Annual Report 2010: A summary of arthroplasty procedures and their outcomes for patients operated on during 2009, 2010.

Serra-Sutton V, Allepuz A, Espallargues M: Arthroplasty registers: A review of international experiences. *Int J Technol Asses Health Care* 2009, 25: 1, 63–72.

Sharma S, Dreghorn CR: registry of shoulder arthroplasty: The Scottish experience. *Ann R Coll Surg Engl* 2006, 88: 122–126.

Smith AJ, Dieppe P, Vernon K, Porter M, Blom AW: Failure rates of stemmed metal-no-metal hip replacements: Analysis of data from the National Joint Registry of England and Wales. *Lancet* 2012, 379: 1199–1204.

Söderman P, Malchau H, Herberts P. Outcome after total hip arthroplasty—Part I. General health evaluation in relation to definition of failure in the Swedish National Total Hip Arthroplasty Register. *Acta Orthop Scand* 2000, 71 (4): 354–359.

SoFCOT Total Hip Arthroplasty Register. Annual Report 2011.

Sorenson C, Tarricone R, Siebert M, Drummmond M. Applying health economics for policy decision making: Do devices differ from drugs? *Europace* 2011, 13, ii54–ii58.

Srivastav AK, Nadkarni B, Srivastav S, Mittal V, Agarwal S. Prophylactic use of antibiotic-loaded bone cement in primary total knee arthroplasty: Justified or not? *Indian J Orthop* 2009, 43(3): 259–263.

Stea S, Bordini B, De Clerico M, Petropulacos K, Toni A. First hip arthroplasty register in Italy: 55,000 cases and 7 year follow-up, *Int Orthop* (SICOT) 2009, 33: 339–346.

Swedish Hip Arthroplasty Register. Annual Report 2010.

Swedish Knee Arthroplasty Register. Annual Report 2011.

Torrado S, Frutos P, Frutos G. Gentamicin bone cements: Characterization and release (in vitro and in vivo assays). *Int J Pharm* 2001, 217 (1–2): 57–69.

Trampuz A, Zimmerli W. Antimicrobial agents in orthopaedic surgery: Prophylaxis and treatment. *Drugs* 2006, 66 (8): 1089–1105.

Unnanuntana A, Dimitroulias A, Bolognesi MP, Hwang KL, et al. Cementless femoral prostheses cost more to implant than cemented femoral prostheses. *Clin Orthop Relat Res* 2009, 467 (6): 1546–1551.

Willert H G, Buchhorn G H. Osseointegration of cemented and noncemented implants in artificial hip replacement: long-term findings in man. *J Long Term Eff Med Implants* 1999, 9: 113–130.

Zimmerli W, Trampuz A, Ochsner PE. Prosthetic-joint infections. *N Engl J Med* 2004, 351 (16): 1645–1654.

Index

acquired resistance 142, 144, 146
active ingredients 131, 134, 138, 142, 149–51, 157, 159–60, 171–73, 175–76, 254
active spectrum 138–39
adhered bacteria 99, 102
adhering microorganisms 83, 85, 87, 89, 91
adhesion 28–29, 31, 37, 45, 62, 64, 68, 74, 79, 92, 97–99, 110–12, 114–18, 133, 160
adsorbed proteins 208
advanced wound care 252, 254, 256, 258, 262–64
ALBC *see* antibiotic-loaded bone cement
alcohols 136, 139
amino acids 23, 53, 192–93, 204
AMPs *see* antimicrobial peptides
angiogenesis 214, 219, 252, 2 55–57, 264, 268
anti-infective coatings 86, 130, 185
antiadhesive properties 86–87
antibacterial coatings 89, 92, 120
antibacterial effect 38, 42, 88, 90, 114
antibiotic cement 301–2
antibiotic-loaded bone cement (ALBC) 130, 184, 295, 300–2, 313
antibiotic-loaded bone cements 130, 184, 295, 301
antibiotic release 92, 152, 156, 167, 184
antibiotics 37–38, 81–83, 89–90, 122, 124, 140–45, 149–52, 155–56, 159–60, 164, 170, 172–73, 181–84, 302, 307–8
  soluble 155–56
antibodies 18, 20, 23, 49–50, 119, 195, 203, 207, 209–10, 234–36, 242, 244, 249, 281–82, 284–86
antifouling concepts 83–84, 89, 92
antigen/autoantibody Interactions 241–43
antigen microarrays 245–46, 248
antigenicity 21–22, 230
antigens 21, 225, 227, 230, 235, 239–40, 243–46, 270–71, 277, 281–82
antimicrobial activity 37–39, 83, 91, 93
antimicrobial agents 89, 103–4, 124, 130, 136, 158, 164, 169, 313
antimicrobial coatings 67, 129–30, 163–64
antimicrobial implant coating 121–22, 124, 126, 128, 130, 132, 134, 136, 138, 140, 142, 144, 146, 148, 184
antimicrobial peptides (AMPs) 37, 83, 91, 120
antimicrobial protection of biomaterials 147
antiseptics 136, 138–39, 155, 172, 185, 188

aptamers 207–12, 214, 216–20, 222
ARs *see* arthroplasty registries
arthroplasty registries (ARs) 291–92, 294–95, 297, 299–303, 306–7, 310
aseptic revision 179, 301
autoantibodies 233–38, 240, 242–48
autoantigens 235, 238, 240, 243
autoimmune diseases 233–34, 236–37, 243, 246
autoimmune profile 242–45
autologous endothelial cells 214

bacteria 28, 37–39, 76, 79–81, 84–85, 87, 89–91, 102–4, 115, 133–34, 137–38, 140–41, 143–48, 162–63, 255
  dead 102–3
  living 102–3
bacteria cells 143
bacterial adhesion 37, 73–74, 76, 84–88, 90, 92, 102, 105, 109, 111, 122
bacterial biofilms 96, 104, 136
bacterial contamination 22, 121, 123, 214, 254
bacterial growth 172–73
bacterial load 252, 254
bacterial load reduction 254
bacterial monocultures 98
bacterial strains 38, 81, 99, 102, 107
bead-based protein microarrays 239–40
beta-lactam antibiotics 144–45
biocompatibility 6, 50, 73, 101, 192, 208–9
biofilm colonizers 81
biofilm communities 77–78, 81
biofilm formation 38, 71–73, 76–82, 84, 86, 92–94, 96–99, 102–5, 107–9, 113, 116–18, 121, 133, 180, 183–84
biofilm-formative bacteria 183
biofilm growth 79, 97, 106
biofilm investigations 96, 98
biofilm matrix 77, 91, 109, 111
biofilm models 96, 98
biofilm propagation 96–97
biofilm research 77
biofilm testing 93, 95, 97, 99
biofilms 39, 71–72, 76–84, 90–92, 96–100, 102–4, 106–8, 110–16, 118, 130–31, 133–36, 144–46, 179–81, 183–84, 186–87
  stable matured 78
biofouling 77, 85, 109, 112–13, 115, 117–19
biofunctional medical devices 191, 202
biofunctionalized wound dressings for advanced wound care 252, 254, 256, 258, 262, 264
biologic-device combination products 19, 192, 199, 202, 252
biological environment 73, 75, 86
biological products 1–2
biological response 73, 75, 86, 93
biological tissues 48–49, 51, 62
biomarkers 218, 233–35, 238–39, 241, 244, 246, 248–49
biomaterial-associated infections 94, 104
biomaterial coatings 176–77
biomaterial surfaces 72, 75, 84, 86–87, 92–93, 96, 101, 103, 111, 119, 122, 130, 148, 208

biomaterials 33, 35, 41–45, 48–49, 51, 53, 62–64, 66, 71–73, 96–97, 111, 113–19, 147, 203, 219–20
biomedical applications 28, 36, 48–49, 51, 57, 90, 103
biomolecules 11–17, 19–22, 48, 191–92, 203, 262
  immobilized 8, 12, 14, 191, 193, 202
biotinylated beads 282, 284
blood cells 72, 211–12, 215, 220, 277
blood stream 143, 148, 214, 217–18, 268
bone 131–32, 150, 160, 162, 185, 187, 299, 309–10
bone cement 124, 151–52, 166–68, 181, 184, 188, 300, 302–3, 307–8
bovine serum albumin (BSA) 278, 281–83
breast cancer 24, 244, 247, 286–87
BSA *see* bovine serum albumin

calcium phosphate layers 159
cancer 140, 233, 239, 244–45, 247, 249, 268, 284, 286–89
cancer cells 285, 289
carcinoma cells 288
catheter-associated urinary tract infections (CAUTIs) 104, 110, 119
catheter-related infections 104, 106, 111
CAUTIs *see* Catheter-associated urinary tract infections
cell adhesion 28, 39, 48, 67, 88–89, 118, 242
cellular uptake 34, 36
cemented implants 296–300
central nervous system (CNS) 139, 243
chemotherapeutics 139–40
chitosan 32, 37, 42, 53, 59, 88, 114, 157
chloramphenicol 140, 142
chlorhexidine 89–90, 113, 115, 130, 138, 172
chronic wounds 251, 253, 256–57
circulating tumor cells (CTCs) 8, 267–73, 275–80, 282, 284–89
CNS *see* central nervous system
combi products 3–5
combination devices 11, 14, 205
corneal epithelial cells 31
CTCs *see* circulating tumor cells
cytokeratin 270–71, 284
cytokines 19, 235, 255–57, 262

defibrillators 125, 158, 174–75
degradation products 16, 18, 157, 160
delayed infections 170
delayed wound healing 251–53, 257, 263
dendritic cells 223–24, 235
dental biomaterials 100, 103
dermal fibroblasts 256–57, 262
desthiobiotin 278–79
diabetes 136, 244, 247, 251, 265
diagnostic markers 235–38, 289
dip coating 56, 162, 165, 172, 225
drug products 13, 15–16, 24

EGFP *see* enhanced green fluorescent protein
electrostatic interactions 52, 54, 66, 74–75, 85
endothelial cells 219, 255, 257
endothelial progenitor cells (EPCs) 207, 213–22
endothelialization 216, 218

enhanced green fluorescent protein (EGFP) 33
enzymes 19, 49–50, 63, 68, 81, 91, 101, 134, 141, 143–45, 162
EpCAM *see* epithelial cell adhesion molecule
EpCAM antigen 278
EPCs *see* endothelial progenitor cells
epidermidis 88–89, 105, 107, 111, 147, 163, 170
epithelial cell adhesion molecule (EpCAM) 270–71, 273–74, 277, 286, 288
epithelial cells 42, 133, 255, 286
EPS *see* extracellular polymeric substances
extracellular polymeric substances (EPS) 79–81, 115

ferrofluid-labeled cells 274
ferrofluids 274, 278–79
fibroblasts 28–31, 39, 43, 163, 255–57, 262–65
fibronectin 31, 45, 136, 256
fibronectin-coated multilayer polyelectrolyte nanofilms 31, 43
fixation techniques 296, 298, 305–6

gelatin 31, 43
gelatine coatings 169–70
gentamicin 89, 140, 151, 159, 161, 164–65, 168, 170–72, 175, 184, 187–88
gentamicin palmitate 165–68, 170–71, 173, 183
gentamicin sulfate 151, 155, 157, 159, 164, 166, 168, 170
germ invasion 131–32, 134
glass 99–100, 203, 282
glycyrrhizic acid 21, 193, 195, 204
gold 135, 203, 210, 219–21, 225, 291, 297

heavy metal ions 136–37, 162–63
heavy metal salts 161–62
heavy metals 137, 143, 161–62
heparin 31, 37, 42
hip replacement 308–11
human proteins 156, 233–34, 240
human umbilical vein endothelial cells (HUVEC) 31
HUVEC *see* human umbilical vein endothelial cells
hybrid fixation 296–98
hydrophobic surfaces 57, 74–75

IgG antibodies 19, 194, 203
IgM molecule 195, 197, 199–201
immune system 132, 134, 145, 196, 234
immunomagnetic enrichment 267, 277, 279
implant-associated infections 37, 72, 100, 104, 134, 136, 147–48
implant coatings 32, 130
implant material 32, 152, 192
implant-related infections 122, 129
implant surfaces 32, 50, 91, 105, 121, 130–33, 135, 166, 177–78, 209
implants 3, 31–32, 48–51, 62, 121, 130–35, 146–48, 157, 159–60, 162–63, 168–69, 175–78, 181–82, 209, 305–6
indwelling medical devices 104–5
infections 37, 105–6, 117, 122–25, 129, 133–34, 136, 146–49, 159–60, 169, 175, 179, 181, 184–88, 301–2
infectious biofilms 77, 81–82, 179
inflammation 105, 212, 255, 257, 263–64
intravascular stents 65–67
irradiation 12, 14–22, 192–94, 197, 202–3, 230

keratinocytes 255, 257, 262–63
knee 293, 295, 301, 312

layer-by-layer assembly 63, 66–67, 69
ligands 36, 207, 209–10, 221, 242
local antibiotic administration 148–50
lyophilization 15, 17, 19, 23–24, 192, 204

macrophages 29, 143, 212, 235, 255, 257
mass spectrometry 239, 241
medical device scaffolds 191
medical devices 1–4, 6–9, 11–12, 20, 37, 40, 104, 106–7, 122, 129–30, 211, 253–54, 291–92, 306, 308
medical implants 50, 82, 121–22, 130, 182, 185
medicinal products 1, 3–4, 23
mesenchymal stem cells (MSCs) 29, 45, 264
metallic implants 124, 135, 147, 151–53, 155, 164, 167, 182, 185
metastatic breast 268, 271–72, 286
metastatic carcinomas 268–69, 287, 289
microbial biofilms 104, 110, 114–15
microcolonies 78–79
microneedles 16, 21–22, 203, 223–28, 230–32
microorganisms 6, 28, 45, 58, 74, 76–78, 83, 90, 96–99, 106, 111, 131–34, 136–38, 140–43, 147
microprojections 225, 227–29
mixed bacterial cultures 71, 101, 105, 108
modified Robbins device (MRD) 94
molecular integrity 18–20
MRD *see* modified robbins device
MSCs *see* mesenchymal stem cells
multilayer films 38, 42, 61, 64–65, 68
multiple sclerosis 234, 240, 243, 247–48
multispecies biofilms 74, 108
myofibroblast differentiation 263, 265
myofibroblasts 252, 256–57, 262–64

nano-coating 19–20, 24, 27, 192–97, 199–203, 206
  functionality of 202–3
nanoparticles 34, 36, 50, 61, 63, 161
nanopatches 21–22, 223–26, 228, 230, 232
nucleic acids 31, 33, 36, 53

oral cavity 81, 94, 96, 100–1, 104, 118
organized biofilms 130, 136, 143
osteocalcin 34–35
osteopontin 34–35
oxygen 14, 89–91, 93, 144, 192

pacemakers 122, 158, 174–75, 181, 183
patient-reported outcome measures (PROMs) 294, 306
penicillin 140–41, 143, 145
peripheral blood 217, 284–86, 288
periprosthetic infections 300, 302
phenols 89, 136, 139
plaque accumulation 101, 103–4
plasma proteins 208
PLL *see* poly-L-lysine
poly-L-lysine (PLL) 28, 31–32, 34–35, 40

polyamide tissue 258
polyelectrolyte blends 51, 59, 67
polyelectrolyte chains 53, 55, 58
polyelectrolyte multilayers 27–28, 30, 32, 34, 36, 38, 40–45, 47–48, 50, 52, 54, 56, 58, 62–64, 66–69
polyelectrolytes 27, 42–43, 50–55, 57–61, 64–68
  natural 53, 57
  weak 55, 61, 68
polyhexanide 90, 139
polyions 29, 56
polylactide 155, 227
polymer-layer-forming carrier system 155
polyoxazolines 88, 119
polyurethane 19, 108, 191, 196, 202–3, 258
positive biofilms 77
PROMs *see* patient-reported outcome measures
prostate cancer 240, 245, 248–49, 268, 270
prostheses 45, 152, 160, 178, 181–82, 213–14, 220, 294, 304, 313
protein adsorption 45, 48, 59, 73, 84–85, 87, 110, 115, 217
protein arrays 235, 239–40, 244, 247
protein microarrays 239, 241, 243–44, 246
protein resistance 86, 88
protein-resistant surfaces 72, 91, 114
protein stability 24, 206
protein stabilization 20, 194–95
protein synthesis 140, 153–54
proteins 14–20, 22–25, 28, 31, 53, 73, 79–81, 83–86, 139, 192–96, 199–201, 204–6, 239, 241–43, 245–46
  immobilized 192–93, 196, 199
proteomics 77, 233, 247

QACs *see* quaternary ammonium compounds
quaternary ammonium compounds (QACs) 89, 91, 138

radiation 6, 11–15, 17, 19, 21, 199–201, 204–5
radiation sterilization 14–15, 23
relapse-remitting multiple sclerosis (RRMS) 243–44
resistance genes 143–45
resorbable polymer 158–59
rheumatoid arthritis 234, 237, 240, 243, 246–47
rifampicin 140, 142, 159, 170, 186, 188
RRMS *see* relapse-remitting multiple sclerosis

SAL *see* sterility assurance level
salivary proteins 79
septic revisions 300–1
serum autoantibodies 242, 248–49
serum proteins 215, 217
silver 38, 45, 89–90, 143, 156, 161, 170, 179, 183, 219, 252, 254, 264
silver coatings 253–54
silver ions 37–38, 40, 42, 89, 137, 156, 162
silver nanoparticles 38, 89, 92, 114
SLE *see* systemic lupus erythematosus
small-angle X-ray scattering 196–97, 199, 204

small-angle X-ray spectroscopy 191–92, 194, 196, 198, 200, 202, 204, 206
small-diameter artificial vascular prostheses 212–13, 215, 217
SPS *see* stabilizing and protecting solution
stabilizing and protecting solution (SPS) 13, 15–19
Staphylococcus epidermidis 38, 75, 84, 113, 118, 121, 170, 181, 183–84
stent coating 215–16
stents 66, 168, 203, 209, 212, 215–16, 218–22
sterility assurance level (SAL) 12, 14, 21
sterilization 6, 11, 15, 20, 22–23, 136, 191–92, 194, 196, 204, 223
  terminal 11–12, 16, 19, 202, 230
sterilization of health care products 6, 12, 205
sterilization of medical devices 6
stimulation of myofibroblasts 256–57, 262
streptavidin 278–82, 284
sutures 121, 124, 158, 172, 186
syringes 8, 21, 224, 281–82
systemic antibiotic administration 148–49
systemic antibiotics 148, 300–1
systemic lupus erythematosus (SLE) 234, 236–37, 240, 243, 246–48

TAAs *see* tumor-associated antigens
THA *see* total hip arthroplasty
therapeutic antibodies 15–16, 18–19
TJA *see* total joint arthroplasty
TKA *see* total knee arthroplasty
tobramycin 140, 150, 153, 164, 187, 307
total hip arthroplasty (THA) 292, 300–1, 305, 307–8, 310–11, 313
total joint arthroplasty (TJA) 292, 294, 302, 305–6, 310
total knee arthroplasty (TKA) 292, 297, 301–2, 304, 307, 311
transdermal vaccination 21, 223, 225, 227, 229
trastuzumab 17–19
tumor-associated antigens (TAAs) 234, 239, 244–45
tumor cells 8, 29, 267–68, 270, 284–86, 288
tumor tissue 239–40, 270

ultrathin coatings 220
uncemented implants 296, 299–300
uncemented systems 297–99
urinary catheters 103–4, 107, 124, 130
urinary tract infections 107–8, 186
urinary tract infections (UTIs) 104, 107, 119
UTIs *see* urinary tract infections

vaccination 223–25, 229, 231
vaccines 15–16, 22, 223–25, 229–31
vascular endothelial growth factor (VEGF) 210, 215, 252, 262, 264
VEGF *see* vascular endothelial growth factor
venous catheters 104, 130, 164, 188

vicinal water 71, 73–74, 86, 93

wound dressings 112, 138–39, 252–54, 258, 263
wound healing 138–39, 254–58, 263, 265
wound-healing phases 255
wound infections 136, 172, 180, 183
wounds 138, 164, 169, 252–57, 262–64